First Aid & Health Service Support Operations

U.S. Army, Navy, Air Force, and Marine Corps

Tactics, Techniques, and Procedures

C1, FM 4-25.11 (FM 21-11)

NTRP 4-02.1.1

AFMAN 44-163(I)

MCRP 3-02G

MCWP 4-11.1

First Aid & Health Service Support Operations: U.S. Army, Navy, Air Force, and Marine Corps Tactics, Techniques, and Procedures

PharmaLogika

PharmaLogika, Inc.
PO Box 461
Willow Springs, NC 27592

www.pharmalogika.com

PharmaLogika Books is an imprint of PharmaLogika, Inc. PharmaLogika and its logos are trademarks of PharmaLogika, Inc. All other trademarks used herein are the properties of their respective owners and are used for identification purposes only.

Author / Editor: Mindy J. Allport-Settle

Published by PharmaLogika, Inc.

Printed in the United States of America.

ISBN 1-9372580-8-4
ISBN-13 978-1-937258-08-5

Contents

First Aid & Health Service Support Operations

U.S. Army, Navy, Air Force, and Marine Corps Tactics, Techniques, and Procedures

C1, FM 4-25.11 (FM 21-11)

NTRP 4-02.1.1

AFMAN 44-163(I)

MCRP 3-02G

MCWP 4-11.1

Health Service Support Operations

Overview

About this Book

The United States military is recognized internationally as the standard for complete, efficient and effective adult education. The military has a tradition of pioneering training systems (including computer-based training) that then transition into the civilian corporate sector.

This manual has been continuously tested and updated to successfully educate every member of the modern United States military. The needs of the instructor, the student, and the military are perfectly balanced. This is the model all educators strive to follow when developing and delivering training programs.

Included Documents and Features

First Aid

Chapter 1. Fundamental Criteria for First Aid

Chapter 2. Basic Measures for First Aid

Chapter 3. First Aid for Specific Injuries

Chapter 4. First Aid for Fractures

Chapter 5. First Aid for Climatic Injuries

Chapter 6. First Aid for Bites and Stings

Chapter 7. First Aid in a Nuclear, Biological, and Chemical Environment

Chapter 8. First Aid for Psychological Reactions

APPENDIX A. First Aid Case and Kits, Dressings, and Bandages

APPENDIX B. Rescue and Transportation Procedures

Health Service Support Operations

Chapter 1. Fundamentals

Chapter 2. Intelligence

Chapter 3. Operations

Chapter 4. Logistics

Chapter 5. Planning

Chapter 6. Command and Control

Chapter 7. Preventive Medicine

Chapter 8. Patient Movement

Chapter 9. Nuclear, Biological, and Chemical Defense

Chapter 10. Combat Casualty Reporting

Chapter 11. Training

References, Index, Appendices and Glossary Supporting Each Section

Introduction

Joint Military First Aid Training

Basic battlefield and military first aid training responsibilities are shared by the United States Army, Navy, Air Force, and Marines. Injuries, wounds, and casualties are similar at the basic level. Additional specialties are addressed as necessary in each individual branch.

First Aid

First aid is the provision of initial care for an illness or injury. It is usually performed by non-expert, but trained personnel to a sick or injured person until definitive medical treatment can be accessed. Certain self-limiting illnesses or minor injuries may not require further medical care past the first aid intervention. It generally consists of a series of simple and in some cases, potentially life-saving techniques that an individual can be trained to perform with minimal equipment.

History

The instances of recorded first aid were provided by religious knights, such as the Knights Hospitaller, formed in the 11th century, providing care to pilgrims and knights, and training other knights in how to treat common battlefield injuries.[1] The practice of first aid fell largely in to disuse during the High Middle Ages, and organized societies were not seen again until in 1859 Jean-Henri Dunant organized local villagers to help victims of the Battle of Solferino, including the provision of first aid. Four years later, four nations met in Geneva and formed the organization which has grown into the Red Cross, with a key stated aim of "aid to sick and wounded soldiers in the field." This was followed by the formation of St. John Ambulance in 1877, based on the principles of the Knights Hospitaller, to teach first aid, and numerous other organizations joined with them. The term first aid was first coined in 1878 as civilian ambulance services spread as a combination of "first treatment" and "national aid" in large railway centres and mining districts as well as with police forces. In 1878

[1] First Aid: From Witchdoctors & Religious Knights to Modern Doctors available at http://www.medicinenet.com/script/main/art.asp?articlekey=52749

Surgeon-Major Peter Shepherd, together with Colonel Francis Duncan established the concept of teaching first aid skills to civilians. Shepherd, together with a Dr Coleman, conducted the first class in the hall of the Presbyterian school in Woolwich using a comprehensive first aid curriculum that he had developed. It was Shepherd who first used the English term "first aid for the injured."[2] First aid training began to spread through the British empire through organisations such as St. John, often starting (as in the United Kingdom) with high risk activities such as ports and railways.[3]

Many developments in first aid and many other medical techniques have been driven by wars, such as in the case of the American Civil War, which prompted Clara Barton to organize the American Red Cross.[4] Today, there are several groups that promote first aid, such as the military and the Scouting movement. New techniques and equipment have helped make today's first aid simple and effective.

Aims

The key aims of first aid can be summarized in three key points:[5]

- **Preserve life:** the overriding aim of all medical care, including first aid, is to save lives
- **Prevent further harm:** also sometimes called prevent the condition from worsening, or danger of further injury, this covers both external factors, such as moving a patient away from any cause of harm, and applying first aid techniques to prevent worsening of the condition, such as applying pressure to stop a bleed becoming dangerous.
- **Promote recovery:** first aid also involves trying to start the recovery process from the illness or injury, and in some cases might involve completing a treatment, such as in the case of applying a plaster to a small wound

First aid training also involves the prevention of initial injury and responder safety, as well as the treatment phases defined in specific training regimens.

---

[2] The earliest days of first aid. John Pearn BMJ 1994;309:1718 20

[3] Industrial Revolution: St. John Ambulance available at http://www.sja.org.uk/sja/about-us/our-history.aspx?utm_source=NHQ&utm_campaign=2012-Feb.

[4] American Red Cross – Museum available at http://www.redcross.org.

[5] "Accidents and first aid." NHS Direct. Archived from the original: http://web.archive.org/web/20080503201513/http://www.nhsdirect.nhs.uk/articles/article.aspx?articleId=450

Specific disciplines

There are several types of first aid which require additional specialized training. These are usually undertaken to fulfill the demands of the work or activity undertaken.

- **Aquatic/Marine first aid**—Usually practiced by professionals such as lifeguards, professional mariners or in diver rescue, and covers the specific problems which may be faced after water-based rescue and/or delayed MedEvac.

- **Battlefield first aid**—This takes in to account the specific needs of treating wounded combatants and non-combatants during armed conflict.

- **Hyperbaric first aid**—Which may be practiced by SCUBA diving professionals, who need to treat conditions such as the bends.

- **Oxygen first aid**—Providing oxygen to casualties who suffer from conditions resulting in hypoxia.

- **Wilderness first aid**—Provision of first aid under conditions where the arrival of emergency responders or the evacuation of an injured person may be delayed due to constraints of terrain, weather, and available persons or equipment. It may be necessary to care for an injured person for several hours or days.

- **Hydrofluoric Acid first aid**—Taught to first aiders in the chemical industry where hydrofluoric acid may be used. Instructs the first aider how to initially treat (with calcium gluconate) any skin that has been splashed with the acid.

Symbols

Although commonly associated with first aid, the symbol of a red cross is an official protective symbol of the Red Cross. According to the Geneva Conventions and other international laws, the use of this and similar symbols is reserved for official agencies of the International Red Cross and Red Crescent, and as a protective emblem for medical personnel and facilities in combat situations. Use by any other person or organization is illegal, and may lead to prosecution.

The internationally accepted symbol for first aid is the white cross on a green background shown below.

Some organizations may make use of the Star of Life, although this is usually reserved for use by ambulance services, or may use symbols such as the Maltese Cross, like the Order of Malta Ambulance Corps and St. John Ambulance. Other symbols may also be used.

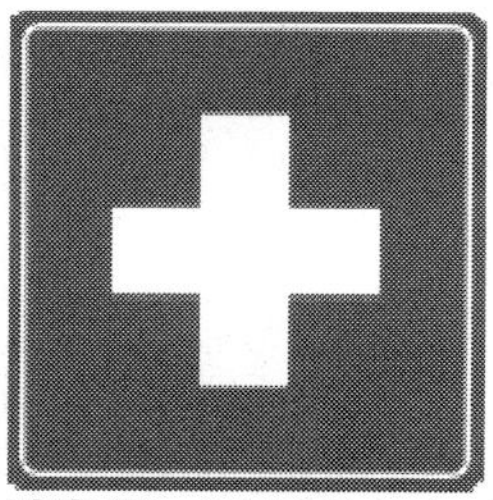

ISO First Aid Symbol

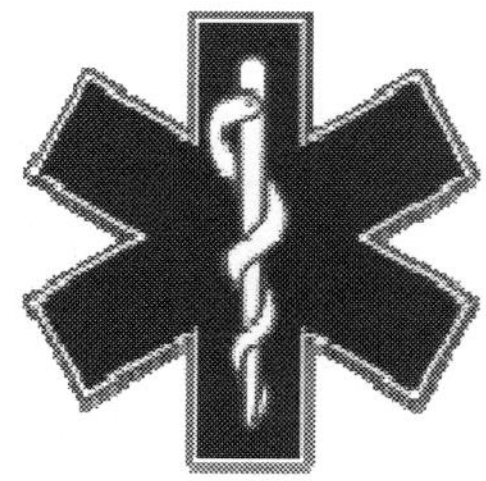

Star of life

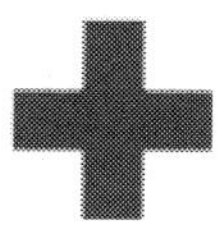

Symbol of the Red Cross

Maltese or Amalfi Cross

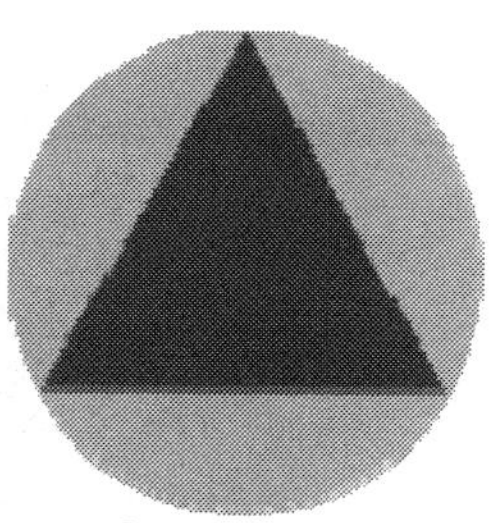

Civil defence

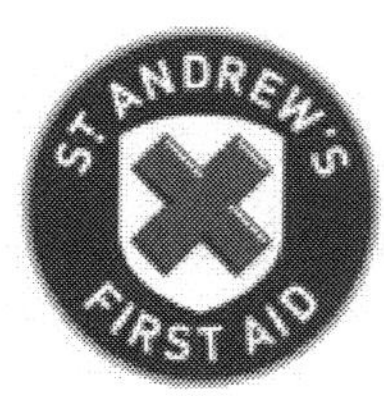

St. Andrew's First Aid Badge

United States Marine Corps

The United States Marine Corps (USMC) is a branch of the United States Armed Forces responsible for providing power projection from the sea,[6] using the mobility of the United States Navy to deliver combined-arms task forces rapidly. It is one of seven uniformed services of the United States. In the civilian leadership structure of the United States military, the Marine Corps is a component of the United States Department of the Navy,[7, 8] often working closely with U.S. naval forces for training, transportation, and logistic purposes; however, in the military leadership structure the Marine Corps is a separate branch.[9]

Captain Samuel Nicholas formed two battalions of Continental Marines on 10 November 1775 in Philadelphia as naval infantry.[10] Since then, the mission of the Marine Corps has evolved with changing military doctrine and American foreign policy. The Marine Corps has served in every American armed conflict and attained prominence in the 20th century when its theories and practices of amphibious warfare proved prescient and ultimately formed the cornerstone of the Pacific campaign of World War II.[11] By the mid-20th century, the Marine Corps had become the dominant theorist and practitioner of amphibious warfare.[12, 13, 14] Its ability to rapidly respond on short notice to expeditionary

---

[6] Gen. Charles C. Krulak (1996) (PDF). Operational Maneuver from the Sea. Headquarters Marine Corps.

[7] "U.S. Navy Organization: An Overview." Available from the United States Navy website at http://www.navy.mil/navydata/organization/org-over.asp.

[8] "National Security Act of 1947, SEC. 206. (a) (50 U.S.C. 409(b))." Available at http://intelligence.senate.gov/nsaact1947.pdf.

[9] "National Security Act of 1947, SEC. 606. (50 U.S.C. 426)." Available at http://intelligence.senate.gov/nsaact1947.pdf.

[10] "Naval Orientation." Chapter 14: United States Marine Corps. Integrated Publishing. pp. 14–1 to 14–11.

[11] Warren, James A. (2005). American Spartans: The U.S. Marines: A Combat History From Iwo Jima to Iraq. New York: Free Press, Simon & Schuster.

[12] Hough, Col Frank O. (USMCR); Ludwig, Maj Verle E. (USMC), and Henry I. Shaw, Jr.. "Part I, Chapter 2: Evolution of Modern Amphibious Warfare, 1920–1941." Pearl Harbor to Guadalcanal. History of U.S. Marine Corps Operations in World War II, Volume I. Historical Branch, HQMC, United States Marine Corps.

[13] Garand, George W. and Truman R. Strobridge (1971). "Part II, Chapter 1: The Development of FMFPac." Western Pacific Operations. History of U.S. Marine Corps Operation in World War II, Volume IV. Historical Branch, HQMC, United States Marine Corps.

[14] Frank, Benis M and Henry I. Saw, Jr. (1968). "Part VI, Chapter 1: Amphibious Doctrine in World War II." Victory and Occupation. History of U.S. Marine Corps Operations in World War II, Volume V. Historical Branch, HQMC, United States Marine Corps.

crises gives it a strong role in the implementation and execution of American foreign policy.[15]

Organization

The Department of the Navy, led by the Secretary of the Navy, is the Federal Government Agency which both the Marine Corps and the Navy are organized within. The most senior Marine officer is the Commandant of the Marine Corps, responsible to the Secretary of the Navy for organizing, recruiting, training, and equipping the Marine Corps so that its forces are ready for deployment under the operational command of the Combatant Commanders. The Marine Corps is organized into four principal subdivisions: Headquarters Marine Corps (HQMC), the Operating Forces, the Supporting Establishment, and the Marine Forces Reserve (MARFORRES or USMCR).

The Operating Forces are further subdivided into three categories: Marine Corps Forces (MARFOR) assigned to unified commands, Marine Corps Security Forces guarding high-risk naval installations, and Marine Corps Security Guard detachments at American embassies. Under the "Forces for Unified Commands" memo, in accordance with the Unified Command Plan approved by the President, Marine Corps Forces are assigned to each of the Combatant Commands at the discretion of the Secretary of Defense. Since 1991, the Marine Corps has maintained component headquarters at each of the regional unified combatant commands.[16] Marine Corps Forces are further divided into Marine Forces Command (MARFORCOM) and Marine Forces Pacific (MARFORPAC), each headed by a Lieutenant General. MARFORCOM has operational control of the II Marine Expeditionary Force; MARFORPAC has operational control of the I Marine Expeditionary Force and III Marine Expeditionary Force.[17]

Relationship with other services

In general, the Marine Corps shares many resources with the other branches of the United States military. However, the Corps has consistently sought to maintain its own identity with regards to mission, funding, and assets, while utilizing the support available from the larger branches. While the Marine Corps has far fewer installations both in the U.S. and worldwide than the other

[15] John Howard Dalton, Secretary of the Navy; Jeremy Michael Boorda, Chief of Naval Operations; Carl E. Mundy, Commandant of the Marine Corps (9 November 1994). Forward... From the Sea. United States Department of the Navy.

[16] United States Marine Corps (2007). Marine Corps Operations. Cosimo, Inc. p. 19.

[17] Chenoweth, USMCR (Ret.), Colonel H. Avery; Colonel Brooke Nihart, USMC (ret) (2005). Semper fi: The Definitive Illustrated History of the U.S. Marines. New York: Main Street.

branches, many Army posts, Naval stations, and Air Force bases have a Marine presence.

United States Army

The Marine Corps combat capabilities in some ways overlap those of the United States Army, the latter having historically viewed the Corps as encroaching on the Army's capabilities and competing for funding, missions, and renown. The attitude dates back to the founding of the Continental Marines, when General George Washington refused to allow the initial Marine battalions to be drawn from among his Continental Army. Most significantly, in the aftermath of World War II, Army efforts to restructure the American defense establishment included the dissolution of the Corps and the folding of its capabilities into the other services. Leading this movement were such prominent Army officers as General Dwight D. Eisenhower and Army Chief of Staff George C. Marshall.[18] With most of the 2000s spent in operations in Afghanistan and Iraq, Secretary of Defense Robert Gates has voiced concerns that the Marines are becoming a "second Army."[19]

Doctrinally, Marine Corps' focus is on being expeditionary and independent, and places emphasis on amphibious mobility and combined arms; these make it a much lighter force than many units of the Army. A larger percentage of the Marine Corps' personnel and assets are in the combat arms (infantry, artillery, armor, and close air support) than the Army. However, the Army maintains much larger and diverse combat arms (infantry, armor, artillery, special operations), ground transport, logistics, while the Marines have a more diverse aviation arm (which constitutes a larger percentage of forces), and is usually organic to the MAGTF. Marines operate as expeditionary units and are completely amphibious. The Marine Corps focus on standardized infantry units with the other arms in support roles as the "Every Marine's a rifleman" creed shows. This commitment to standardized units can be seen in the short-lived experiment of the Marine Raiders, which was controversial, while the U.S. Army's 75th Ranger Regiment, born in World War II, enjoys high prestige to this day. While the Army has a longer continuous tradition of special operations forces, Marines joined the Special Operations Command with the establishment of MCSOCOM Detachment One in 2003.[20]

---

[18] Krulak, Victor H. (1984). First To Fight: An Inside View of the U.S. Marine Corps. Annapolis, Maryland: Naval Institute Press. ISBN 0-87021-785-2. Chapter 7, The Marines' Push Button 113–119

[19] Kevin Baron (August 12, 2010). "Gates: Time has come to re-examine future of Marine Corps."

[20] Priddy, Maj. Wade (2006). "Marine Detachment 1: Opening the door for a Marine force contribution to USSOCom." Marine Corps Gazette (Marine Corps Association) 90 (6): 58–59.

The Marines often leverage the Army's acquisition of ground equipment (as well as benefiting from Army research and development resources), training resources, and other support concepts. The majority of vehicles and weapons are shared with, modified, or inherited from Army programs.

Culturally, Marines and soldiers share most of the common U.S. military slang and terminology, but the Corps utilizes a large number of naval terms and traditions incompatible with the Army lifestyle, as well as their own unique vernacular. Many Marines regard their culture to have a deeper warrior tradition, with the ethos that every Marine is a rifleman and emphasis on cross-training and combat readiness despite actual job, be it infantry or otherwise. One source states Marines tend to decentralize and push leadership to lower levels, while fostering initiative to a greater degree.[21]

United States Navy

The Marine Corps' counterpart under the Department of the Navy is the United States Navy. As a result, the Navy and Marine Corps have a close relationship, more so than with other branches of the military. Whitepapers and promotional literature have commonly used the phrase "Navy-Marine Corps Team," [22, 23]or refer to "the Naval Service." Both the Chief of Naval Operations (CNO) and Commandant of the Marine Corps report directly to the Secretary of the Navy.

Cooperation between the two services really begins with the training and instruction of Marines. The Corps receives a significant portion of its officers from the United States Naval Academy and Naval Reserve Officer Training Corps (NROTC). NROTC staff includes Marine instructors, while Marine drill instructors contribute to training of officers in the Navy's Officer Candidate School. Marine aviators are trained in the Naval Aviation training pipeline and are winged as Naval Aviators.

Training alongside each other is viewed as critical, as the Navy provides transport, logistical, and combat support to put Marine units into the fight, for example, the Maritime Prepositioning ships and naval gunfire support. Most Marine aviation assets ultimately derive from the Navy, with regard to acquisition, funding, and testing, and Navy aircraft carriers typically deploy with a Marine squadron alongside Navy squadrons. Marines do not recruit or train

---

[21] Connable, Maj Ben (2008). "Culture Warriors: Marine Corps Organizational Culture and Adaptation to Cultural Terrain." Small Wars Journal (Small Wars Foundation).
[22] Clark, Adm. Vern; Hinton, Don (October 2002). "Sea Power 21." Proceedings (Naval Institute Press) 130 (October 2002): 3005.
[23] Lt. Col. James Kuhn (2 November 2005). Enduring Freedom (Film). Department of the Navy.

noncombatants such as chaplains or medical/dental personnel; naval personnel fill these roles. Some of these sailors, particularly Hospital Corpsmen and Religious Programs Specialists, generally wear Marine uniforms emblazoned with Navy insignia. Conversely, the Marine Corps is responsible for conducting land operations to support naval campaigns, including the seizure of naval and air bases. Both services operate a network security team in conjunction.

Marines and Sailors share many naval traditions, especially terminology and customs. Marine Corps Medal of Honor recipients wear the Navy variant of this and other awards; and with few exceptions, the awards and badges of the Navy and Marine Corps are identical. Much of testing for new Marine Corps aircraft is done at NAS Patuxent River. The Navy's Blue Angels flight demonstration team is staffed by both Navy and Marine officers and enlisted men, and includes a Marine C-130 Hercules aircraft.[24]

In 2007, the Marine Corps joined with the Navy and Coast Guard to adopt a new maritime strategy called *A Cooperative Strategy for 21st Century Seapower* that raises the notion of prevention of war to the same philosophical level as the conduct of war.[25] This new strategy charts a course for the Navy, Coast Guard and Marine Corps to work collectively with each other and international partners to prevent regional crises, man-made or natural, from occurring or reacting quickly should one occur to avoid negative impacts to the United States.

United States Air Force

While the majority of Marine aviation assets ultimately derive from the Navy, some support is drawn from the United States Air Force. The Marine Corps makes extensive use of the USAF Air Mobility Command to airlift Marines and equipment.

The Air Force traditionally provides the Joint Force Air Component Commander who controls "sorties for air defense, and long range interdiction and reconnaissance" while the MAGTF commander retains control of the Marines' organic aviation assets.[26, 27]

---

24 Lawliss, Chuck (1988). *The Marine Book: A Portrait of America's Military Elite*. New York: Thames and Hudson.
25 Jim Garamone (17 October 2007). "Sea Services Unveil New Maritime Strategy." Navy News Service.
26 Purpose of JFACC (archived). U.S. Air Force.
27 United States Marine Corps (2005). *Expeditionary Operations (Marine Corps Doctrinal Publication 3)*. Willside Press LLC. p. 83.

The Marines provide some ground training for Air Force ground personnel, but most is handled by the Army.[28]

United States Navy Hospital Corpsman

A Hospital Corpsman (HM) is frequently the only medical care-giver available in many fleet or Marine units on extended deployment. Hospital Corpsmen serve as enlisted medical specialists for the United States Navy and the United States Marine Corps. The Hospital Corpsman works in a wide variety of capacities and locations, including shore establishments such as naval hospitals and clinics, aboard ships, as the primary medical caregivers for sailors while underway. Hospital Corpsman perform duties as assistants in the prevention and treatment of disease and injury and assist health care professionals in providing medical care to Navy people and their families. They may function as clinical or specialty technicians, medical administrative personnel and health care providers at medical treatment facilities. They also serve as battlefield corpsmen with the Marine Corps, rendering emergency medical treatment to include initial treatment in a combat environment. Qualified hospital corpsmen may be assigned the responsibility of independent duty aboard ships and submarines; Fleet Marine Force, Special Forces and Seabee units, and at isolated duty stations where no medical officer is available.

The colloquial form of address for a Hospital Corpsman is "Doc." In the U.S. Marine Corps, this term is generally used as a sign of respect.

Organization

Because of the need for Hospital Corpsmen in a vast array of foreign, domestic, and shipboard duty stations, as well as with United States Marine Corps units, the Hospital Corps is the largest rating in the United States Navy.

The basic training for Hospital Corpsmen is Naval Hospital Corps School, located in Great Lakes, IL, one of the Navy's "A" schools (primary rating training). Upon graduation, the Hospital Corpsman is given the Navy Enlisted Classification (NEC) code of HM-0000, or "quad-zero" in common usage. NECs are analogous to MOS in the United States Army and Marine Corps, or AFSC in the Air Force. There are primary NECs, and secondary NECs. For example, a Hospital Corpsman who completes Field Medical Training Battalion (FMTB) and earns the NEC HM-8404, moves that NEC to primary and has a secondary NEC of HM-0000. If that Hospital Corpsman attends a "C" School, then the NEC earned at the "C" School becomes their primary and HM-8404

[28] Sloan, Dennis L. "Marines vote JB MDL Airman 'Gung Ho': USAF EC instructor first Airman to graduate Marine PME." USAF.

becomes the secondary. Some Hospital Corpsmen go on to receive more specialized training in roles such as Medical Laboratory Technician, Radiology Technician, Aviation/Aerospace Medicine Specialist, Pharmacy Technician, Operating Room Technician, etcetera. This advanced education is done through "C" schools, which confer additional NECs. Additionally, Hospital Corpsmen E-5 and above may attend Surface Force Independent Duty training, qualifying for independent duty in surface ships and submarines, with diving teams, and Fleet Marine Force Recon teams, as well as at remote shore installations. In addition to advanced medical training, these Hospital Corpsmen receive qualification in sanitation and public health.

Hospital Corpsmen who have received the warfare designator of Enlisted Fleet Marine Force Warfare Specialist are highly trained members of the Hospital Corps who specialize in all aspects of working with the United States Marine Corps operating forces. Attainment of this designation is highly prized among all Corpsmen. The Enlisted Fleet Marine Force Warfare designation for Hospital Corpsmen is the only US Navy warfare device awarded solely by a US Marine Corps General Officer. This awarding authority cannot be delegated to US Navy Officers. However, obtaining the title of "FMF" is a rigorous procedure and not every Hospital Corpsman who has been with a Marine Corps unit will wear the FMF warfare device. U.S. Navy officers in the medical community(Medical Corps (Doctor), Nurse Corps, Dental Corps) can earn and wear the officer equivalent to this insignia. Additionally any sailor attached to a Marine unit can earn and wear an FMF warfare device. (Example, administrative rates such as Logistic Specialists).

The first Physician Assistants were selected from Navy Corpsmen who had combat experience in Vietnam. The Navy trained its own Physician Assistants drawing from the ranks of qualified Independent Duty Hospital Corpsmen at the Naval School of Health Sciences in Portmouth, VA until 1985, then at San Diego, CA. Navy Hospital Corpsmen are also represented in many medical disciplines, as Physicians, Nurses, Medical Administrators and other walks of life.

Be they assigned to hospital ships, reservist installations, recruiter offices, or Marine Corps combat units, the rating of Hospital Corpsman is the most decorated in the United States Navy with 22 Medals of Honor, 174 Navy Crosses, 31 Distinguished Service Medals, 946 Silver Stars, and 1,582 Bronze Stars.[29] There have been 20 naval ships that have been named after hospital corpsmen.

[29] BMC Mayport (2003-06-19). "Happy 105th Birthday To The Hospital Corps"

Hospital Corpsman Pledge

"I solemnly pledge myself before God and these witnesses to practice faithfully all of my duties as a member of the Hospital Corps. I hold the care of the sick and injured to be a privilege and a sacred trust and will assist the Medical Officer with loyalty and honesty. I will not knowingly permit harm to come to any patient. I will not partake of nor administer any unauthorized medication. I will hold all personal matters pertaining to the private lives of patients in strict confidence. I dedicate my heart, mind and strength to the work before me. I shall do all within my power to show in myself an example of all that is honorable and good throughout my naval career."

Rate / Rating Structure

- HR -Hospitalman Recruit (E-1)
- HA -Hospitalman Apprentice (E-2)
- HN -Hospitalman (E-3) (See USN Apprenticeships)
- HM3 -Hospital Corpsman Third Class (E-4)
- HM2 -Hospital Corpsman Second Class (E-5)
- HM1 -Hospital Corpsman First Class (E-6)
- HMC -Chief Hospital Corpsman (E-7)
- HMCS-Senior Chief Hospital Corpsman (E-8)
- HMCM-Master Chief Hospital Corpsman (E-9)

Army Medical Command

The U.S. Army Medical Command (MEDCOM) is a major command of the U.S. Army that provides command and control of the Army's fixed-facility medical, dental, and veterinary treatment facilities, providing preventive care, medical research and development and training institutions.

Structure and Subordinate Commands

MEDCOM is divided into Regional Medical Commands that oversee day-to-day operations in military treatment facilities, exercising command and control over the medical treatment facilities in their regions. There are currently five of these regional commands:

- Europe Regional Medical Command
- Southern Regional Medical Command

- Northern Regional Medical Command
- Pacific Regional Medical Command
- Western Regional Medical Command.

Additional subordinate commands of MEDCOM include:

- Army Medical Department Center & School (AMEDDC&S)
- U.S. Army Public Health Command (Provisional), (known as the U.S. Army Center for Health Promotion & Preventive Medicine prior to 1 October 2009 {USACHPPM or CHPPM})
- U.S. Army Medical Research and Materiel Command (USAMRMC)
- Warrior Transition Command (WTC)
- U.S. Army Dental Command (DENCOM)

Operations

In Garrison (Peacetime)

MEDCOM maintains day-to-day health care for soldiers, retired soldiers and the families of both. Despite the wide range of responsibilities involved in providing health care in traditional settings as well as on the battlefield, the Army Medical Department's quality of care compares very favorably with that of civilian health organizations, when measured by civilian standards. Many Army medical facilities report on their own quality-of-care standards on their individual Internet sites.

Deployments

When Army field hospitals deploy, most clinical professional and support personnel come from MEDCOM's fixed facilities. In addition to support of combat operations, deployments can be for humanitarian assistance, peacekeeping, and other stability and support operations. Under the Professional Officer Filler System (PROFIS), up to 26 percent of MEDCOM physicians and 43 percent of MEDCOM nurses are sent to field units during a full deployment. To replace PROFIS losses, Reserve units and Individual Mobilization Augmentees (non-unit reservists) are mobilized to work in medical treatment facilities. The department also provides trained medical specialists to the Army's combat medical units, which are assigned directly to combatant commanders.

Many Army Reserve and Army National Guard units deploy in support of the Army Medical Department. The Army depends heavily on its Reserve component for medical support—about 63 percent of the Army's medical forces are in the Reserve component.

Army Medical Department

The Army Medical Department of the U.S. Army (AMEDD) comprises the Army's six medical Special Branches (or "Corps") of officers and medical enlisted soldiers. It was established as the "Army Hospital" in July 1775 to coordinate the medical care required by the Continental Army during the Revolutionary War. The AMEDD is led by the Surgeon General of the U.S. Army, a lieutenant general.

The AMEDD is the U.S. Army's healthcare organization, not a U.S. Army command. The AMEDD is found in all three components of the Army: the Active Army, the U.S. Army Reserve, and the Army National Guard. Its headquarters are at Fort Sam Houston, San Antonio, Texas, which hosts the AMEDD Center and School. Equal numbers of AMEDD senior leaders can be found in Washington D.C., divided between the Pentagon and the Walter Reed Army Medical Center (WRAMC).

The Academy of Health Sciences, under the Army Medical Department Center & School, provides training to the officers and enlisted soldiers of the AMEDD. As a result of BRAC 2005, enlisted medical training was transferred to the new Medical Education and Training Campus, consolidating most military enlisted medical training at Fort Sam Houston.[30]

Medical Special Branches

- Medical Corps (MC)
- Nurse Corps (AN)
- Dental Corps (DC)
- Veterinary Corps (VC)
- Medical Service Corps (MS)

[30] U.S. Army Medical Department AMEDD Center and School Portal available on the Internet at: http://www.cs.amedd.army.mil/. Additional information specific to the Fort Sam Houston consolidation is available n the Internet at: http://www.aetc.af.mil/shared/media/document/AFD-071026-035.pdf

- Medical Specialist Corps (AMSC)

United States Army Training and Doctrine Command

Established 1 July 1973, the United States Army Training and Doctrine Command (TRADOC) is an army command of the United States Army headquartered at Fort Monroe, Virginia. It is charged with overseeing training of Army forces, the development of operational doctrine, and the development and procurement of new weapons systems. TRADOC operates 33 schools and centers at 16 Army installations. TRADOC schools conduct 2,734 courses (81 directly in support of mobilization) and 373 language courses. The 2,734 courses include 503,164 seats for 434,424 soldiers; 34,675 other-service personnel; 7,824 international soldiers; and 26,241 civilians.[31]

TRADOC MissionThe official mission statement for TRADOC states:

> TRADOC develops the Army's Soldiers and Civilian leaders and designs, develops and integrates capabilities, concepts and doctrine in order to build a campaign-capable, expeditionary Army in support of joint warfighting capability through Army Force Generation (ARFORGEN).[32]

TRADOC is the official command component that is responsible for training and developing the United States Army.

TRADOC History

TRADOC was established as a major U.S. Army command on 1 July 1973. The new command, along with the U.S. Army Forces Command (FORSCOM), was created from the Continental Army Command (CONARC) located at Fort Monroe, VA. That action was the major innovation in the Army's post-Vietnam reorganization, in the face of realization that CONARC's obligations and span of control were too broad for efficient focus. The new organization functionally realigned the major Army commands in the continental United States. CONARC, and Headquarters, U.S. Army Combat Developments Command (CDC), situated at Fort Belvoir, VA, were discontinued, with TRADOC and FORSCOM at Fort Belvoir assuming the realigned missions. TRADOC assumed the combat developments mission from CDC, took over the individual training mission formerly the responsibility of CONARC, and assumed command from CONARC of the major Army installations in the

---

31 TRADOC fact sheet available at: http://www.tradoc.army.mil/about.htm

32 TRADOC commander on ARFORGEN, and the US Army available at: http://www.tradoc.army.mil/about.htm

United States housing Army training center and Army branch schools. FORSCOM assumed CONARC's operational responsibility for the command and readiness of all divisions and corps in the continental U.S. and for the installations where they were based.

Joined under TRADOC, the major Army missions of individual training and combat developments each had its own lineage. The individual training responsibility had belonged, during World War II, to Headquarters Army Ground Forces (AGF). In 1946 numbered Army areas were established in the U.S. under AGF command. At that time, the AGF moved from Washington, D.C. to Fort Monroe, VA. In March 1948, the AGR was replaced at Fort Monroe with the new Office, Chief of Army Field Forces (OCAFF). OCAFF, however, did not command the training establishment. That function was exercised by Headquarters, Department of the Army through the numbered Armies to the corps, division, and Army Training Centers. In February 1955, HQ Continental Army Command (CONARC) replaced OCAFF, assuming its missions as well as the training missions from DA. In January, HQ CONARC was redesignated U.S. Continental Army Command. Combat developments emerged as a formal Army mission in the early 1950s, and OCAFF assumed that role in 1952. In 1955, CONARC assumed the mission. In 1962, HQ U.S. Army Combat Development Command (CDC) was established to bring the combat developments function under one major Army command.[33]

TRADOC Priorities

1. Leader Development
2. Initial Military Training
3. Concepts and Capabilities Integration
4. Human Capital Enterprise
5. Army Training and Learning Concept
6. Doctrine

The Role of Education in the Military

Military education and training is a process which intends to establish and improve the capabilities of military personnel in their respective roles.

Military education can be voluntary or compulsory duty. Before any person gets authorization to operate technical equipment or be on the battle field, they must

[33] TRADOC history available at: http://www.tradoc.army.mil/about.htm

take a medical and often a physical test. If passed, they may begin primary training. The primary training is recruit training. Recruit training attempts to teach the basic information and training in techniques necessary to be an effective service member. To achieve this, service members are drilled physically, technically and psychologically. The drill instructor has the task of making the service members fit for military use.

After finishing basic training, many service members undergo advanced training more in line with their chosen or assigned specialties. This range from navy training to studies of explosives. In advanced training, military technology and equipment is often taught.

Many large countries have several military academies, one for each branch of the service, that offer college degrees in a variety of subjects, similar to other colleges. However, academy graduates usually rank as officers, and as such have many options besides civilian work in their major subject. Higher ranking officers also have further educational opportunities.

Personnel Resocialization

While regulated industry does not seek to create soldiers and certainly does not want to employ all of the standard military training techniques, it does need to make certain personnel are trained to follow directions precisely and respect the authority of the regulatory agencies as well as their internal command chain (supervisors, managers, and executives).

Resocialization is an important aspect of inducting a civilian into a military team. Resocialization is a sociological concept dealing with the process of mentally and emotionally "re-training" a person so they can operate in an environment other than what they are accustomed to. Successful resocialization into a total institution involves changes to an individual's personality.

Key examples include the process of resocializing new recruits into the military so that they can operate as soldiers – or, in other words, as members of a cohesive unit. Another example is the reverse process, in which those who have become accustomed to such roles return to society after military discharge.

Resocialization from the life of a combat soldier to a civilian member of society is often difficult because of what that soldier saw and did in his military experience. In the transition from civilian to soldier, the individual is trained to solely follow the command of his superiors. In some cases commands would go against certain natural aversions (such as killing) of the individual based on one's moral and ethical principles.

A leading expert in military training methods, Grossman(2001) gives four types of training techniques used; brutalization, classical conditioning, operant conditioning and role modeling.[34] According to Grossman (2001), these techniques were meant to break down barriers to embrace a new set of norms and way of life (brutalization), condition them to pair killing with something more enjoyable and pleasurable (Classical Conditioning), repeat the stimulus-response reaction to develop a reflex (Operant Conditioning), and finally the use of a role model of a superior to provide action by example.

While leaders effectively train their soldiers to accomplish the goal of battle preparedness, these techniques increase psychological trauma experienced in veterans post-combat.[35] It is because of the evident psychological problems in post-combat situations (i.e. Post Traumatic Stress Disorder) that pose a threat to public safety because of the conditioning of the individual who might be made unstable because of his actions. Resocialization following such intense training and conditioning should be further researched and developed to better aide those discharged from the military service.

---

[34] Grossman, D. (2001) Trained to Kill. *Professorenforum-Journal*,2(2).

[35] Kilner, P. (2002, March). Military Leaders' Obligation to Justify Killing in War. *Military Review*, 32(2).

First Aid

C1, FM 4-25.11 (FM 21-11)

NTRP 4-02.1.1

AFMAN 44-163(I)

MCRP 3-02G

This page intentionally left blank.

C1, FM 4-25.11 (FM 21-11)
★NTRP 4-02.1.1
AFMAN 44-163(I)
★MCRP 3-02G

FIRST AID

★HEADQUARTERS, DEPARTMENTS OF THE ARMY, THE NAVY, AND THE AIR FORCE AND COMMANDANT, MARINE CORPS

DECEMBER 2002

DISTRIBUTION RESTRICTION: Approved for public release; distribution is unlimited.

C1, FM 4-25.11 (FM 21-11)
NTRP 4-02.1.1
AFMAN 44-163(I)
MCRP 3-02G

Change 1

HEADQUARTERS
DEPARTMENTS OF THE ARMY,
THE NAVY, AND THE AIR FORCE
AND COMMANDANT, MARINE CORPS
Washington, DC, 15 July 2004

FIRST AID

1. Change FM 4-25.11/NTRP 4-02.1/AFMAN 44-163(I), 23 December 2002, as follows:

Remove old pages	Insert new pages
Cover	Cover
Back cover	Back cover

2. New or changed material is indicated by a star (★).

3. File this transmittal sheet in front of the publication.

DISTRIBUTION RESTRICTION: Approved for public release; distribution is unlimited.

By Order of the Secretary of the Army:

PETER J. SCHOOMAKER
General, United States Army
Chief of Staff

Official:

JOEL B. HUDSON
Administrative Assistant to the Secretary of the Army
0417001

By Direction of the Chief of Naval Operations:

Official:

R.G. SPRIGG
Rear Admiral, USN
Navy Warfare Development Command

By Order of the Secretary of the Air Force:

Official:

GEORGE PEACH TAYLOR, JR.
Lieutenant General, USAF, MC, CFS
Surgeon General

By Direction of the Commandant of the Marine Corps:

Official:

EDWARD HANLON, JR.
Lieutenant General, U.S. Marine Corps
Commanding General
Marine Corps Combat Development Command

DISTRIBUTION:

US Army:	*Active Army, USAR, and ARNG*: To be distributed in accordance with the initial distribution number 110161, requirements for FM 4-25.11.
US Navy:	All Ships and Stations having Medical Department Personnel.
US Air Force:	F
US Marine Corps:	PCN: 144 000037 00

*FIELD MANUAL
NO. 4-25.11
NAVY TACTICAL
REFERENCE
PUBLICATION
NO. 4-02.1
AIR FORCE MANUAL
NO. 44-163(I)

HEADQUARTERS
DEPARTMENT OF THE ARMY,
THE NAVY, AND THE AIR FORCE
Washington, DC, 23 December 2002

FIRST AID

TABLE OF CONTENTS

Page

*This publication supersedes FM 21-11, 27 October 1988

PREFACE

This manual meets the first aid training needs of individual service members. Because medical personnel will not always be readily available, the nonmedical service members must rely heavily on their own skills and knowledge of life-sustaining methods to survive on the integrated battlefield. This publication outlines both self-aid and aid to other service members (buddy aid). More importantly, it emphasizes prompt and effective action in sustaining life and preventing or minimizing further suffering and disability. First aid is the emergency care given to the sick, injured, or wounded before being treated by medical personnel. The term *first aid* can be defined as "urgent and immediate lifesaving and other measures, which can be performed for casualties by nonmedical personnel when medical personnel are not immediately available." Nonmedical service members have received basic first aid training and should remain skilled in the correct procedures for giving first aid. This manual is directed to *all* service members. The procedures discussed apply to all types of casualties and the measures described are for use by both male and female service members.

This publication is in consonance with the following North Atlantic Treaty Organization (NATO) International Standardization Agreements (STANAGs) and American, British. Canadian, and Australian Quadripartite Standardization Agreements (QSTAGs).

TITLE	STANAG	QSTAG
Medical Training in First Aid, Basic Hygiene and Emergency Care	2122	535
First Aid Kits and Emergency Medical Care Kits	2126	
Medical First Aid and Hygiene Training in NBC Operations	2358	
First Aid Material for Chemical Injuries	2871	

These agreements are available on request, using Department of Defense (DD) Form 1425 from the Standardization Documents Order Desk, 700 Robins Avenue, Building 4, Section D, Philadelphia, Pennsylvania 19111-5094.

Unless this publication states otherwise, masculine nouns and pronouns do not refer exclusively to men.

Use of trade or brand names in this publication is for illustrative purposes only and does not imply endorsement by the Department of Defense (DOD).

The proponent for this publication is the US Army Medical Department Center and School. Submit comments and recommendations for the improvement of this publication directly to the **Commander, US Army Medical Department Center and School, ATTN: MCCS-FCD-L, 1400 East Grayson Street, Fort Sam Houston, Texas 78234-5052**.

CHAPTER 1

FUNDAMENTAL CRITERIA FOR FIRST AID

"The fate of the wounded rests in the hands of the ones who apply the first dressing."

Nicholas Senn (1898) (49th President of the American Medical Association)

1-1. General

When a nonmedical service member comes upon an unconscious or injured service member, he must accurately evaluate the casualty to determine the first aid measures needed to prevent further injury or death. He should seek medical assistance as soon as possible, but he should not interrupt the performance of first aid measures. To interrupt the first aid measures may cause more harm than good to the casualty. Remember that in a chemical environment, the service member should not evaluate the casualty until the casualty has been masked. After performing first aid, the service member must proceed with the evaluation and continue to monitor the casualty for development of conditions which may require the performance of necessary basic lifesaving measures, such as clearing the airway, rescue breathing, preventing shock, and controlling bleeding. He should continue to monitor the casualty until relieved by medical personnel.

Service members may have to depend upon their first aid knowledge and skills to save themselves (self-aid) or other service members (buddy aid/ combat lifesaver). They may be able to save a life, prevent permanent disability, or reduce long periods of hospitalization by knowing **WHAT** to do, **WHAT NOT** to do, and **WHEN** to seek medical assistance.

NOTE

The prevalence of various body armor systems currently fielded to US service members, and those in development for future fielding, may present a temporary obstacle to effective evaluation of an injured service member. You may have to *carefully remove* the body armor from the injured service member to complete the evaluation or administer first aid. Begin by removing the outer–most hard or soft body armor components (open, unfasten or cut the closures, fasteners, or straps), then remove any successive layers in the same manner. Be sure to follow other notes, cautions and warnings regarding procedures in contaminated situations and when a broken back or neck is suspected. Continue to evaluate.

1-2. Terminology

To enhance the understanding of the material contained in this publication, the following terms are used—

- *Combat lifesaver*. This is a US Army program governed by Army Regulation (AR) 350-41. The combat lifesaver is a member of a nonmedical unit selected by the unit commander for additional training beyond basic first aid procedures (referred to as *enhanced first aid*). A minimum of one individual per squad, crew, team, or equivalent-sized unit should be trained. The primary duty of this individual does not change. The additional duty of combat lifesaver is to provide enhanced first aid for injuries based on his training before the trauma specialist (military occupational specialty [MOS] 91W) arrives. The combat lifesaver's training is normally provided by medical personnel assigned, attached, or in direct support (DS) of the unit. The senior medical person designated by the commander manages the training program.

- *Trauma Specialist (US Army) or Hospital Corpsman (HM)*. A medical specialist trained in emergency medical treatment (EMT) procedures and assigned or attached in support of a combat or combat support unit or marine forces.

- *Casualty evacuation*. Casualty evacuation (CASEVAC) is a term used by nonmedical units to refer to the movement of casualties aboard nonmedical vehicles or aircraft. See also the term *transported* below. Refer to FM 8-10-6 for additional information.

CAUTION

Casualties transported in this manner do not receive en route medical care.

- *Enhanced first aid (US Army)*. Enhanced first aid is administered by the combat lifesaver. It includes measures, which require an additional level of training above self-aid and buddy aid, such as the initiation of intravenous (IV) fluids.

- *Medical evacuation*. Medical evacuation is the timely, efficient movement of the wounded, injured, or ill service members from the battlefield and other locations to medical treatment facilities (MTFs). Medical personnel provide en route medical care during the evacuation. Once the casualty has entered the medical stream (trauma specialist, hospital corpsman, evacuation crew, or MTF), the role of first aid in the care of the casualty ceases and the casualty becomes the responsibility of the health service support (HSS) chain. Once he has entered the HSS chain he is referred to as a *patient*.

- *First aid measures*. Urgent and immediate lifesaving and other measures, which can be performed for casualties (or performed by the casualty himself) by nonmedical personnel when medical personnel are not immediately available.

- *Medical treatment*. Medical treatment is the care and management of wounded, injured, or ill service members by medically trained (MOS-trained) HM, and area of concentration (AOC) personnel. It may include EMT, advanced trauma management (ATM), and resuscitative and surgical intervention.

- *Medical treatment facility*. Any facility established for the purpose of providing medical treatment. This includes battalion aid stations, Level II facilities, dispensaries, clinics, and hospitals.

- *Self-aid/buddy aid*. Each individual service member is trained to be proficient in a variety of specific first aid procedures. This training enables the service member or a buddy to apply immediate first aid measures to alleviate a life-threatening situation.

- *Transported*. A casualty is moved to an MTF in a nonmedical vehicle without en route care provided by a medically-trained service member (such as a Trauma Specialist or HM). First aid measures should be continually performed while the casualty is being transported. If the casualty is acquired by a dedicated medical vehicle with a medically-trained crew, the role of first aid ceases and the casualty becomes the responsibility of the HSS chain, and is then referred to as a *patient*. This method of transporting a casualty is also referred to as *CASEVAC*.

1-3. Understanding Vital Body Functions for First Aid

In order for the service member to learn to perform first aid procedures, he must have a basic understanding of what the vital body functions are and what the result will be if they are damaged or not functioning.

a. *Breathing Process*. All humans must have oxygen to live. Through the breathing process, the lungs draw oxygen from the air and put it into the blood. The heart pumps the blood through the body to be used by the cells that require a constant supply of oxygen. Some cells are more dependent on a constant supply of oxygen than others. For example, cells of the brain may die within 4 to 6 minutes without oxygen. Once these cells die, they are lost forever since they do not regenerate. This could result in permanent brain damage, paralysis, or death.

b. Respiration. Respiration occurs when a person inhales (oxygen is taken into the body) and then exhales (carbon dioxide [CO_2] is expelled from the body). Respiration involves the—

- *Airway.* The airway consists of the nose, mouth, throat, voice box, and windpipe. It is the canal through which air passes to and from the lungs.

- *Lungs.* The lungs are two elastic organs made up of thousands of tiny air spaces and covered by an airtight membrane. The *bronchial tree* is a part of the lungs.

- *Rib cage.* The rib cage is formed by the muscle-connected ribs, which join the spine in back, and the breastbone in front. The top part of the rib cage is closed by the structure of the neck, and the bottom part is separated from the abdominal cavity by a large dome-shaped muscle called the *diaphragm* (Figure 1-1). The diaphragm and rib muscles, which are under the control of the respiratory center in the brain, automatically *contract* and *relax*. *Contraction* increases and *relaxation* decreases the size of the rib cage. When the rib cage increases and then decreases, the air pressure in the lungs is first less and then more than the atmospheric pressure, thus causing the air to rush into and out of the lungs to equalize the pressure. This cycle of inhaling and exhaling is repeated about 12 to 18 times per minute.

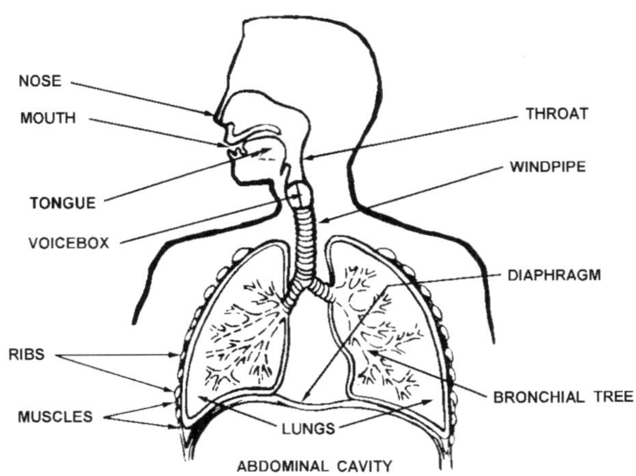

Figure 1-1. Airway, lungs, and rib cage.

c. *Blood Circulation.* The heart and the blood vessels (arteries, veins, and capillaries) circulate blood through the body tissues. The heart is divided into two separate halves, each acting as a pump. The left side pumps oxygenated blood (bright red) through the arteries into the capillaries; nutrients and oxygen pass from the blood through the walls of the capillaries into the cells. At the same time waste products and CO_2 enter the capillaries. From the capillaries the oxygen poor blood is carried through the veins to the right side of the heart and then into the lungs where it expels the CO_2 and picks up oxygen. Blood in the veins is dark red because of its low oxygen content. Blood does not flow through the veins in spurts as it does through the arteries. The entire system of the heart, blood vessels, and lymphatics is called the *circulatory system.*

(1) *Heartbeat.* The heart functions as a pump to circulate the blood continuously through the blood vessels to all parts of the body. It contracts, forcing the blood from its chambers; then it relaxes, permitting its chambers to refill with blood. The rhythmical cycle of contraction and relaxation is called the *heartbeat.* The normal heartbeat is from 60 to 80 beats per minute.

(2) *Pulse.* The heartbeat causes a rhythmical expansion and contraction of the arteries as it forces blood through them. This cycle of expansion and contraction can be felt (monitored) at various points in the body and is called the *pulse.* The common points for checking the pulse are at the—

- Side of the neck (*carotid*).
- Groin (*femoral*).
- Wrist (*radial*).
- Ankle (*posterior tibial*).

(*a*) *Carotid pulse.* To check the carotid pulse, feel for a pulse on the side of the casualty's neck closest to you. This is done by placing the tips of your first two fingers beside his Adam's apple (Figure 1-2).

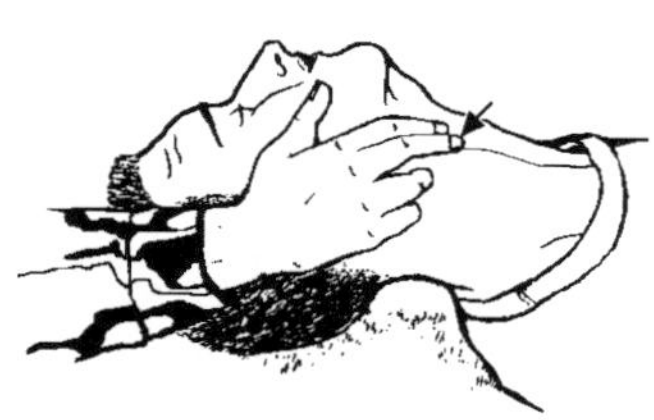

Figure 1-2. Carotid pulse.

(*b*) *Femoral pulse*. To check the femoral pulse, press the tips of your first two fingers into the middle of the groin (Figure 1-3).

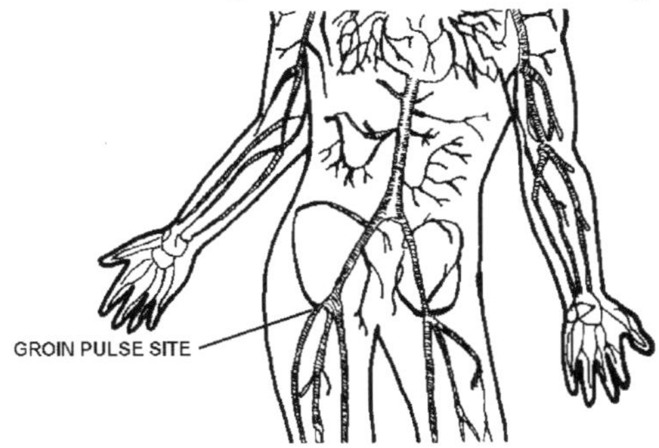

Figure 1-3. Femoral pulse.

(*c*) *Radial pulse*. To check the radial pulse, place your first two fingers on the thumb side of the casualty's wrist (Figure 1-4).

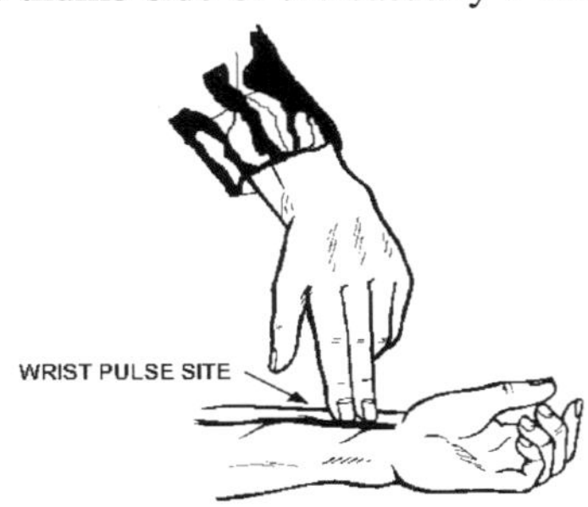

Figure 1-4. Radial pulse.

(*d*) *Posterior tibial pulse*. To check the posterior tibial pulse, place your first two fingers on the inside of the ankle (Figure 1-5).

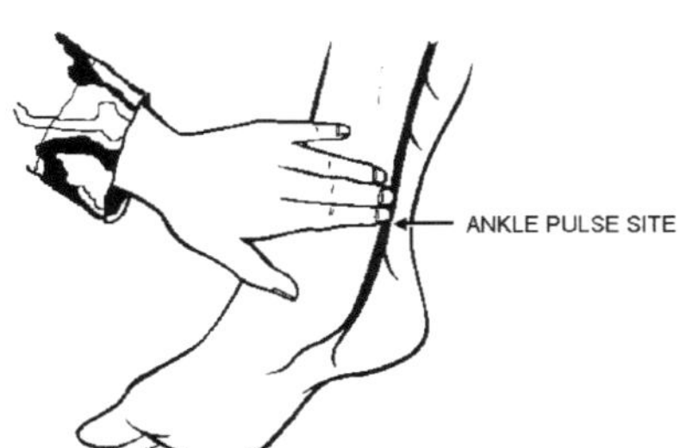

Figure 1-5. Posterior tibial pulse.

NOTE

DO NOT use your thumb to check a casualty's pulse because you may confuse the beat of your pulse with that of the casualty.

1-4. Adverse Conditions

a. Lack of Oxygen. Human life cannot exist without a continuous intake of oxygen. Lack of oxygen rapidly leads to death. First aid involves knowing how to open the airway and restore breathing.

b. Bleeding. Human life cannot continue without an adequate volume of blood circulating through the body to carry oxygen to the tissues. An important first aid measure is to stop the bleeding to prevent the loss of blood.

c. Shock. Shock means there is an inadequate blood flow to the vital tissues and organs. Shock that remains uncorrected may result in death even though the injury or condition causing the shock would not otherwise be fatal. Shock can result from many causes, such as loss of blood, loss of fluid from deep burns, pain, and reaction to the sight of a wound or blood. First aid includes preventing shock, since the casualty's chances of survival are much greater if he does not develop shock. Refer to paragraphs 2-21 through 2-24 for a further discussion of shock.

d. Infection. Recovery from a severe injury or a wound depends largely upon how well the injury or wound was initially protected. Infections result from the multiplication and growth (spread) of harmful microscopic organisms (sometimes referred to as germs). These harmful microscopic organisms are in the air, water, and soil, and on the skin and clothing. Some of these organisms will immediately invade (contaminate) a break in the skin or an open wound. The objective is to keep wounds clean and free of these organisms. A good working knowledge of basic first aid measures also includes knowing how to dress a wound to avoid infection or additional contamination.

1-5. Basics of First Aid

Most injured or ill service members are able to return to their units to fight or support primarily because they are given appropriate and timely first aid followed by the best medical care possible. Therefore, all service members must remember the basics.

- Check for **BREATHING**: Lack of oxygen intake (through a compromised airway or inadequate breathing) can lead to brain damage or death in very few minutes.

- Check for **BLEEDING**: Life cannot continue without an adequate volume of blood to carry oxygen to tissues.

- Check for **SHOCK**: Unless shock is prevented, first aid performed, and medical treatment provided, death may result even though the injury would not otherwise be fatal.

1-6. Evaluating a Casualty

a. The time may come when you must instantly apply your knowledge of first aid measures. This could occur during combat operations, in training situations, or while in a nonduty status. Any service member observing an unconscious and/or ill, injured, or wounded person must carefully and skillfully evaluate him to determine the first aid measures required to prevent further injury or death. He should seek help from medical personnel as soon as possible, but must not interrupt his evaluation of the casualty or fail to administer first aid measures. A second service member may be sent to find medical help. One of the cardinal principles for assisting a casualty is that you (the initial rescuer) must continue the evaluation and first aid measures, as the tactical situation permits, until another individual relieves you. If, during any part of the evaluation, the casualty exhibits the conditions (such as shock) for which the service member is checking, the service member must stop the evaluation and immediately administer first aid. In a chemical environment, the service member should not evaluate the casualty until both the individual and the casualty have been masked. If it is suspected that a nerve agent was used, administer the casualty's own nerve agent antidote autoinjector. After providing first aid, the service member must proceed with the evaluation and continue to monitor the casualty for further complications until relieved by medical personnel.

WARNING

Do not use your own nerve agent antidote autoinjector on the casualty.

NOTE

Remember, when evaluating and/or administering first aid to a casualty, you should seek medical aid as soon as possible. **DO NOT** stop first aid measures, but if the situation allows, send another service member to find medical aid.

b. To evaluate a casualty, perform the following steps:

(1) *Check the casualty for responsiveness.* This is done by gently shaking or tapping him while calmly asking, "Are you OK?" Watch for a response. If the casualty does not respond, go to step (2). If the casualty responds, continue with the evaluation.

(*a*) If the casualty is conscious, ask him where he feels different than usual or where it hurts. Ask him to identify the location of pain if he can, or to identify the area in which there is no feeling.

(*b*) If the casualty is conscious but is choking and cannot talk, stop the evaluation and begin first aid measures. Refer to paragraphs 2-10 and 2-11 for specific information on opening the airway.

WARNING

If a broken back or neck is suspected, do not move the casualty unless his life is in immediate danger (such as close to a burning vehicle). Movement may cause permanent paralysis or death.

(2) *Check for breathing.* (Refer to paragraph 2-6 for this procedure.)

(*a*) If the casualty is breathing, proceed to step (3).

(*b*) If the casualty is not breathing, stop the evaluation and begin first aid measures to attempt to ventilate the casualty. Attempt to open the airway, if an airway obstruction is apparent, clear the airway obstruction, then ventilate (see paragraphs 2-10 and 2-11).

(*c*) After successfully ventilating the casualty, proceed to step (3).

(3) *Check for pulse.* (Refer to paragraph 1-3*c*(2) for specific methods.) If a pulse is present and the casualty is breathing, proceed to step (4).

(*a*) If a pulse is present, but the casualty is still not breathing, start rescue breathing.

(*b*) If a pulse is not present, seek medical personnel for help.

(4) *Check for bleeding.* Look for spurts of blood or blood-soaked clothes. Also check for *both* entry and exit wounds. If the casualty is bleeding from an open wound, stop the evaluation and begin first aid procedures as follows for a—

(*a*) Wound of the arm or leg (refer to paragraphs 2-16 through 2-18 for information on putting on a field or pressure dressing).

(*b*) Partial or complete amputation, apply dressing (refer to paragraph 2-16 to 2-18) and then apply tourniquet if bleeding is not stopped (refer to paragraph 2-20 for information on putting on a tourniquet).

(*c*) Open head wound (refer to paragraph 3-10 for information on applying a dressing to an open head wound).

(*d*) Open chest wound (refer to paragraph 3-5 for information on applying a dressing to an open chest wound).

(*e*) Open abdominal wound (refer to paragraph 3-7 for information on applying a dressing to an open abdominal wound).

WARNING

In a chemically contaminated area, do not expose the wounds. Apply field dressing and then pressure dressing over wound area as needed.

(5) *Check for shock.* (Refer to paragraph 2-24 for first aid measures for shock.) If the signs and symptoms of shock are present, stop the evaluation, and begin first aid measures immediately. The following are the nine signs and symptoms of shock.

(*a*) Sweaty but cool skin (clammy skin).

(*b*) Paleness of skin. (In dark-skinned service members look for a grayish cast to the skin.)

(*c*) Restlessness or nervousness.

(*d*) Thirst.

(*e*) Loss of blood (bleeding).

(*f*) Confusion (does not seem aware of surroundings).

(*g*) Faster than normal breathing rate.

(*h*) Blotchy or bluish skin, especially around the mouth.

(*i*) Nausea or vomiting.

WARNING

Leg fractures must be splinted before elevating the legs as a first aid measure for shock.

(6) *Check for fractures.*

(*a*) Check for the following signs and symptoms of a back or neck injury and perform first aid procedures as necessary.

- Pain or tenderness of the back or neck area.
- Cuts or bruises on the back or neck area.
- Inability of a casualty to move or decreased sensation to extremities (paralysis or numbness).
  - Ask about ability to move (paralysis).
  - Touch the casualty's arms and legs and ask whether he can feel your hand (numbness).
- Unusual body or limb position.

(*b*) Immobilize any casualty suspected of having a back or neck injury by doing the following:

- Tell the casualty not to move.
- If a back injury is suspected, place padding (rolled or folded to conform to the shape of the arch) under the natural arch of the casualty's back. (For example, a blanket/poncho may be used as padding.)

> **WARNING**
>
> **Do not move casualty to place padding.**

- If a neck injury is suspected, immediately immobilize (manually) the head and neck. Place a roll of cloth under the casualty's neck, and put weighted boots (filled with dirt or sand) or rocks on both sides of his head.

(*c*) Check the casualty's arms and legs for open or closed fractures.

- Check for *open* fractures by looking for—
  - Bleeding.
  - Bones sticking through the skin.
  - Check for pulse.
- Check for *closed* fractures by looking for—
  - Swelling.
  - Discoloration.
  - Deformity.
  - Unusual body position.
  - Check for pulse.

(*d*) Stop the evaluation and begin first aid measures if a fracture to an arm or leg is suspected. Refer to Chapter 4 for information on splinting a suspected fracture.

(*e*) Check for signs/symptoms of fractures of other body areas (for example, shoulder or hip) and provide first aid as necessary.

(7) *Check for burns.* Look carefully for reddened, blistered, or charred skin; also check for singed clothing. If burns are found, stop the evaluation and begin first aid procedures. Refer to paragraph 3-9 for information on giving first aid for burns.

NOTE

Burns to the upper torso and face may cause respiratory complications. When evaluating the casualty, look for singed nose hair, soot around the nostrils, and listen for abnormal breath sounds or difficulty breathing.

(8) *Check for possible head injury.*

(*a*) Look for the following signs and symptoms:

- Unequal pupils.
- Fluid from the ear(s), nose, mouth, or injury site.
- Slurred speech.
- Confusion.
- Sleepiness.
- Loss of memory or consciousness.
- Staggering in walking.
- Headache.
- Dizziness.
- Nausea or vomiting.
- Paralysis.
- Convulsions or twitches.
- Bruising around the eyes and behind the ears.

(*b*) If a head injury is suspected, continue to watch for signs which would require performance of rescue breathing, first aid measures for shock, or control of bleeding; seek medical aid. Refer to paragraph 3-10 for information on first aid measures for head injuries.

CHAPTER 2

BASIC MEASURES FOR FIRST AID

2-1. General

Several conditions that require immediate attention are an inadequate airway, lack of breathing, and excessive loss of blood (circulation). A casualty without a clear airway or who is not breathing may die from lack of oxygen. Excessive loss of blood may lead to shock, and shock can lead to death; therefore, you must act immediately to control the loss of blood. All wounds are considered to be contaminated, since infection-producing organisms (germs) are always present on the skin and clothing, and in the soil, water, and air. Any missile or instrument (such as a bullet, shrapnel, knife, or bayonet) causing a wound pushes or carries the germs into that wound. Infection results as these organisms multiply. That a wound is contaminated does not lessen the importance of protecting it from further contamination. You must dress and bandage a wound as soon as possible to prevent further contamination.

NOTE

It is also important that you attend to any airway, breathing, or bleeding problems **IMMEDIATELY** because these problems, if left unattended, may become life threatening.

Section I. OPEN THE AIRWAY AND RESTORE BREATHING

2-2. Breathing Process

All humans must have oxygen to live. Through the breathing process, the lungs draw oxygen from the air and put it into the blood. The heart pumps the blood through the body to be used by the cells that require a constant supply of oxygen. Some cells are more dependent on a constant supply of oxygen than others. For example, cells of the brain may die within 4 to 6 minutes without oxygen. Once these cells die, they are lost forever since they do not regenerate. This could result in permanent brain damage, paralysis, or death.

2-3. Assessment of and Positioning the Casualty

a. **CHECK** for responsiveness (Figure 2-1A)—establish whether the casualty is conscious by gently shaking him and asking, “Are you OK?”

b. **CALL** for help (Figure 2-1B).

c. **POSITION** the unconscious casualty so that he is lying on his back and on a firm surface (Figure 2-1C).

> **WARNING**
>
> **If the casualty is lying on his chest (prone position), cautiously roll the casualty as a unit so that his body does not twist (which may further complicate a back, neck, or spinal injury).**

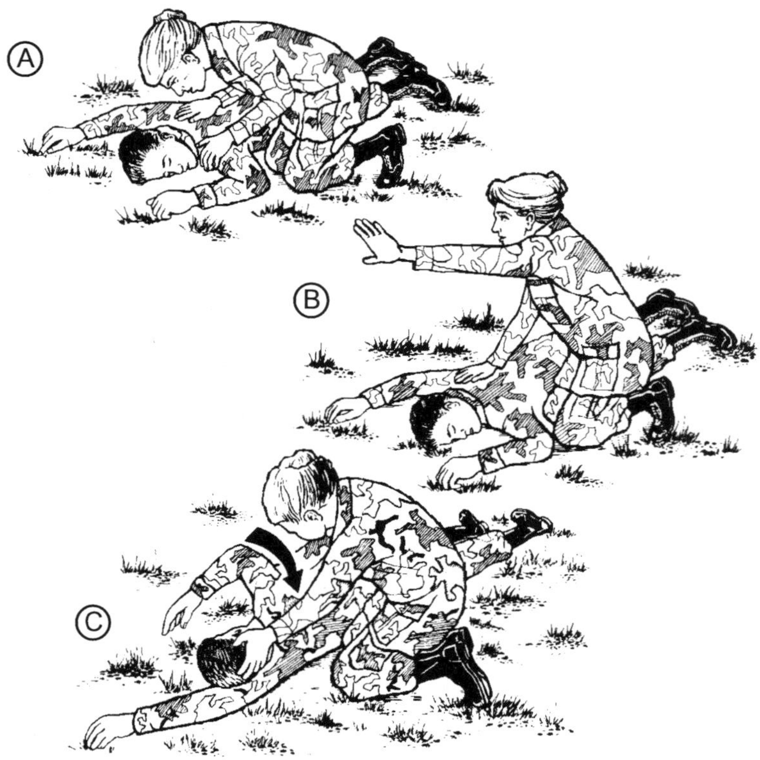

Figure 2-1. Assessment (Illustrated A—C).

(1) Straighten the casualty's legs. Take the casualty's arm that is nearest to you and move it so that it is straight and above his head. Repeat the procedure for the other arm.

(2) Kneel beside the casualty with your knees near his shoulders (leave space to roll his body) (Figure 2-1B). Place one hand behind his head and neck for support. With your other hand, grasp the casualty under his far arm (Figure 2-1C).

(3) Roll the casualty towards you using a steady, even pull. His head and neck should stay in line with his back.

(4) Return the casualty's arms to his side. Straighten his legs. Reposition yourself so that you are now kneeling at the level of the casualty's shoulders. However, if a neck injury is suspected and the jaw-thrust technique will be used, kneel at the casualty's head, looking towards his feet.

2-4. Opening the Airway of an Unconscious or Not Breathing Casualty

The tongue is the single most common cause of an airway obstruction (Figure 2-2). In most cases, simply using the head-tilt/chin-lift technique can clear the airway. This action pulls the tongue away from the air passage in the throat (Figure 2-3).

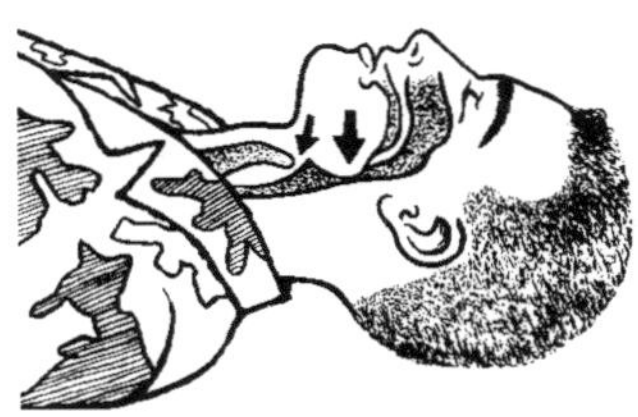

Figure 2-2. Airway blocked by tongue.

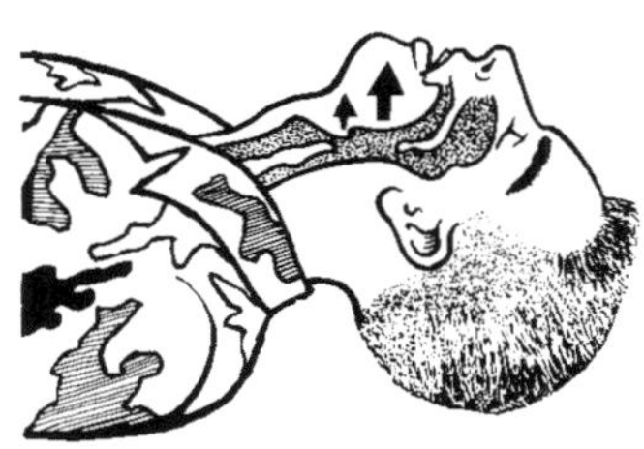

Figure 2-3. Airway opened by extending neck.

a. Call for help and then position the casualty. Move (roll) the casualty onto his back (Figure 2-1C). (Refer to paragraph 2-3*c* for information on positioning the casualty.)

NOTE

Perform finger sweep. If foreign material or vomitus is visible in the mouth, it should be removed, but do not spend an excessive amount of time doing so.

b. Open the airway using the jaw-thrust or head-tilt/chin-lift technique.

CAUTION

The head-tilt/chin-lift technique is an important procedure in opening the airway; however, use extreme care because excess force in performing this maneuver may cause further spinal injury. In a casualty with a suspected neck injury or severe head trauma, the safest approach to opening the airway is the jaw-thrust technique because in most cases it can be accomplished without extending the neck.

(1) *Perform the jaw-thrust technique*. The jaw-thrust may be accomplished by the rescuer grasping the angles of the casualty's lower jaw and lifting with both hands, one on each side, displacing the jaw forward and up (Figure 2-4). The rescuer's elbows should rest on the surface on which the casualty is lying. If the lips close, the lower lip can be retracted with the thumb. If mouth-to-mouth breathing is necessary, close the nostrils by placing your cheek tightly against them. The head should be carefully supported without tilting it backwards or turning it from side to side. If this is unsuccessful, the head should be tilted back very slightly. The jaw-thrust is the safest first approach to opening the airway of a casualty who has a suspected neck injury because in most cases it can be accomplished without extending the neck.

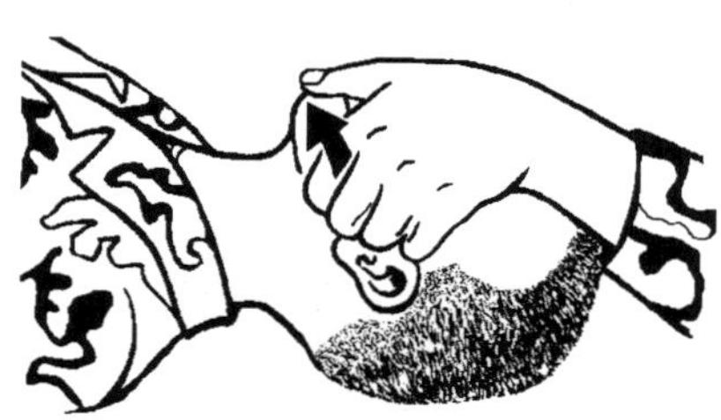

Figure 2-4. Jaw-thrust technique of opening airway.

(2) *Perform the head-tilt/chin-lift technique.* Place one hand on the casualty's forehead and apply firm, backward pressure with the palm to tilt the head back. Place the fingertips of the other hand under the bony part of the lower jaw and lift, bringing the chin forward. The thumb should not be used to lift the chin (Figure 2-5).

NOTE

The fingers should not press deeply into the soft tissue under the chin because the airway may be obstructed.

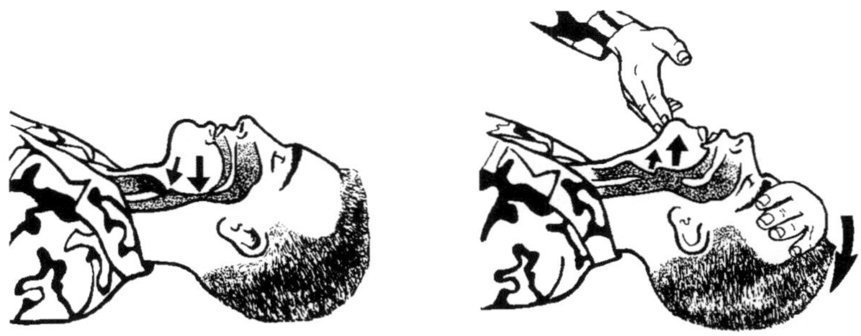

Figure 2-5. Head-tilt/chin-lift technique of opening airway.

(3) *Check for breathing (while maintaining an airway).* After establishing an open airway, it is important to maintain that airway in an open position. Often the act of just opening and maintaining the airway will allow the casualty to breathe properly. Once the rescuer uses one of the techniques to open the airway (jaw-thrust or head-tilt/chin-lift), he should maintain that head position to keep the airway open. Failure to maintain the open airway will prevent the casualty from receiving an adequate supply of oxygen. Therefore, while maintaining an open airway the rescuer should check for breathing by observing the casualty's chest and performing the following actions within 3 to 5 seconds:

(*a*) **LOOK** for the chest to rise and fall.

(*b*) **LISTEN** for air escaping during exhalation by placing your ear near the casualty's mouth.

(*c*) **FEEL** for the flow of air on your cheek (see Figure 2-6).

(*d*) **PERFORM** rescue breathing if the casualty does not resume breathing spontaneously.

NOTE

If the casualty resumes breathing, monitor and maintain the open airway. He should be transported to an MTF, as soon as practical.

2-5. Rescue Breathing (Artificial Respiration)

a. If the casualty does not promptly resume adequate spontaneous breathing after the airway is open, rescue breathing (artificial respiration) must be started. Be calm! Think and act quickly! The sooner you begin rescue breathing, the more likely you are to restore the casualty's breathing. If you are in doubt whether the casualty is breathing, give artificial respiration, since it can do no harm to a person who is breathing. If the casualty is breathing, you can feel and see his chest move. If the casualty is breathing, you can feel and hear air being expelled by putting your hand or ear close to his mouth and nose.

b. There are several methods of administering rescue breathing. The mouth-to-mouth method is preferred; however, it cannot be used in all situations. If the casualty has a severe jaw fracture or mouth wound or his jaws are tightly closed by spasms, use the mouth-to-nose method.

2-6. Preliminary Steps—All Rescue Breathing Methods

a. Establish unresponsiveness. Call for help. Turn or position the casualty.

b. Open the airway.

c. Check for breathing by placing your ear over the casualty's mouth and nose, and looking toward his chest.

(1) **LOOK** for rise and fall of the casualty's chest (Figure 2-6).

(2) **LISTEN** for sounds of breathing.

(3) **FEEL** for breath on the side of your face. If the chest does not rise and fall and no air is exhaled, then the casualty is not breathing.

(4) **PERFORM** rescue breathing if the casualty is not breathing.

NOTE

Although the rescuer may notice that the casualty is making respiratory efforts, the airway may still be obstructed and opening the airway may be all that is needed. If the casualty resumes breathing, the rescuer should continue to maintain an open airway.

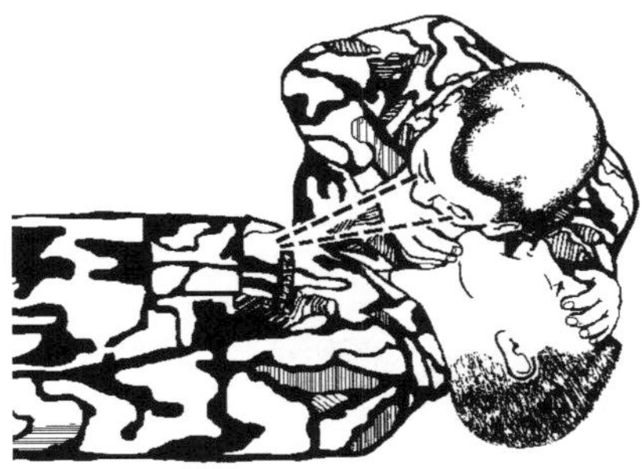

Figure 2-6. Check for breathing.

2-7. Mouth-to-Mouth Method

In this method of rescue breathing, you inflate the casualty's lungs with air from your lungs. This can be accomplished by blowing air into the person's mouth. The mouth-to-mouth rescue breathing method is performed as follows:

a. If the casualty is not breathing, place your hand on his forehead, and pinch his nostrils together with the thumb and index finger of this hand. Let this same hand exert pressure on his forehead to maintain the backward head tilt and maintain an open airway. With your other hand, keep your fingertips on the bony part of the lower jaw near the chin and lift (Figure 2-7).

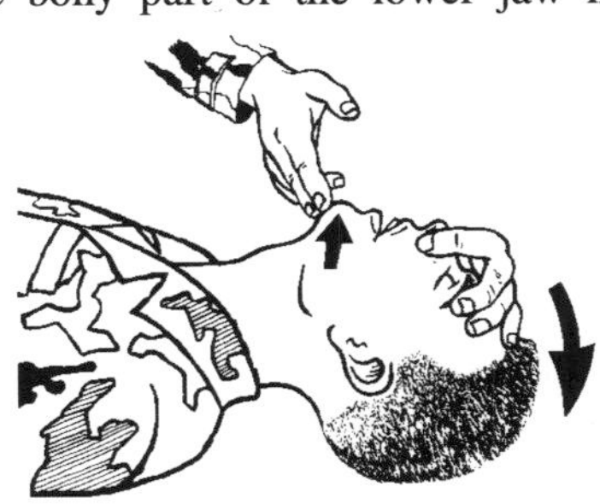

Figure 2-7. Head tilt/chin lift.

NOTE

If you suspect the casualty has a neck injury and you are using the jaw-thrust technique, close the nostrils by placing your cheek tightly against them.

b. Take a deep breath and place your mouth (in an airtight seal) around the casualty's mouth (Figure 2-8). (If the injured person is small, cover both his nose and mouth with your mouth, sealing your lips against the skin of his face.)

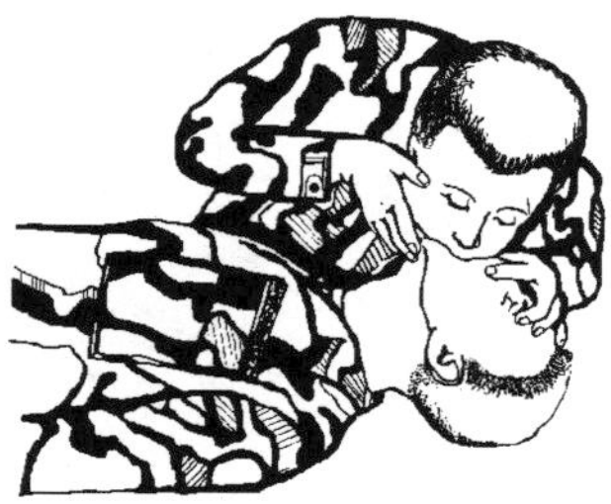

Figure 2-8. Rescue breathing.

c. Blow two full breaths into the casualty's mouth (1 to 1 1/2 seconds per breath), taking a breath of fresh air each time before you blow. Watch out of the corner of your eye for the casualty's chest to rise. If the chest rises, sufficient air is getting into the casualty's lungs. Therefore, proceed as described in step (1). If the chest does not rise, do the following (*a*, *b*, and *c* below) and then attempt to ventilate again.

(1) Take corrective action immediately by reestablishing the airway. Make sure that air is not leaking from around your mouth or out of the casualty's pinched nose.

(2) Reattempt to ventilate.

(3) If the chest still does not rise, take the necessary action to open an obstructed airway (paragraph 2-10).

NOTE

If the initial attempt to ventilate the casualty is unsuccessful, reposition the casualty's head and repeat rescue breathing. Improper chin and head positioning is the most common cause of difficulty with ventilation. If the casualty cannot be ventilated after repositioning the head, proceed with foreign-body airway obstruction maneuvers (see paragraph 2-10).

(4) After giving two slow breaths, which cause the chest to rise, attempt to locate a pulse on the casualty. Feel for a pulse on the side of the casualty's neck closest to you by placing the first two fingers (index and middle fingers) of your hand on the groove beside the casualty's Adam's apple (carotid pulse) (Figure 2-9). (Your thumb should not be used for pulse taking because you may confuse your pulse beat with that of the casualty.) Maintain the airway by keeping your other hand on the casualty's forehead. Allow 5 to 10 seconds to determine if there is a pulse.

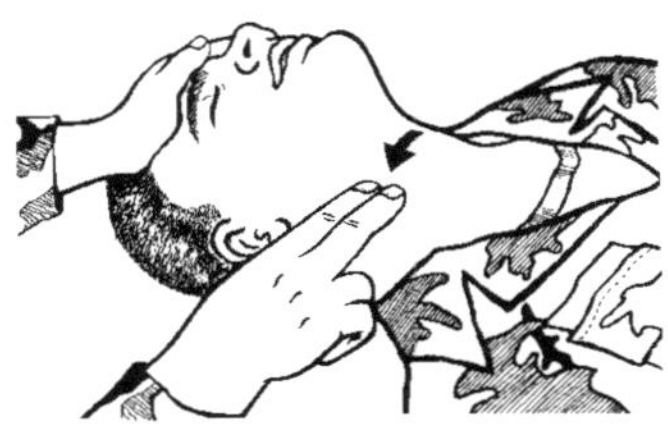

Figure 2-9. Placement of fingers to detect pulse.

(*a*) If signs of circulation are present and a pulse is found and the casualty is breathing—**STOP**; allow the casualty to breathe on his own. If possible, keep him warm and comfortable.

(*b*) If a pulse is found and the casualty is not breathing, continue rescue breathing.

(*c*) If a pulse is not found, seek medically trained personnel for help as soon as possible.

2-8. Mouth-to-Nose Method

Use this method if you cannot perform mouth-to-mouth rescue breathing because the casualty has a severe jaw fracture or mouth wound or his jaws are tightly closed by spasms. The mouth-to-nose method is performed in the same way as the mouth-to-mouth method except that you blow into the nose while you hold the lips closed with one hand at the chin. You then remove your mouth to allow the casualty to exhale passively. It may be necessary to separate the casualty's lips to allow the air to escape during exhalation.

2-9. Heartbeat

If a casualty's heart stops beating, you must immediately seek medical help. **SECONDS COUNT!** Stoppage of the heart is soon followed by cessation of respiration unless it has occurred first. Be calm! Think and act! When a casualty's heart has stopped, there is no pulse at all; the person is unconscious and limp, and the pupils of his eyes are open wide. When evaluating a casualty or when performing the preliminary steps of rescue breathing, feel for a pulse. If you DO NOT detect a pulse, seek medical help.

2-10. Airway Obstructions

In order for oxygen from the air to flow to and from the lungs, the upper airway must be unobstructed.

a. Upper airway obstructions often occur because—

(1) The casualty's tongue falls back into his throat while he is unconscious. The tongue *falls back* and *obstructs* the airway, it is not swallowed by the casualty.

NOTE

Ensure the correct positioning and maintenance of the open airway for an injured or unconscious casualty.

(2) Foreign bodies become lodged in the throat. These obstructions usually occur while eating. Choking on food (usually meat) is associated with—

- Attempting to swallow large pieces of poorly chewed food.
- Drinking alcohol.
- Slipping dentures.

(3) The contents of the stomach are regurgitated and may block the airway.

(4) Blood clots may form as a result of head and facial injuries.

b. Upper airway obstruction may cause either partial or complete airway blockage.

(1) *Partial airway obstruction.* The casualty may still have an air exchange. A good air exchange means that the casualty can cough

forcefully, though he may be wheezing between coughs. You, the rescuer, should not interfere, and should encourage the casualty to cough up the object obstructing his airway on his own. A poor air exchange may be indicated by weak coughing with a high pitched noise between coughs. Further, the casualty may show signs of shock (paragraph 1-6*b*[5]) indicating a need for oxygen. You should assist the casualty and treat him as though he had a complete obstruction.

(2) *Complete airway obstruction.* A complete obstruction (no air exchange) is indicated if the casualty cannot speak, breathe, or cough at all. He may be clutching his neck and moving erratically. In an unconscious casualty, a complete obstruction is also indicated if after opening his airway you cannot ventilate him.

2-11. Opening the Obstructed Airway—Conscious Casualty

Clearing a conscious casualty's airway obstruction can be performed with the casualty either standing or sitting and by following a relatively simple procedure.

WARNING

Once an obstructed airway occurs, the brain will develop an oxygen deficiency resulting in unconsciousness. Death will follow rapidly if breathing is not promptly restored.

a. Ask the casualty if he can speak or if he is choking. Check for the universal choking sign (Figure 2-10).

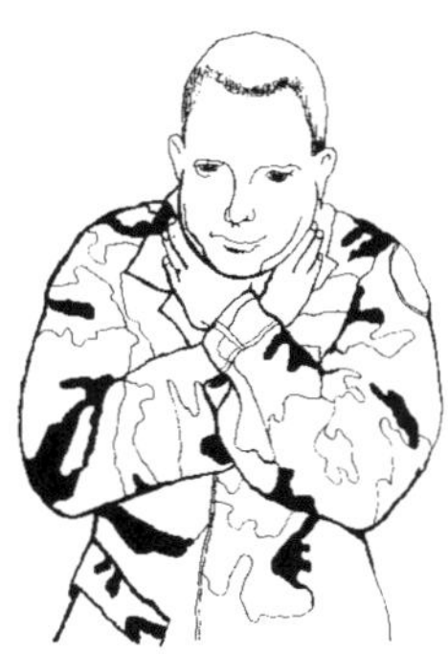

Figure 2-10. Universal sign of choking.

b. If the casualty can speak, encourage him to attempt to cough; the casualty still has a good air exchange. If he is able to speak or cough effectively, DO NOT interfere with his attempts to expel the obstruction.

c. Listen for high pitched sounds when the casualty breathes or coughs (poor air exchange). If there is poor air exchange or no breathing, CALL FOR HELP and immediately deliver manual thrusts (either an abdominal or chest thrust).

NOTE

The manual thrust with the hands centered between the waist and the rib cage is called an abdominal thrust (or Heimlich maneuver). The chest thrust (the hands are centered in the middle of the breastbone) is used only for an individual in the advanced stages of pregnancy, in the markedly obese casualty, or if there is a significant abdominal wound.

(1) Apply abdominal thrusts. This can be accomplished by using the following procedures:

(*a*) Stand behind the casualty and wrap your arms around his waist.

(*b*) Make a fist with one hand and grasp it with the other. The thumb side of your fist should be against the casualty's abdomen, in the midline and slightly above the casualty's navel, but well below the tip of the breastbone (Figure 2-11).

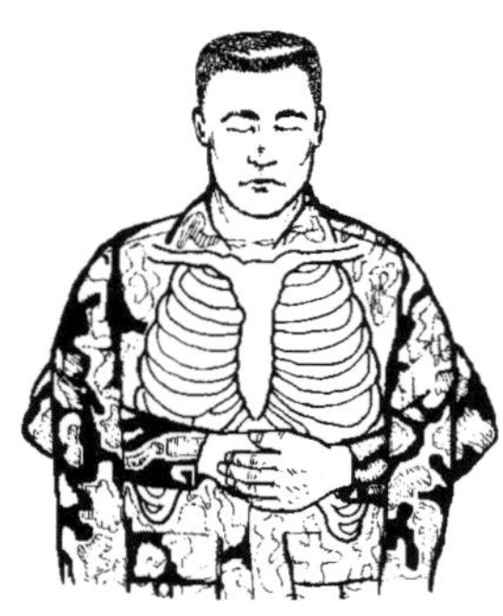

Figure 2-11. Anatomical view of abdominal thrust procedure.

(*c*) Press the fists into the abdomen with a quick backward and upward thrust (Figure 2-12).

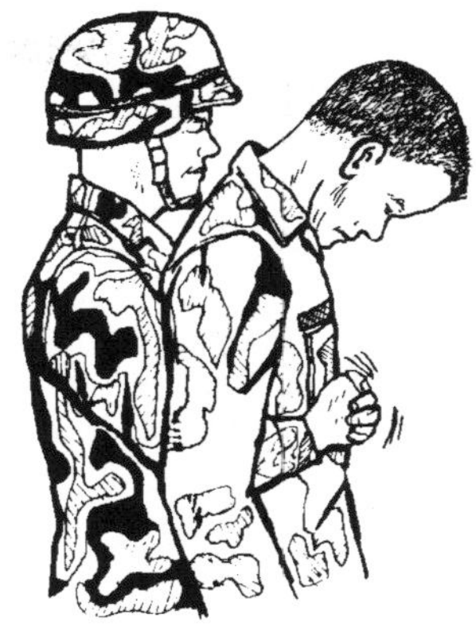

Figure 2-12. Profile view of abdominal thrust.

(*d*) Each thrust should be a separate and distinct movement.

NOTE

Continue performing abdominal thrusts until the obstruction is expelled or the casualty becomes unresponsive.

(*e*) If the casualty becomes unresponsive, call for help as you proceed with steps to open the airway, and perform rescue breathing. (Refer to paragraph 2-7 for information on how to perform mouth-to-mouth resuscitation.)

(2) Apply chest thrusts. An alternate technique to the abdominal thrust is the chest thrust. This technique is useful when the casualty has an abdominal wound, when the casualty is pregnant, or when the casualty is so large that you cannot wrap your arms around the abdomen. To apply chest thrusts with casualty sitting or standing:

(*a*) Stand behind the casualty and wrap your arms around his chest with your arms under his armpits.

(*b*) Make a fist with one hand and place the thumb side of the fist in the middle of the breastbone (take care to avoid the tip of the breastbone and the margins of the ribs).

(*c*) Grasp the fist with the other hand and exert thrusts (Figure 2-13).

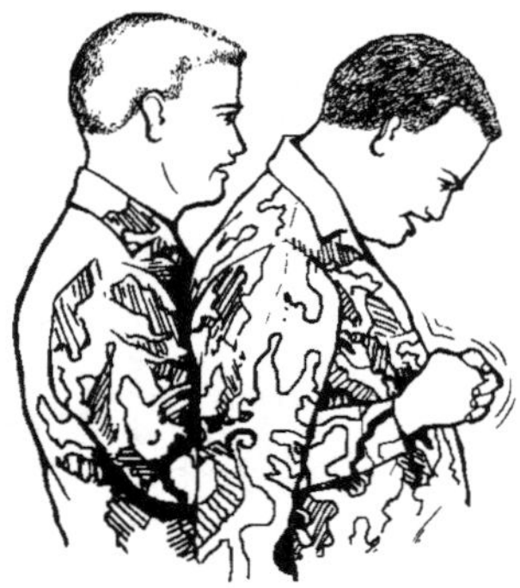

Figure 2-13. Profile view of chest thrust.

(*d*) Each thrust should be delivered slowly, distinctly, and with the intent of relieving the obstruction.

(*e*) Perform chest thrusts until the obstruction is expelled or the casualty becomes unresponsive.

(*f*) If the casualty becomes unresponsive, call for help as you proceed with steps to open the airway and perform rescue breathing.

2-12. Opening the Obstructed Airway—Casualty Lying Down or Unresponsive

The following procedures are used to expel an airway obstruction in a casualty who is lying down, who becomes unconscious, or who is found unconscious (the cause unknown):

- If a conscious casualty who is choking becomes unresponsive, call for help, open the airway, perform a finger sweep, and attempt rescue breathing (paragraphs 2-4 through 2-8). If you still cannot administer rescue breathing due to an airway blockage, then remove the airway obstruction using the procedures as in *b* below.

- If a casualty is unresponsive when you find him (the cause unknown), assess or evaluate the situation, call for help, position the casualty on his back, open the airway, establish breathlessness, and attempt to perform rescue breathing (paragraphs 2-4 through 2-8).

a. Open the airway and attempt rescue breathing (refer to paragraph 2-7 for information on how to perform mouth-to-mouth resuscitation).

b. If still unable to ventilate the casualty, perform 6 to 10 manual (abdominal or chest) thrusts.

(1) To perform the abdominal thrusts:

(*a*) Kneel astride the casualty's thighs (Figure 2-14).

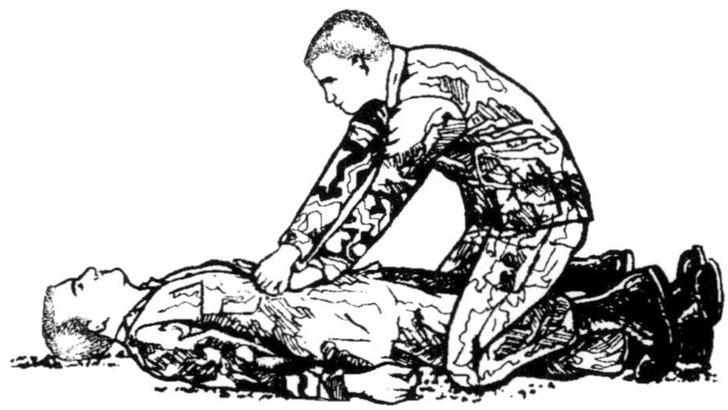

Figure 2-14. Abdominal thrust on unresponsive casualty.

(*b*) Place the heel of one hand against the casualty's abdomen (in the midline slightly above the navel but well below the tip of the breastbone). Place your other hand on top of the first one. Point your fingers toward the casualty's head.

(*c*) Press into the casualty's abdomen with a quick, forward and upward thrust. You can use your body weight to perform the maneuver. Deliver each thrust quickly and distinctly.

(*d*) Repeat the sequence of abdominal thrusts, finger sweep, and rescue breathing (attempt to ventilate) as long as necessary to remove the object from the obstructed airway.

(*e*) If the casualty's chest rises, proceed to feeling for pulse.

(2) To perform chest thrusts:

(*a*) Place the unresponsive casualty on his back, face up, and open his mouth. Kneel close to the side of the casualty's body.

1. Locate the lower edge of the casualty's ribs with your fingers. Run the fingers up along the rib cage to the notch (Figure 2-15A).

2. Place the middle finger on the notch and the index finger next to the middle finger on the lower edge of the breastbone. Place the heel of the other hand on the lower half of the breastbone next to the two fingers (Figure 2-15B).

3. Remove the fingers from the notch and place that hand on top of the positioned hand on the breastbone, extending or interlocking the fingers (Figure 2-15C).

4. Straighten and lock your elbows with your shoulders directly above your hands without bending the elbows, rocking, or allowing the shoulders to sag. Apply enough pressure to depress the breastbone 1 1/2 to 2 inches, then release the pressure completely (Figure 2-15D). Do this 6 to 10 times. Each thrust should be delivered quickly and distinctly. See Figure 2-16 for another view of the breastbone being depressed.

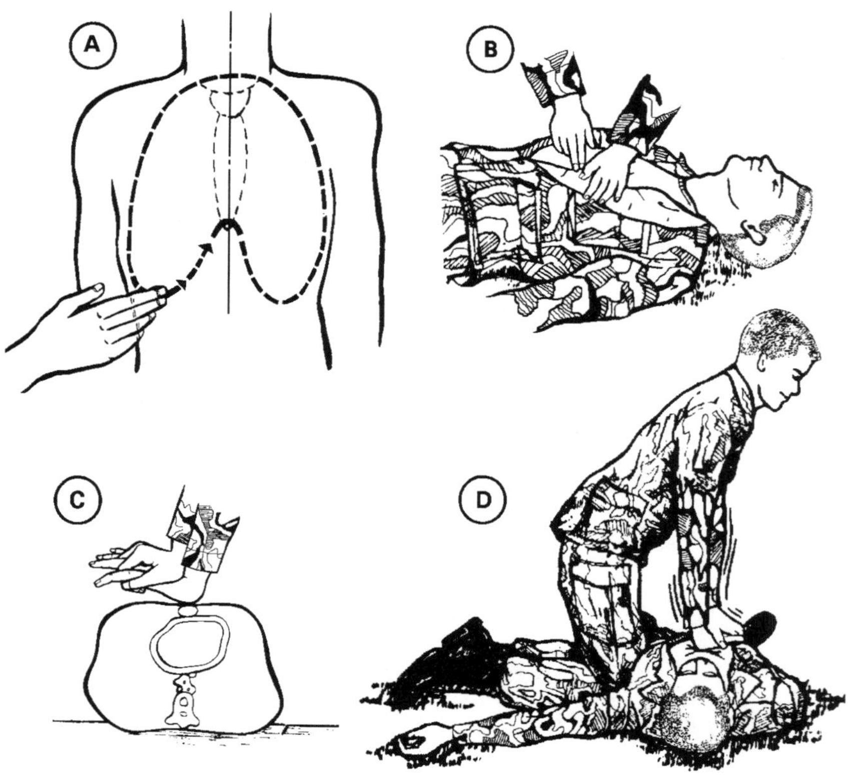

Figure 2-15. Hand placement for chest thrust (Illustrated A-D).

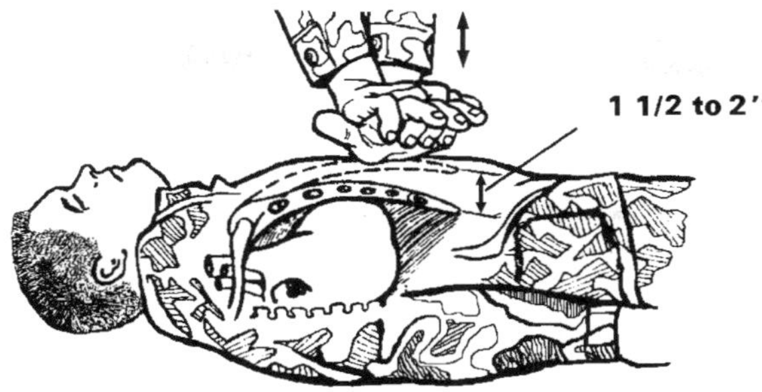

Figure 2-16. Breastbone depressed 1 1/2 to 2 inches.

(*b*) Repeat the sequence of chest thrust, finger sweep, and rescue breathing as long as necessary to clear the object from the obstructed airway. See paragraph (3) below.

(*c*) If the casualty's chest rises, proceed to feeling for his pulse.

(3) If you still cannot administer rescue breathing due to an airway obstruction, then remove the airway obstruction using the procedures in steps (*a*) and (*b*) below.

(*a*) Place the casualty on his back, face up, turn the unresponsive casualty as a unit, and call out for help.

(*b*) Perform finger sweep, keep casualty face up, use tongue-jaw lift to open mouth.

1. Open the casualty's mouth by grasping both his tongue and lower jaw between your thumb and fingers and lifting (tongue-jaw lift) (Figure 2-17). If you are unable to open his mouth, cross your fingers and thumb (crossed-finger method) and push his teeth apart (Figure 2-18) by pressing your thumb against his upper teeth and pressing your finger against his lower teeth.

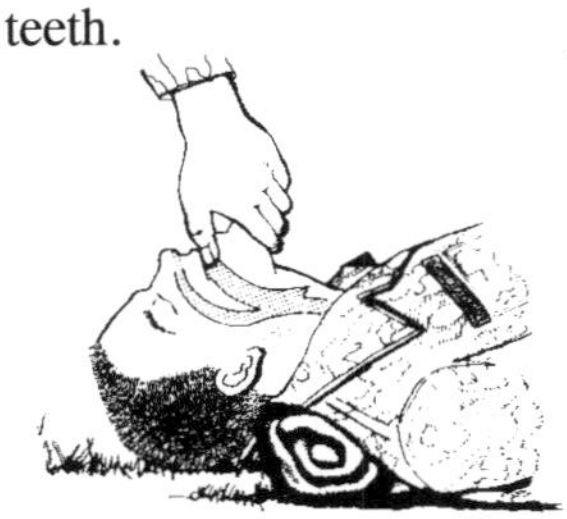

Figure 2-17. Opening casualty's mouth (tongue-jaw lift).

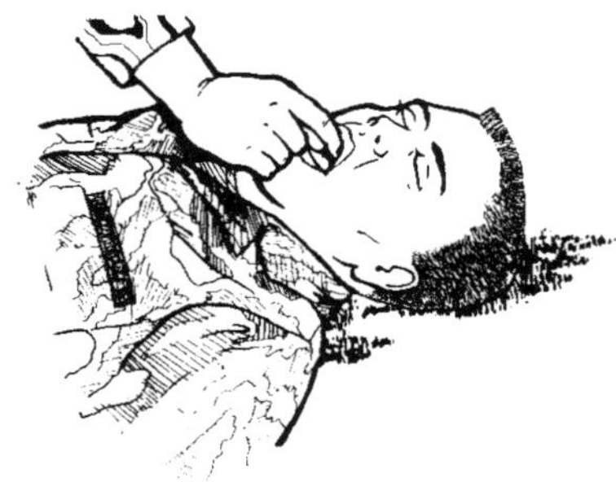

Figure 2-18. Opening casualty's mouth (crossed-finger method).

2. Insert the index finger of the other hand down along the inside of his cheek to the base of the tongue. Use a hooking motion from the side of the mouth toward the center to dislodge the foreign body (Figure 2-19).

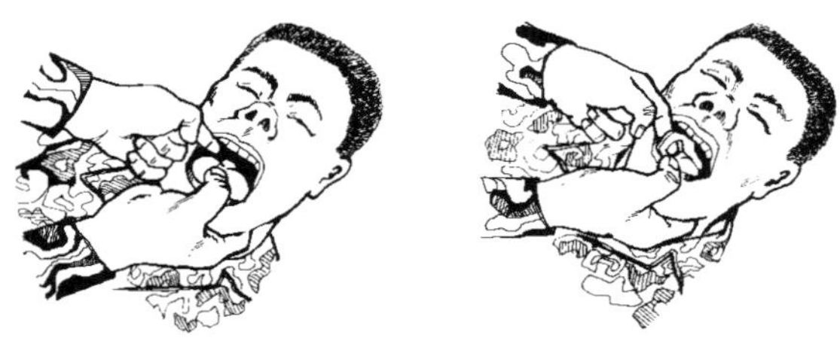

Figure 2-19. Using finger to dislodge a foreign body.

WARNING

Take care not to force the object deeper into the airway by pushing it with the finger.

Section II. STOP THE BLEEDING AND PROTECT THE WOUND

2-13. General

The longer a service member bleeds from a major wound, the less likely he will be able to survive his injuries. It is, therefore, important that the first aid provider promptly stop the external bleeding.

2-14. Clothing

In evaluating the casualty for location, type, and size of the wound or injury, cut or tear his clothing and carefully expose the entire area of the wound. This procedure is necessary to properly visualize injury and avoid further contamination. Clothing stuck to the wound should be left in place to avoid further injury. DO NOT touch the wound; keep it as clean as possible.

WARNING

DO NOT REMOVE protective clothing in a chemical environment. Apply dressings over the protective clothing.

2-15. Entrance and Exit Wounds

Before applying the dressing, carefully examine the casualty to determine if there is more than one wound. A missile may have entered at one point and exited at another point. The *EXIT* wound is usually *LARGER* than the entrance wound.

WARNING

The casualty should be continually monitored for development of conditions which may require the performance of necessary basic lifesaving measures, such as clearing the airway and mouth-to-mouth resuscitation. All open (or penetrating) wounds should be checked for a point of entry and exit and first aid measures applied accordingly.

WARNING

If the missile lodges in the body (fails to exit), DO NOT attempt to remove it or probe the wound. Apply a dressing. If there is an object extending from (impaled in) the wound, DO NOT remove the object. Apply a dressing around the object and use additional improvised bulky materials/dressings (use the cleanest material available) to build up the area around the object to stabilize the object and prevent further injury. Apply a supporting bandage over the bulky materials to hold them in place.

2-16. Field Dressing

a. Use the casualty's field dressing; remove it from the wrapper and grasp the tails of the dressing with both hands (Figure 2-20).

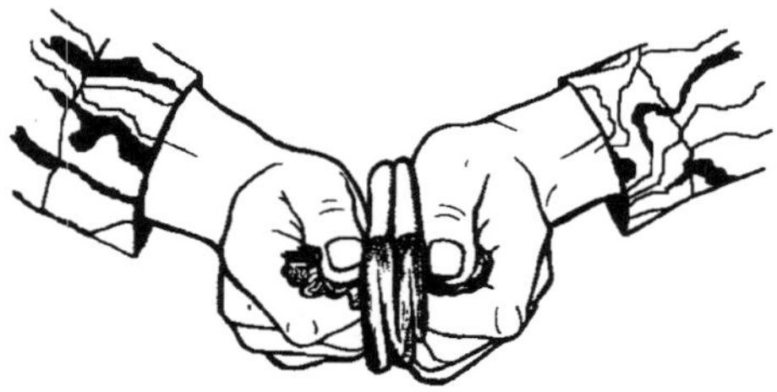

Figure 2-20. Grasping tails of dressing with both hands.

> **WARNING**
>
> **DO NOT touch the white (sterile) side of the dressing, and DO NOT allow it to come in contact with any surface other than the wound.**

b. Hold the dressing directly over the wound with the white side down. Pull the dressing open (Figure 2-21) and place it directly over the wound (Figure 2-22).

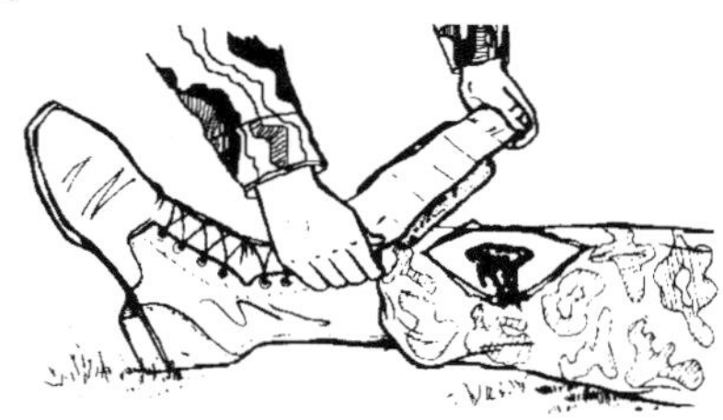

Figure 2-21. Pulling dressing open.

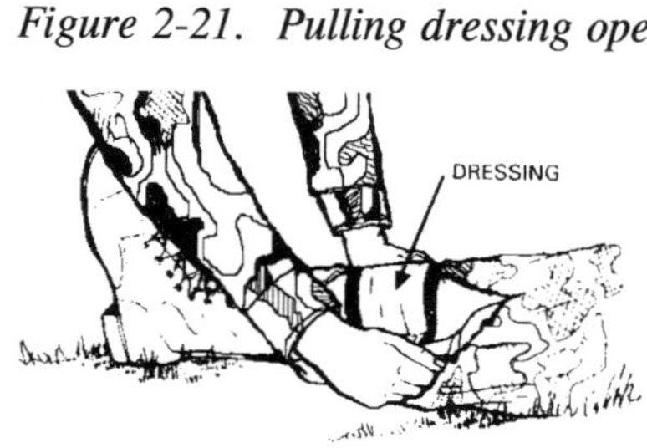

Figure 2-22. Placing dressing directly on wound.

c. Hold the dressing in place with one hand. Use the other hand to wrap one of the tails around the injured part, covering about one-half of the dressing (Figure 2-23). Leave enough of the tail for a knot. If the casualty is able, he may assist by holding the dressing in place.

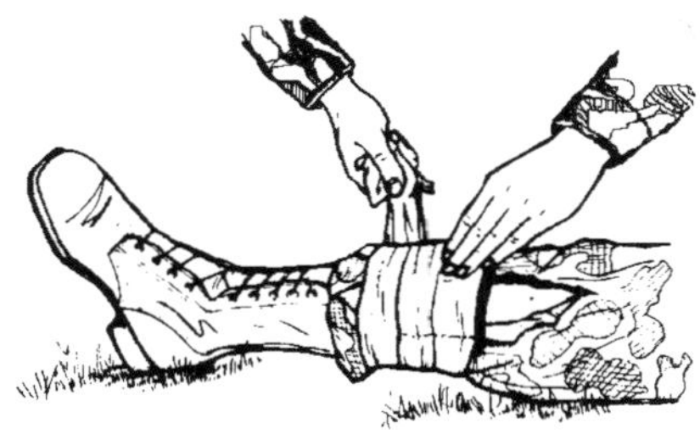

Figure 2-23. Wrapping tail of dressing around injured part.

d. Wrap the other tail in the opposite direction until the remainder of the dressing is covered. The tails should seal the sides of the dressing to keep foreign material from getting under it.

e. Tie the tails into a nonslip knot over the outer edge of the dressing (Figure 2-24). **DO NOT TIE THE KNOT OVER THE WOUND.** In order to allow blood to flow to the rest of an injured limb, tie the dressing firmly enough to prevent it from slipping but without causing a tourniquet-like effect; that is, the skin beyond the injury should not becomes cool, blue, or numb.

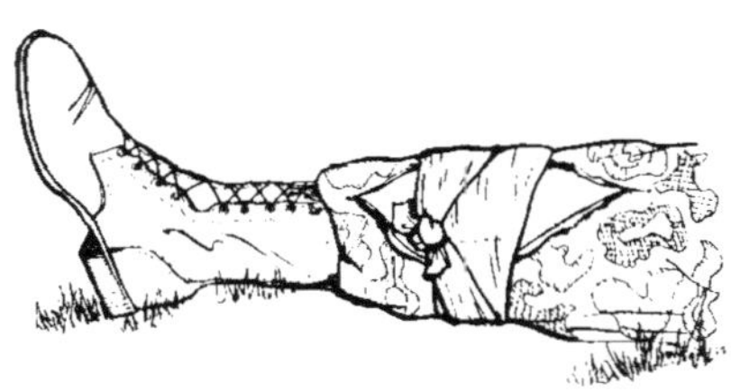

Figure 2-24. Tails tied into nonslip knot.

2-17. Manual Pressure

a. If bleeding continues after applying the sterile field dressing, direct manual pressure may be used to help control bleeding. Apply such pressure by placing a hand on the dressing and exerting firm pressure for 5 to 10 minutes (Figure 2-25). The casualty may be asked to do this himself if he is conscious and can follow instructions.

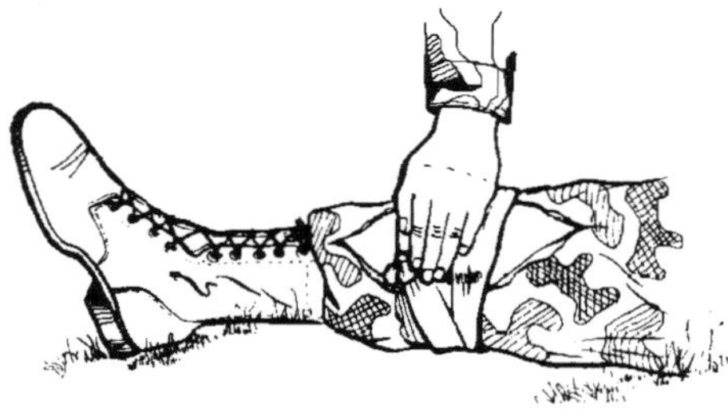

Figure 2-25. Direct manual pressure applied.

b. Elevate an injured limb slightly above the level of the heart to reduce the bleeding (Figure 2-26).

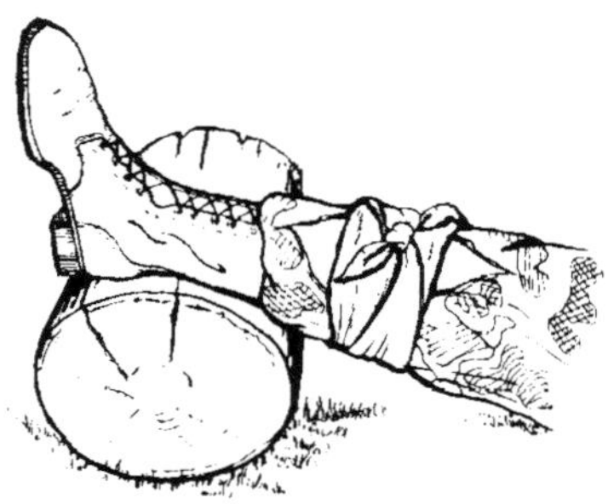

Figure 2-26. Injured limb elevated.

WARNING

DO NOT elevate a suspected fractured limb unless it has been properly splinted.

c. If the bleeding stops, check shock; administer first aid for shock as necessary. If the bleeding continues, apply a pressure dressing.

2-18. Pressure Dressing

Pressure dressings aid in blood clotting and compress the open blood vessel. If bleeding continues after the application of a field dressing, manual pressure, and elevation, then a pressure dressing must be applied as follows:

a. Place a wad of padding on top of the field dressing, directly over the wound (Figure 2-27). Keep the injured extremity elevated.

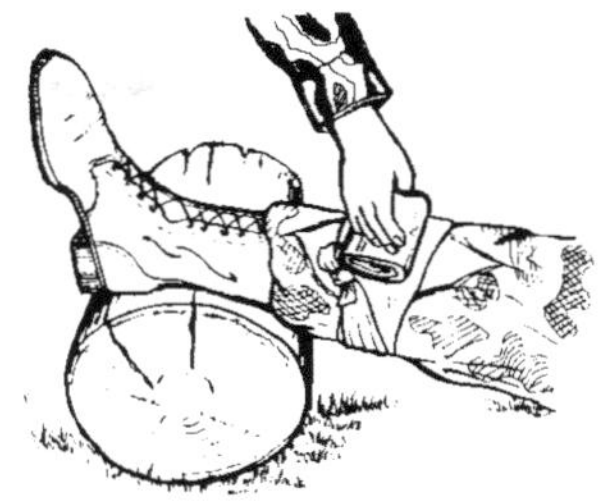

Figure 2-27. Wad of padding on top of field dressing.

NOTE

Improvised bandages may be made from strips of cloth. These strips may be made from T-shirts, socks, or other garments.

b. Place an improvised dressing (or cravat, if available) over the wad of padding (Figure 2-28). Wrap the ends tightly around the injured limb, covering the previously placed field dressing (Figure 2-29).

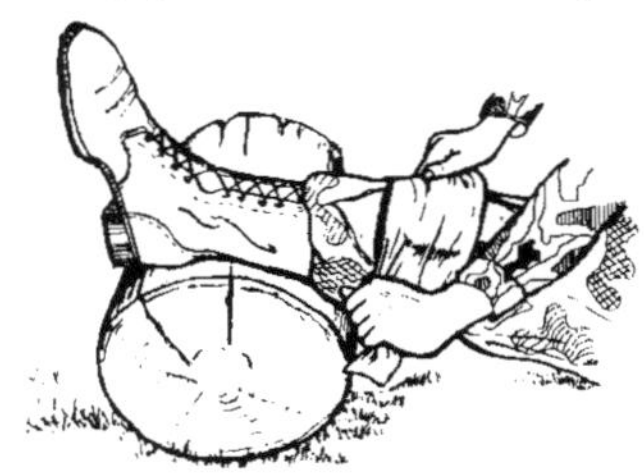

Figure 2-28. Improvised dressing over wad of padding

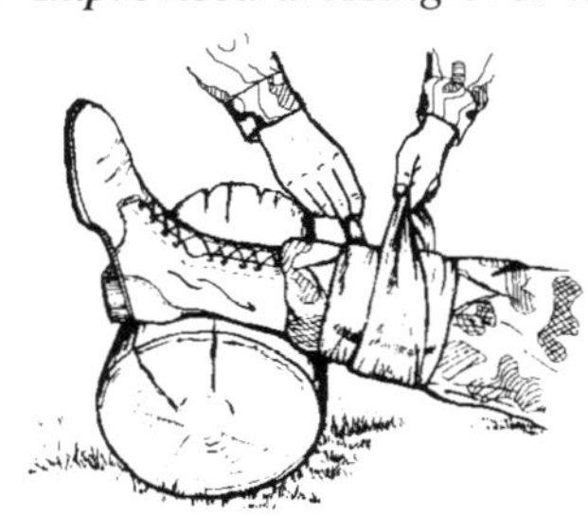

Figure 2-29. Ends of improvised dressing wrapped tightly around limb.

c. Tie the ends together in a nonslip knot, directly over the wound site (Figure 2-30). DO NOT tie so tightly that it has a tourniquet-like effect. If bleeding continues and all other measures have failed, or if the limb is severed, then apply a tourniquet. Use the tourniquet as a **LAST RESORT**. When the bleeding stops, check for shock; administer first aid for shock as necessary.

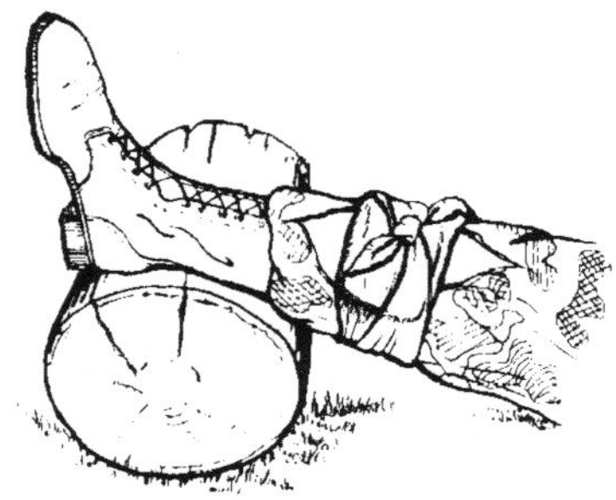

Figure 2-30. Ends of improvised dressing tied together in nonslip knot.

NOTE

Distal end of wounded extremities (fingers and toes) should be checked periodically for adequate circulation. The dressing must be loosened if the extremity becomes cool, blue, or numb.

NOTE

If bleeding continues and all other measures have failed (dressings and covering wound, applying direct manual pressure, elevating the limb above the heart level, and applying a pressure dressing while maintaining limb elevation) *then apply digital pressure* (see paragraph 2-19).

2-19. Digital Pressure

Digital pressure (often called "pressure points") is an alternative method to control bleeding. This method uses pressure from the fingers, thumbs, or hands to press at the site or point where a main artery supplying the wounded area lies near the skin surface or over bone (Figure 2-31). This pressure may help shut off or slow down the flow of blood from the heart to the wound and is used in combination with direct pressure and elevation. It may help in instances where bleeding is not easily controlled, where a pressure dressing has not yet been applied, or where pressure dressings are not readily available.

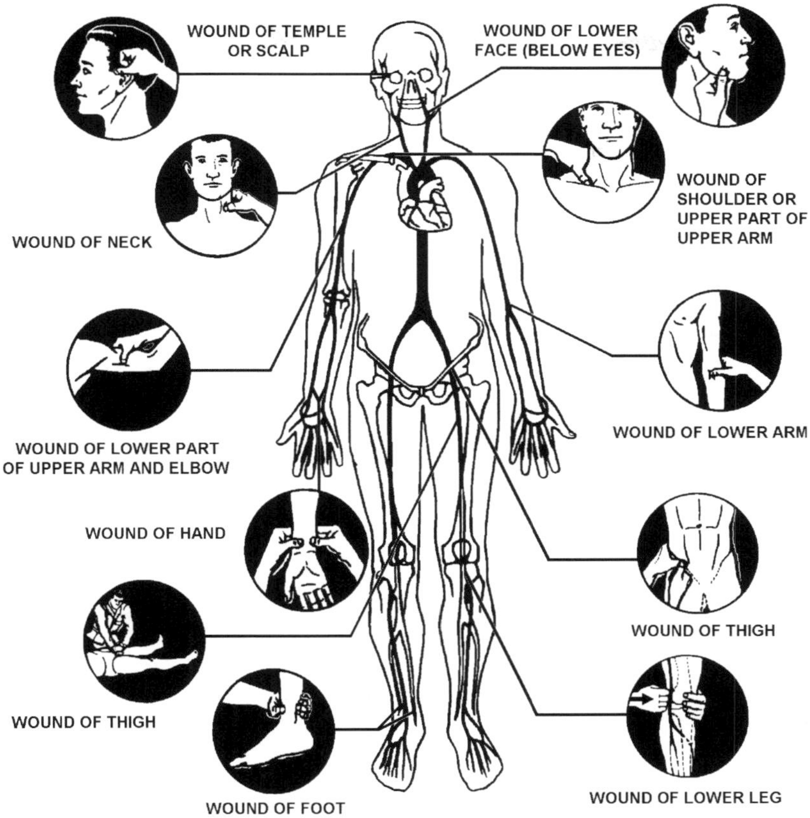

Figure 2-31. Digital pressure (pressure with fingers, thumbs or hands).

2-20. Tourniquet

DANGER

A tourniquet is only used on an arm or leg where there is a danger of the casualty losing his life (bleeding to death).

A tourniquet is a constricting band placed around an arm or leg to control bleeding. A service member whose arm or leg has been completely amputated may not be bleeding when first discovered, but a tourniquet should be applied anyway. This absence of bleeding is due to the body's normal defenses (contraction or clotting of blood vessels) as a result of the amputation, but after a period of time bleeding will start as the blood vessels relax or the clot may be knocked loose by moving the casualty. Bleeding from a major artery of the thigh, lower leg, or arm and bleeding from multiple arteries (which occurs in a traumatic amputation) may prove to be beyond control by manual pressure. If the pressure dressing (see paragraph 2-18, above) under firm hand pressure becomes soaked with blood and the wound continues to bleed, apply a tourniquet.

WARNING

Casualty should be continually monitored for development of conditions which may require the performance of necessary basic lifesaving measures, such as: clearing the airway, performing mouth-to-mouth resuscitation, preventing shock, and/or bleeding control. All open (or penetrating) wounds should be checked for a point of entry or exit and treated accordingly.

The tourniquet should not be used unless a pressure dressing has failed to stop the bleeding or an arm or leg has been cut off. On occasion, tourniquets have injured blood vessels and nerves. If left in place too long, a tourniquet can cause loss of an arm or leg. Once applied, it must stay in place, and the casualty must be taken to the nearest MTF as soon as possible. *DO NOT loosen or release a tourniquet after it has been applied as release could precipitate bleeding and potentially lead to shock.*

a. Improvising a Tourniquet. In the absence of a specially designed tourniquet, a tourniquet may be made from a strong, pliable material, such as gauze or muslin bandages, clothing, or cravats. An improvised tourniquet is used with a rigid stick-like object. To minimize skin damage, ensure that the improvised tourniquet is at least 2 inches wide.

WARNING

The tourniquet must be easily identified or easily seen.

WARNING

DO NOT use wire or shoestring for a tourniquet band.

b. Placing the Improvised Tourniquet.

(1) Place the tourniquet around the limb, between the wound and the body trunk (or between the wound and the heart). Never place it directly over a wound, a fracture, or joint. Tourniquets, for maximum effectiveness, should be placed on the upper arm or above the knee on the thigh (Figure 2-32).

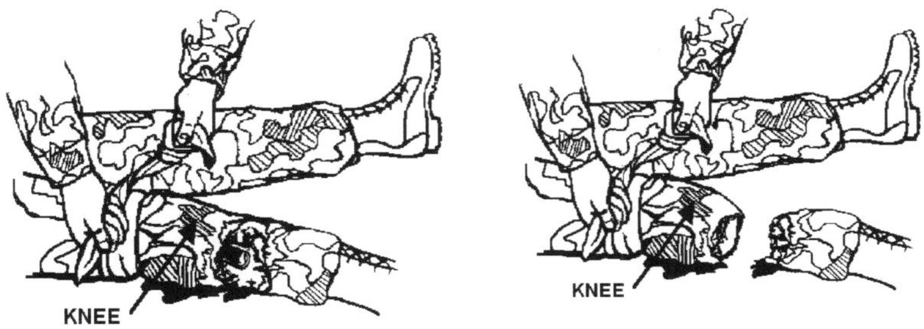

Figure 2-32. Tourniquet above knee.

(2) The tourniquet should be well-padded. If possible, place the tourniquet over the smoothed sleeve or trouser leg to prevent the skin from being pinched or twisted. If the tourniquet is long enough, wrap it around the limb several times, keeping the material as flat as possible. Damaging the skin may deprive the surgeon of skin required to cover an amputation. Protection of the skin also reduces pain.

c. Applying the Tourniquet.

(1) Tie a half-knot. (A half-knot is the same as the first part of tying a shoe lace.)

(2) Place a stick (or similar rigid object) on top of the half-knot (Figure 2-33).

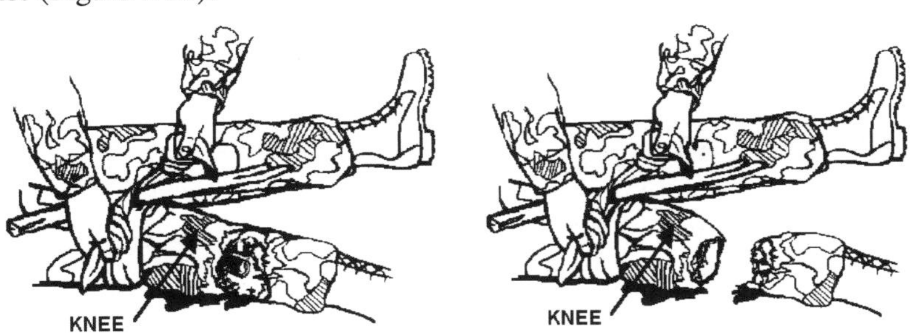

Figure 2-33. Rigid object on top of half-knot.

(3) Tie a full knot over the stick (Figure 2-34).

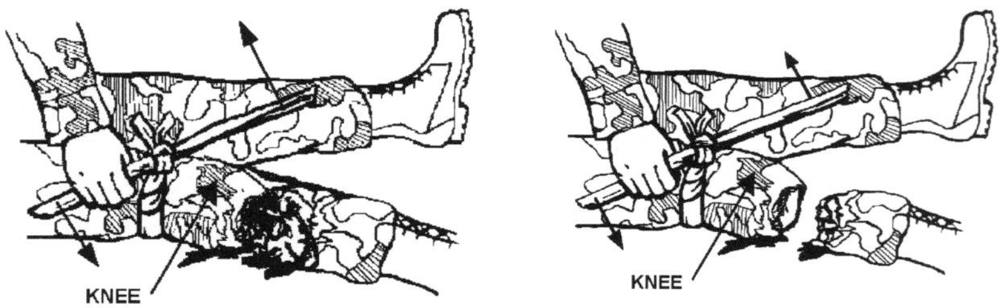

Figure 2-34. Full knot over rigid object.

(4) Twist the stick (Figure 2-35) until the tourniquet is tight around the limb and/or the bright red bleeding has stopped. In the case of amputation, dark oozing blood may continue for a short time. This is the blood trapped in the area between the wound and tourniquet.

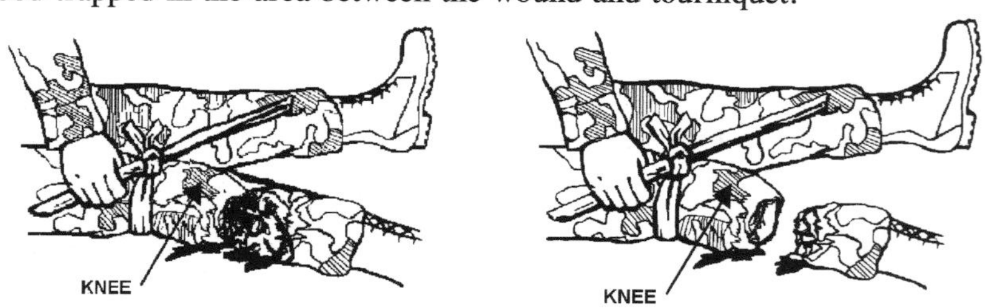

Figure 2-35. Stick twisted.

(5) Fasten the tourniquet to the limb by looping the free ends of the tourniquet over the ends of the stick. Then bring the ends around the limb to prevent the stick from loosening. Tie them together on the side of the limb (Figure 2-36).

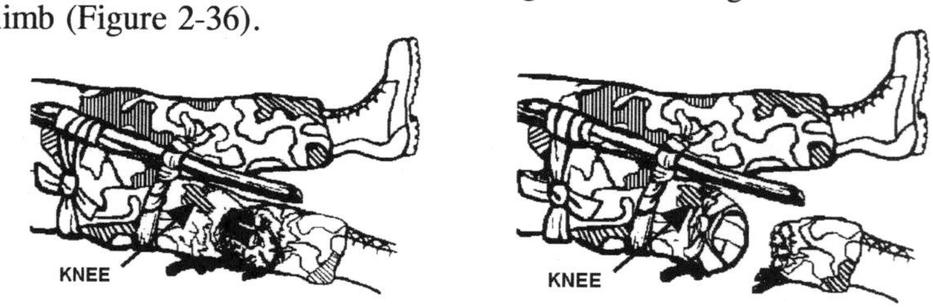

Figure 2-36. Tie free ends on side of limb.

NOTE

Other methods of securing the stick may be used as long as the stick does not unwind and no further injury results.

NOTE

If possible, save and transport any severed (amputated) limbs or body parts with (but out of sight of) the casualty.

(6) DO NOT cover the tourniquet—you should leave it in full view. If the limb is missing (total amputation), apply a dressing to the stump. All wounds should have a dressing to protect the wound from contamination.

(7) Mark the casualty's forehead with a "T" and the time to indicate a tourniquet has been applied. If necessary, use the casualty's blood to make this mark.

(8) Check and treat for shock.

(9) Seek medical aid.

CAUTION

Only appropriately skilled medical personnel may adjust or otherwise remove/release the tourniquet in the appropriate setting.

Section III. CHECK FOR SHOCK AND ADMINISTER FIRST AID MEASURES

2-21. General

The term *shock* has a variety of meanings. In medicine, it refers to a collapse of the body's cardiovascular system which includes an inadequate supply of blood to the body's tissues. Shock stuns and weakens the body. When the normal blood flow in the body is upset, death can result. Early recognition and proper first aid may save the casualty's life.

2-22. Causes and Effects

a. There are three basic mechanisms associated with shock. These are—

- The heart is damaged and fails to work as a pump.
- Blood loss (heavy bleeding) causes the volume of fluid within the vascular system to be insufficient.
- The blood vessels dilate (open wider) so that the blood within the system (even though it is a normal volume [the casualty is not bleeding or dehydrated]) is insufficient to provide adequate circulation within the body.

b. Shock may be the result of a number of conditions. These include—

- Dehydration.
- Allergic reaction to foods, drugs, insect stings, and snakebites.
- Significant loss of blood.
- Reaction to the sight of a wound, blood, or other traumatic scene.
- Traumatic injuries, such as—
  - Burns.
  - Gunshot or shrapnel wounds.
  - Crush injuries.
  - Blows to the body (which can cause broken bones or damage to internal organs).
  - Head injuries.
  - Penetrating wounds (such as from a knife, bayonet, or missile).

2-23. Signs and Symptoms of Shock

Examine the casualty to see if he has any of the following signs and symptoms:

- Sweaty but cool skin (clammy skin).

- Weak and rapid pulse.
- Paleness of skin (in dark-skinned individuals they may have a grayish look to their skin).
- Restlessness, nervousness.
- Thirst.
- Loss of blood (bleeding).
- Confusion (or loss of awareness).
- Faster-than-normal breathing rate.
- Blotchy or bluish skin (especially around the mouth and lips).
- Nausea and/or vomiting.

2-24. First Aid Measures for Shock

In the field, the first aid procedures administered for shock are identical to procedures that would be performed *to prevent shock*. When treating a casualty, assume that shock is present or will occur shortly. By waiting until actual signs and symptoms of shock are noticeable, the rescuer may jeopardize the casualty's life.

a. Position the Casualty. (DO NOT move the casualty or his limbs if suspected fractures have not been splinted. See Chapter 4 for details.)

(1) Move the casualty to cover, if cover is available and the situation permits.

(2) Lay the casualty on his back.

NOTE

A casualty in shock from a chest wound or one who is experiencing breathing difficulty, may breathe easier in a sitting position. If this is the case, allow him to sit upright, but monitor carefully in case his condition worsens.

(3) Elevate the casualty's feet higher than the level of his heart. Use a stable object (field pack or rolled up clothing) so that his feet will not slip off (Figure 2-37).

WARNING

DO NOT elevate legs if the casualty has an unsplinted broken leg, head injury, or abdominal injury.

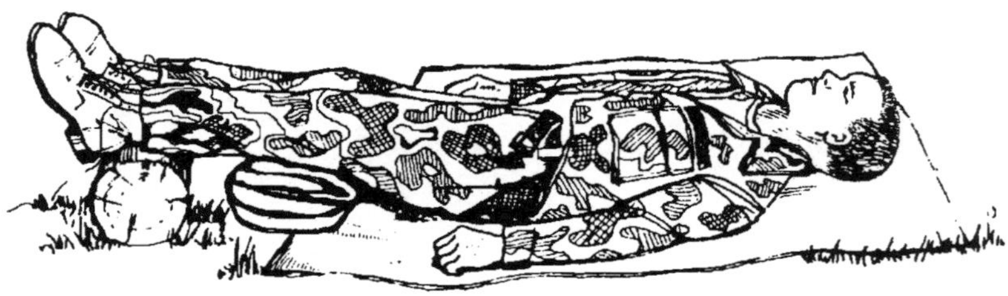

Figure 2-37. Clothing loosened and feet elevated.

WARNING

Check casualty for leg fracture(s) and splint, if necessary, before elevating his feet. For a casualty with an abdominal wound, place his knees in an upright (flexed) position.

(4) Loosen clothing at the neck, waist, or wherever it may be binding.

CAUTION

DO NOT loosen or remove protective clothing in a chemical environment.

(5) Prevent chilling or overheating. The key is to maintain body temperature. In cold weather, place a blanket or other like item over him to keep him warm and under him to prevent chilling (Figure 2-38). However, if a tourniquet has been applied, leave it exposed (if possible). In hot weather, place the casualty in the shade and protect him from becoming chilled; however, avoid the excessive use of blankets or other coverings.

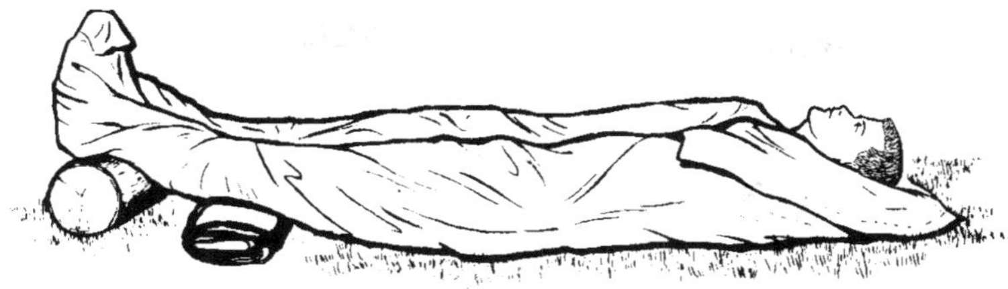

Figure 2-38. Body temperature maintained.

(6) Calm the casualty. Throughout the entire procedure of providing first aid for a casualty, the rescuer should reassure the casualty and keep him calm. This can be done by being authoritative (taking charge) and by showing self-confidence. Assure the casualty that you are there to help him.

(7) Seek medical aid.

b. Food and/or Drink. When providing first aid for shock, DO NOT give the casualty any food or drink. If you must leave the casualty or if he is unconscious, turn his head to the side to prevent him from choking if he vomits (Figure 2-39).

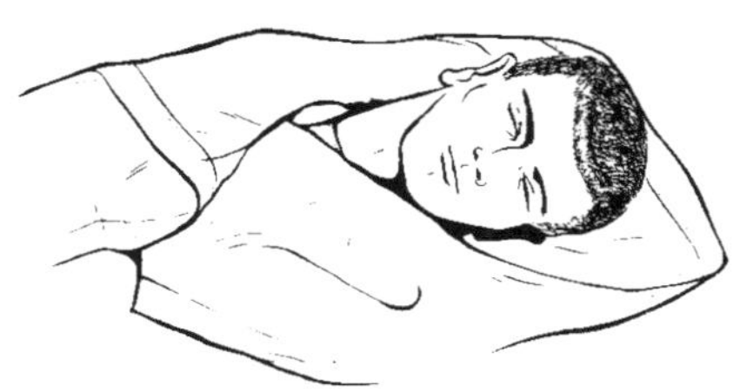

Figure 2-39. Casualty's head turned to side.

c. Evaluate Casualty. Continue to evaluate the casualty until medical personnel arrives or the casualty is transported to an MTF.

CHAPTER 3

FIRST AID FOR SPECIFIC INJURIES

3-1. General

Basic lifesaving steps are discussed in Chapters 1 and 2; they apply to first aid measures for all injuries. Some wounds and burns will require special precautions and procedures when applying these measures. This chapter discusses specific first aid procedures for wounds of the head, face, and neck; chest and stomach wounds; and burns. It also discusses the techniques for applying dressings and bandages to specific parts of the body.

3-2. Head, Neck, and Facial Injuries

a. Head Injuries.

(1) Head injuries range from minor abrasions or cuts on the scalp to severe brain injuries that may result in unconsciousness and sometimes death. Head injuries are classified as open or closed wounds. An open wound is one that is visible, has a break in the skin, and usually has evidence of bleeding. A closed wound may be visible (such as a depression in the skull) or the first aid provider may not be able to see any apparent injury (such as internal bleeding). Some head injuries result in unconsciousness; however, a service member may have a serious head wound and still be conscious. Casualties with head and neck injuries should be treated as though they also have a spinal injury. The casualty should not be moved until the head and neck is stabilized unless he is in immediate danger (such as close to a burning vehicle).

(2) Prompt first aid measures should be initiated for casualties with suspected head and neck injuries. The conscious casualty may be able to provide information on the extent of his injuries. However, as a result of the head injury, he may be confused and unable to provide accurate information. The signs and symptoms a first aid provider might observe are—

- Nausea and vomiting.
- Convulsions or twitches.
- Slurred speech.
- Confusion and loss of memory. (Does he know who he is? Does he know where he is? Does he know what day it is?)
- Recent unconsciousness.

- Dizziness.
- Drowsiness.
- Blurred vision, unequal pupils, or bruising (black eyes).
- Paralysis (partial or full).
- Complaint of headache.
- Bleeding or other fluid discharge from the scalp, nose, or ears.
- Deformity of the head (depression or swelling).
- Staggering while walking.

b. Neck Injuries. Neck injuries may result in heavy bleeding. Apply pressure above and below the injury, *but do not interfere with the breathing process*, and attempt to control the bleeding. Apply a dressing. Always evaluate the casualty for a possible neck fracture/spinal cord injury; if suspected, seek medical treatment immediately.

NOTE

Establish and maintain the airway in cases of facial or neck injuries. If a neck fracture or spinal cord injury is suspected, immobilize the injury and, if necessary, perform basic life support measures.

c. Facial Injuries. Soft tissue injuries of the face and scalp are common. Abrasions (scrapes) of the skin cause no serious problems. Contusions (injury without a break in the skin) usually cause swelling. A contusion of the scalp looks and feels like a lump. Laceration (cut) and avulsion (torn away tissue) injuries are also common. Avulsions are frequently caused when a sharp blow separates the scalp from the skull beneath it. Because the face and scalp are richly supplied with blood vessels (arteries and veins), wounds of these areas usually bleed heavily.

3-3. General First Aid Measures

a. General Considerations. The casualty with a head injury (or suspected head injury) should be continually monitored for the development of conditions that *may require* basic lifesaving measures. After initiating first aid measures, request medical assistance and evacuation. If dedicated medical evacuation assets are not available, transport the casualty to an MTF as soon as the situation permits. The first aid provider should not attempt to remove a protruding object from the head or give the casualty anything to eat or drink. Further, the first aid provider should be prepared to—

- Clear the airway.
- Control bleeding (external).
- Administer first aid measures for shock.
- Keep the casualty warm.
- Protect the wound.

b. *Unconscious Casualty*. An unconscious casualty does not have control of all of his body's functions and may choke on his tongue, blood, vomitus, or other substances. (Refer to Figure 2-39.)

(1) *Breathing*. The brain requires a constant supply of oxygen. A bluish (or in an individual with dark skin—grayish) color of skin around the lips and nail beds indicates that the casualty is not receiving enough oxygen. Immediate action must be taken to clear the airway, to position the casualty on his side, or to initiate rescue breathing.

(2) *Bleeding*. Bleeding from a head injury usually comes from blood vessels within the scalp. Bleeding can also develop inside the skull or within the brain. In most instances visible bleeding from the head can be controlled by application of the field first aid dressing.

CAUTION

DO NOT attempt to put unnecessary pressure on the wound or attempt to push any brain matter back into the head (skull). **DO NOT** apply a pressure dressing.

c. *Concussion*. If an individual receives a heavy blow to the head or face, he may suffer a brain concussion (an injury to the brain that involves a temporary loss of some or all of the brain's ability to function). For example, the casualty may not breathe properly for a short period of time, or he may become confused and stagger when he attempts to walk. Symptoms of a concussion may only last for a short period of time. However, if a casualty is suspected of having suffered a concussion, he should be transported to an MTF as soon as conditions permit.

d. *Convulsions*. Convulsions (seizures/involuntary jerking) may occur even after a mild head injury. When a casualty is convulsing, protect him from hurting himself. Take the following measures:

(1) Ease him to the ground if he is standing or sitting.

(2) Support his head and neck.

(3) Maintain his airway.

(4) Protect him from further injury (such as hitting close-by objects).

NOTE

DO NOT forcefully hold the arms and legs if they are jerking because this can lead to broken bones. **DO NOT** force anything between the casualty's teeth—especially if they are tightly clenched because this may obstruct the casualty's airway. Maintain the casualty's airway if necessary.

e. *Brain Damage*. In *severe* head injuries where brain tissue is protruding, *leave the wound alone*; carefully place a loose moistened dressing (moistened with sterile normal saline if available) and also a first aid dressing over the tissue to protect it from further contamination. ***DO NOT** remove or disturb any foreign matter that may be in the wound*. Position the casualty so that his head is higher than his body. Keep him warm and *seek medical assistance immediately*.

NOTE

If there is an object extending from the wound, **DO NOT** remove the object. Improvise bulky dressings from the cleanest material available and place this material around the protruding object for support, then apply the field dressing.

3-4. Chest Wounds

Blunt trauma, bullet or missile wounds, stab wounds, or falls may cause chest injuries. These injuries can be serious and may cause death quickly if first aid is not administered in a timely manner. A casualty with a chest injury may complain of pain in the chest or shoulder area; he may have difficulty breathing. His chest may not rise normally when he breathes. The injury may cause the casualty to cough up blood and to have a rapid or a weak heartbeat. A casualty with an open chest wound has a punctured chest wall. The sucking sound heard when he breathes is caused by air leaking into his chest cavity. This particular type of wound is dangerous and will collapse the injured lung (Figure 3-1). Breathing becomes difficult for the casualty because the wound is open. The service members life may depend upon how quickly you apply an occlusive dressing over the wound (refer to paragraph 3-5).

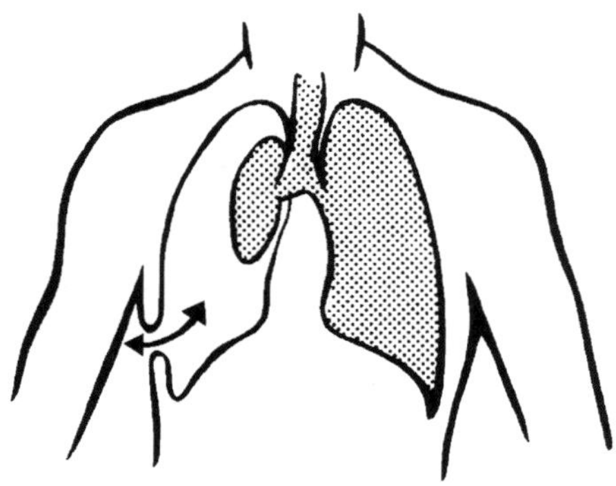

Figure 3-1. Collapsed lung.

3-5. First Aid for Chest Wounds

a. Evaluate the Casualty. Be prepared to perform first aid measures. These measures may include clearing the airway, rescue breathing, treatment for shock, and/or bleeding control.

b. Expose the Wound. If appropriate, cut or remove the casualty's clothing to expose the wound. Remember, **DO NOT** remove clothing that is stuck to the wound because additional injury may result. **DO NOT** attempt to clean the wound.

NOTE

Examine the casualty to see if there is an entry and exit wound. If there are two wounds (entry, exit), perform the same procedure for both wounds. Treat the more serious (heavier bleeding, larger) wound first. It may be necessary to improvise a dressing for the second wound by using strips of cloth, such as a torn T-shirt, or whatever material is available. Also, listen for sucking sounds to determine if the chest wall is punctured.

> **CAUTION**
>
> If there is an object impaled in the wound, **DO NOT** remove it. Apply a dressing around the object and use additional improvised bulky materials/dressings (use the cleanest materials available) to build up the area around the object. Apply a supporting bandage over the bulky materials to hold them in place.

> **CAUTION**
>
> **DO NOT REMOVE** protective clothing in a chemical environment. Apply dressings *over* the protective clothing.

c. Open the Casualty's Field Dressing Plastic Wrapper. In cases where there is a sucking chest wound, the plastic wrapper is used with the field dressing to create an occlusive dressing. If a plastic wrapper is not available, or if an additional wound needs to be treated; cellophane, foil, the casualty's poncho, or similar material may be used. The covering should be wide enough to extend 2 inches or more beyond the edges of the wound in all directions.

(1) Tear open one end of the casualty's plastic wrapper covering the field dressing. Be careful not to destroy the wrapper and **DO NOT** touch the inside of the wrapper.

(2) Remove the inner packet (field dressing).

(3) Complete tearing open the empty plastic wrapper using as much of the wrapper as possible to create a flat surface.

d. Place the Wrapper Over the Wound. Place the inside surface of the plastic wrapper directly over the wound *when the casualty exhales* and hold it in place (Figure 3-2). The casualty may hold the plastic wrapper in place if he is able.

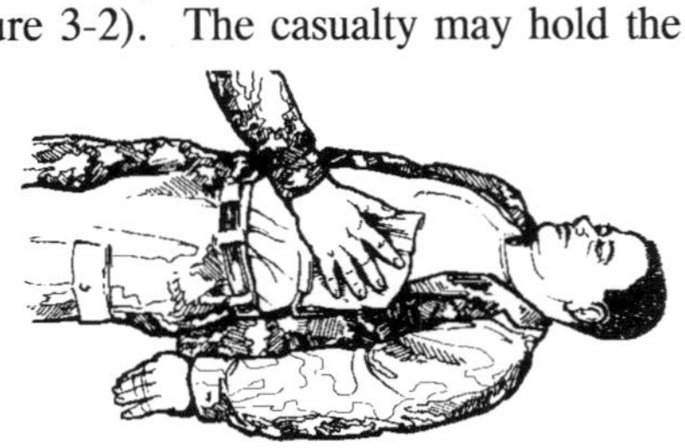

Figure 3-2. Open chest wound sealed with an occlusive dressing.

e. Apply the Dressing to the Wound.

(1) Use your free hand and shake open the field dressing (Figure 3-3).

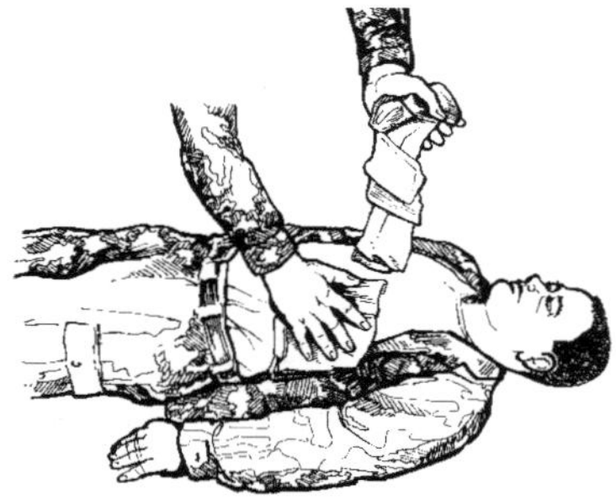

Figure 3-3. Shaking open the field dressing.

(2) Place the white side of the dressing on the plastic wrapper covering the wound (Figure 3-4).

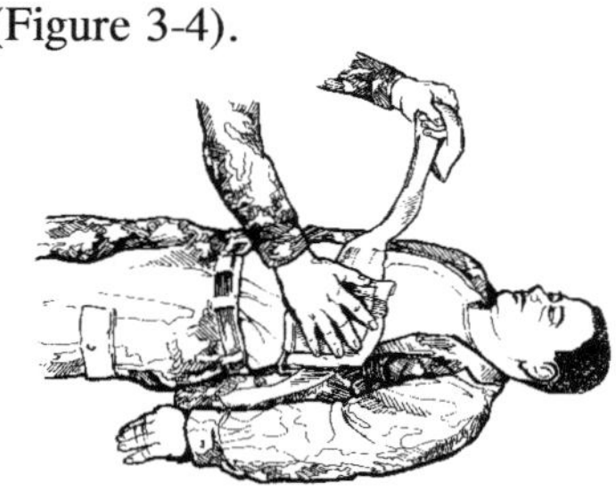

Figure 3-4. Field dressing placed on plastic wrapper.

NOTE

Use the casualty's field dressing, not your own.

(3) Have the casualty breathe normally.

(4) While maintaining pressure on the dressing, grasp one tail of the field dressing with the other hand and wrap it around the casualty's back. If tape is available, tape three sides of the plastic wrapper to the chest wall to provide occlusive type dressing. Leave one side untapped to provide emergency escape for air that may build up in the chest. If tape is not available, secure wrapper on three sides with field dressing leaving the fourth side as a flap.

(5) Wrap the other tail in the opposite direction, bringing both tails over the dressing (Figure 3-5).

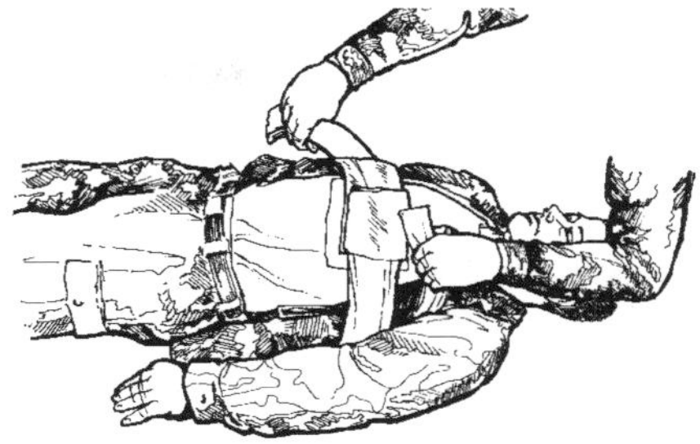

Figure 3-5. Tails of field dressing wrapped around casualty in opposite direction.

(6) Tie the tails into a square knot in the center of the dressing *after* the casualty exhales and *before* he inhales. This will aid in maintaining pressure on the bandage after it has been tied (Figure 3-6). Tie the dressing firmly enough to secure the dressing without interfering with the casualty's breathing.

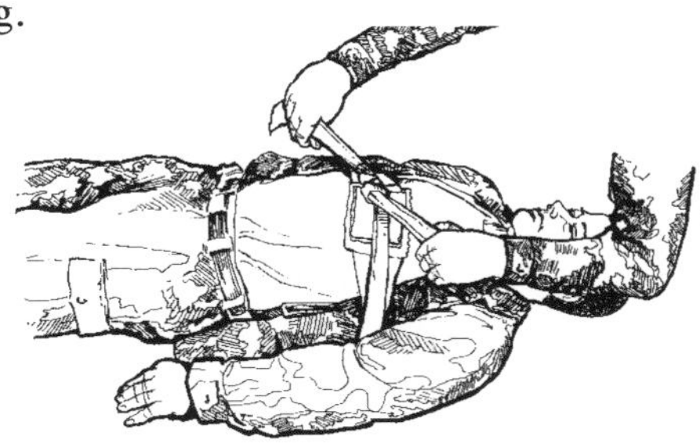

Figure 3-6. Tails of dressing tied into square knot over center of dressing.

NOTE

When practical, apply direct manual pressure over the dressing for 5 to 10 minutes to help control the bleeding.

f. Position the Casualty. Position the casualty on his injured side or in a sitting position, whichever makes breathing easier (Figure 3-7).

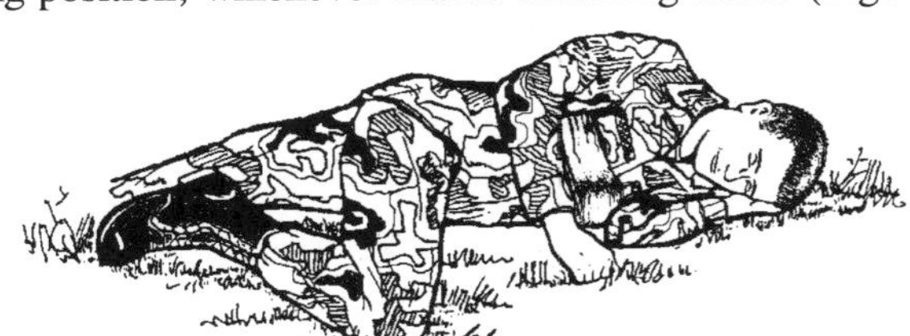

Figure 3-7. Casualty positioned (lying) on injured side.

g. Seek Medical Assistance. Contact medical personnel.

WARNING

If an occlusive dressing has been improperly placed, air may enter the chest cavity with no means of escape. This causes a life-threatening condition called *tension pneumothorax*. If the casualty's condition (for example, difficulty breathing, shortness of breath, restlessness, or blueness/grayness of the skin) worsens after placing the dressing, quickly lift or remove, and then replace the occlusive dressing.

3-6. Abdominal Wounds

The most serious abdominal wound is one in which an object penetrates the abdominal wall and pierces internal organs or large blood vessels. In these instances, bleeding may be severe and death can occur rapidly.

3-7. First Aid for Abdominal Wounds

a. Evaluate the Casualty. Be prepared to perform basic first aid measures. Always check for both entry and exit wounds. If there are two wounds (entry and exit), treat the wound that appears more serious first (for example, the heavier bleeding, protruding organs, larger wound, and so forth). It may be necessary to improvise dressings for the second wound by using strips of cloth, a T-shirt, or the cleanest material available.

b. Position the Casualty. Place and maintain the casualty on his back with his knees in an upright (flexed) position (Figure 3-8). The knees-up position helps relieve pain, assists in the treatment of shock, prevents further exposure of the bowel (intestines) or abdominal organs, and helps relieve abdominal pressure by allowing the abdominal muscles to relax.

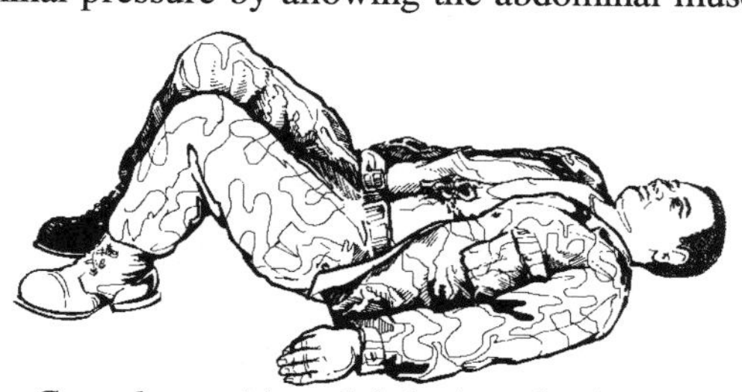

Figure 3-8. Casualty positioned (lying) on back with knees (flexed) up.

c. Expose the Wound.

(1) Remove the casualty's loose clothing to expose the wound. However, **DO NOT** attempt to remove clothing that is stuck to the wound; removing it may cause further injury.

CAUTION

DO NOT REMOVE protective clothing in a chemical environment. Apply dressings *over* the protective clothing.

(2) Gently pick up any organs that may be on the ground. Do this with a clean, dry dressing or with the cleanest available material. Place the organs on top of the casualty's abdomen (Figure 3-9).

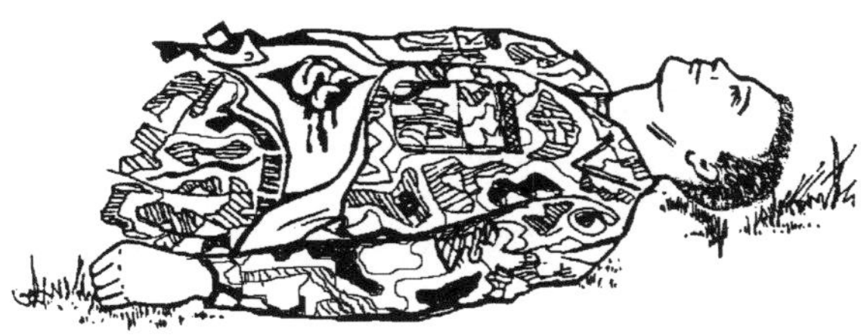

Figure 3-9. Protruding organs placed near wound.

NOTE

DO NOT probe, clean, or try to remove any foreign object from the abdomen. **DO NOT** touch with bare hands any exposed organs. **DO NOT** push organs back inside the body.

d. Apply the Field Dressing. Use the casualty's field dressing, not your own. If the field dressing is not large enough to cover the entire wound, the plastic wrapper from the dressing may be used to cover the wound first (placing the field dressing on top). Open the plastic wrapper carefully without touching the inner surface. If necessary, other improvised dressings may be made from clothing, blankets, or the cleanest materials available.

WARNING

If there is an object extending from the wound, DO NOT remove it. Place as much of the wrapper over the wound as possible without dislodging or moving the object. DO NOT place the wrapper over the object.

(1) Grasp the tails in both hands.

(2) Hold the dressing with the white side down directly over the wound. **DO NOT** touch the white (sterile) side of the dressing or allow anything except the wound to come in contact with it.

(3) Pull the dressing open and place it directly over the wound (Figure 3-10). If the casualty is able, he may hold the dressing in place.

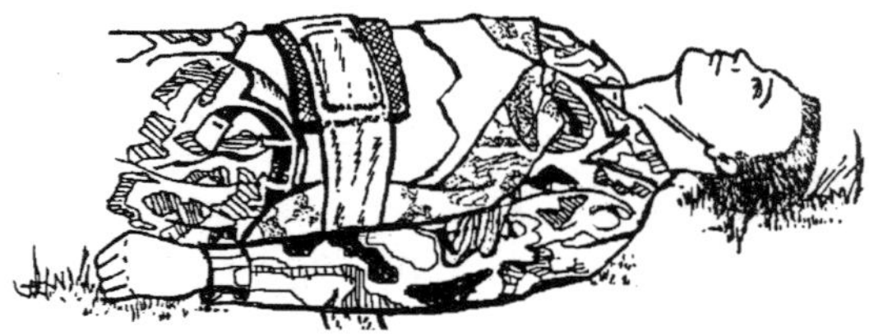

Figure 3-10. Dressing placed directly over the wound.

(4) Hold the dressing in place with one hand and use the other hand to wrap one of the tails around the body.

(5) Wrap the other tail in the opposite direction until the dressing is completely covered. Leave enough of the tail for a knot.

(6) Loosely tie the tails with a square knot at the casualty's side (Figure 3-11).

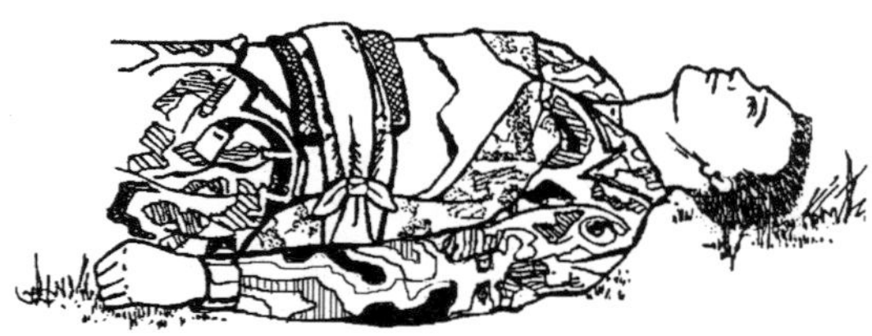

Figure 3-11. Dressing applied and tails tied with a square knot.

WARNING

When the dressing is applied, DO NOT put pressure on the wound or exposed internal parts, because pressure could cause further injury (vomiting, ruptured intestines, and so forth). Therefore, tie the dressing ties (tails) loosely at casualty's side, not directly over the dressing.

(7) Tie the dressing firmly enough to prevent slipping without applying pressure to the wound site (Figure 3-12).

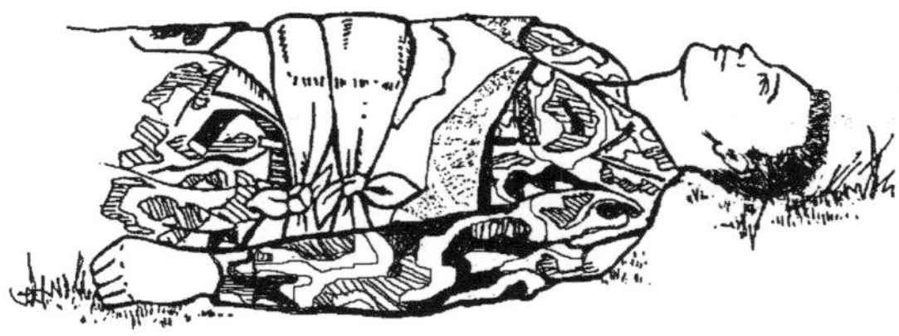

Figure 3-12. Field dressing covered with improvised material and loosely tied.

Field dressings can be covered with improvised reinforcement material (cravats, strips of torn T-shirt, or other cloth) for additional support and protection. Tie improvised bandage on the opposite side of the dressing ties firmly enough to prevent slipping but without applying additional pressure to the wound.

> **CAUTION**
>
> **DO NOT** give casualties with abdominal wounds food or water (moistening the lips is allowed).

e. Seek Medical Assistance. Notify medical personnel.

3-8. Burn Injuries

Burns often cause extreme pain, scarring, or even death. Before administering first aid, you must be able to recognize the type of burn. There are four types of burns:

- Thermal burns caused by fire, hot objects, hot liquids, and gases; or by nuclear blast or fireball.

- Electrical burns caused by electrical wires, current, or lightning.

- Chemical burns caused by contact with wet or dry chemicals or white phosphorus (WP)—from marking rounds and grenades.

- Laser burns (eye [ocular] injury).

3-9. First Aid for Burns

a. Eliminate the Source of the Burn. The source of the burn must be eliminated before any evaluation of the casualty can occur and first aid administered.

(1) Quickly remove the casualty from danger and cover the *thermal burn* with any large nonsynthetic material, such as a field jacket. If the casualty's clothing is still on fire, roll the casualty on the ground to smother (put out) the flames (Figure 3-13).

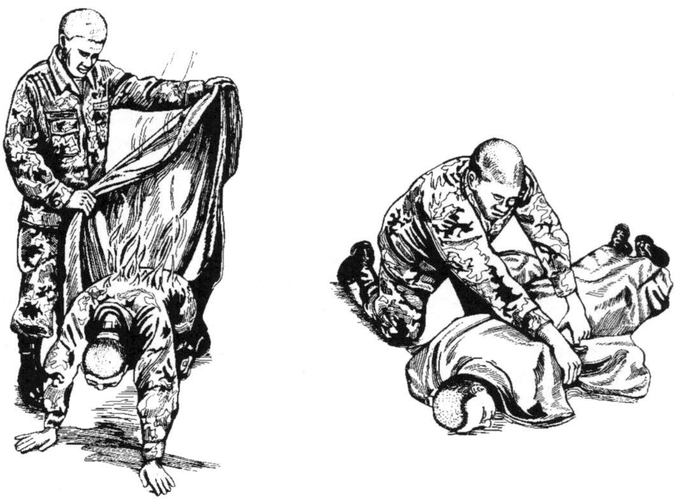

Figure 3-13. Casualty covered and rolled on ground.

> **CAUTION**
>
> Synthetic materials, such as nylon, may melt and cause further injury.

(2) Remove the *electrical burn* casualty from the electrical source by turning off the electrical current. **DO NOT** attempt to turn off the electricity if the source is not close by. Speed is critical, so **DO NOT** waste unnecessary time. If the electricity cannot be turned off, wrap any *nonconductive* material (*dry* rope, clothing, wood, and so forth) around the casualty's back and shoulders and drag the casualty away from the electrical source (Figure 3-14). **DO NOT** make body-to-body contact with the casualty or touch any wires because you could also become an electrical burn casualty.

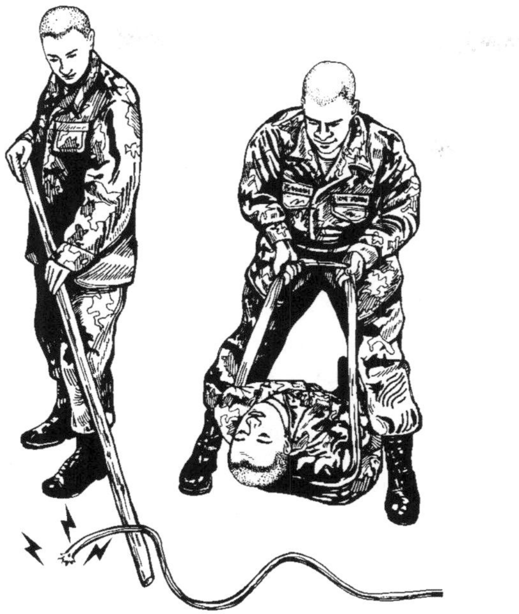

Figure 3-14. Casualty removed from electrical source (using nonconductive material).

> **WARNING**
>
> **High voltage electrical burns may cause temporary unconsciousness, difficulties in breathing, or difficulties with the heart (heartbeat).**

(3) Remove the *chemical* from the *burned casualty*. Remove *liquid* chemicals by flushing with as much water as possible. Remove *dry* chemicals by brushing off loose particles (**DO NOT** use the bare surface of your hand because you could become a chemical burn casualty) and then flush with large amounts of water, if available. If large amounts of water are not available, then **NO** water should be applied because small amounts of water applied to a dry chemical burn may cause a chemical reaction. When WP strikes the skin, smother with a wet cloth or mud. Keep WP covered with a wet material to exclude air; this should help prevent the particles from burning.

(4) Remove the *laser burn* casualty from the source. When removing the casualty from the laser beam source, be careful not to enter the

beam or you may become a casualty. Never look directly at the beam source and if possible, wear appropriate eye protection.

NOTE

After the casualty is removed from the source of the burn, he should be evaluated for conditions requiring basic first aid measures.

b. Expose the Burn. Cut and gently lift away any clothing covering the burned area, without pulling clothing over the burns. Leave in place any clothing that is stuck to the burn. If the casualty's hands or wrists have been burned, remove jewelry if possible without causing further injury (rings, watches, and so forth) and place in his pockets. This prevents the necessity to cut off jewelry since swelling usually occurs as a result of a burn.

CAUTION

DO NOT lift or cut away clothing if in a chemical environment. Apply the dressing directly over the casualty's protective clothing. **DO NOT** attempt to decontaminate skin where blisters have formed.

c. Apply a Field Dressing to the Burn.

(1) Grasp the tails of the casualty's dressing in both hands.

(2) Hold the dressing directly over the wound with the white side down, pull the dressing open, and place it directly over the wound. **DO NOT** touch the white (sterile) side of the dressing or allow anything except the wound to come in contact with it. If the casualty is able, he may hold the dressing in place.

(3) Hold the dressing in place with one hand and use the other hand to wrap one of the tails around the limbs or the body.

(4) Wrap the other tail in the opposite direction until the dressing is completely covered.

(5) Tie the tails into a square knot over the outer edge of the dressing. The dressing should be applied lightly over the burn. Ensure that dressing is applied firmly enough to prevent it from slipping.

NOTE

Use the cleanest improvised dressing material available if a field dressing is not available or if it is not large enough for the entire wound.

d. *Take the Following Precautions*:

- **DO NOT** place the dressing over the face or genital area.
- **DO NOT** break the blisters.
- **DO NOT** apply grease or ointments to the burns.
- For electrical burns, check for both an entry and exit burn from the passage of electricity through the body. Exit burns may appear on any area of the body despite location of entry burn.
- For burns caused by wet or dry chemicals, flush the burns with large amounts of water and cover with a dry dressing.
- For burns caused by WP, flush the area with water, then cover with a wet material, dressing, or mud to exclude the air and keep the WP particles from burning.
- For laser burns, apply a field dressing.
- If the casualty is conscious and not nauseated, give him small amounts of water.

e. *Seek Medical Assistance*. Notify medical personnel.

3-10. Dressings and Bandages

a. *Head Wounds.*

(1) *Position the casualty.*

WARNING

DO NOT move the casualty if you suspect he has sustained a neck, spine, or head injury (which produces any signs or symptoms other than minor bleeding).

- If the casualty has a minor (superficial) scalp wound and is conscious:

  - Have the casualty sit up (unless other injuries prohibit or he is unable to).

  - If the casualty is lying down and is not accumulating fluids or drainage in his throat, elevate his head slightly.

  - If the casualty is bleeding from or into his mouth or throat, turn his head to the side or position him on his side so that the airway will be clear. Avoid putting pressure on the wound and place him on his uninjured side (Figure 3-15).

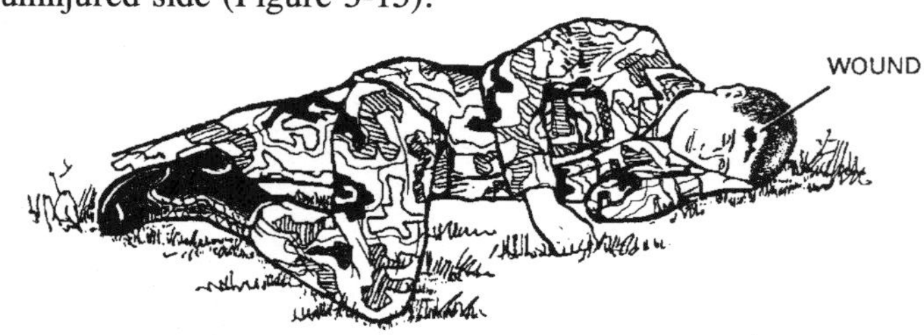

Figure 3-15. Casualty lying on side opposite injury.

- If the casualty is unconscious or has a severe head injury, then suspect and treat him as having a potential neck or spinal injury, *immobilize and **DO NOT** move the casualty.*

NOTE

If the casualty is choking or vomiting or is bleeding from or into his mouth (thus compromising his airway), position him on his uninjured side to allow for drainage and to help keep his airway clear.

WARNING

If it is necessary to turn a casualty with a suspected neck/spine injury; roll the casualty gently onto his side, keeping the head, neck, and body aligned while providing support for the head and neck. DO NOT roll the casualty by yourself but seek assistance. *Move him only if absolutely necessary*, otherwise keep the casualty immobilized to prevent further damage to the neck/spine.

(2) *Expose the wound.* Remove the casualty's helmet (if necessary). In a nuclear, biological, and chemical (NBC) environment, the first aid provider must leave the casualty as much protection (such as protective mask, mission-oriented protective posture [MOPP] overgarments) as possible. What items of protective equipment can be removed is dependent upon the casualty's injuries (where on the body and what type), the MOPP level, integrity of protective equipment (such as tears in the garment or mask seal), availability of chemical protective shelters, and the tactical situation.

WARNING

DO NOT attempt to clean the wound or remove a protruding object.

NOTE

Always use the casualty's field dressing, not your own.

(3) *Apply a dressing to a wound of the forehead or back of head.* To apply a dressing to a wound of the forehead or back of the head—

(*a*) Remove the dressing from the wrapper.

(*b*) Grasp the tails of the dressing in both hands.

(*c*) Hold the dressing (white side down) directly over the wound. **DO NOT** touch the white (sterile) side of the dressing or allow anything except the wound to come in contact with it.

(*d*) Place it directly over the wound.

(*e*) Hold it in place with one hand. If the casualty is able, he may assist.

(*f*) Wrap the first tail horizontally around the head; ensure the tail covers the dressing (Figure 3-16).

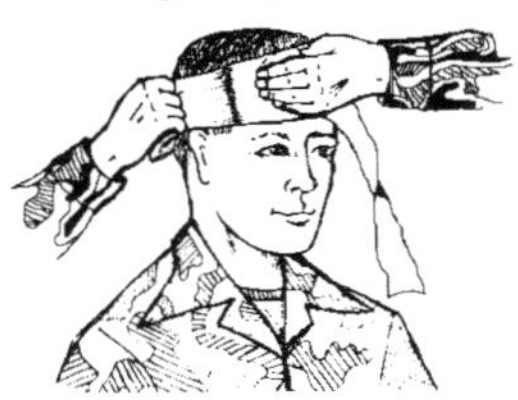

Figure 3-16. First tail of dressing wrapped horizontally around head.

(*g*) Hold the first tail in place and wrap the second tail in the opposite direction, covering the dressing (Figure 3-17).

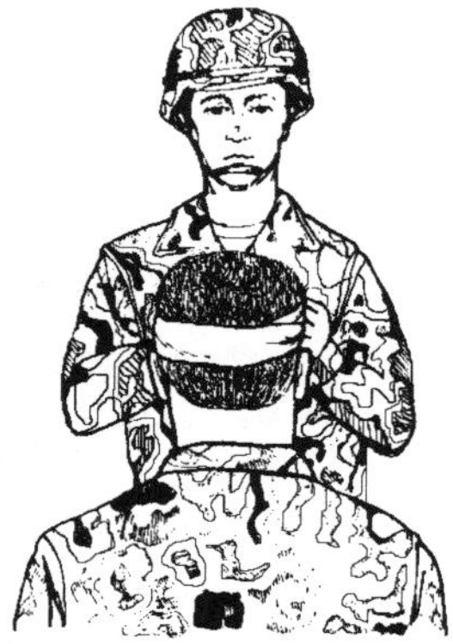

Figure 3-17. Second tail wrapped in opposite direction.

(*h*) Tie a square knot and secure the tails at the side of the head, making sure they **DO NOT** cover the eyes or ears (Figure 3-18).

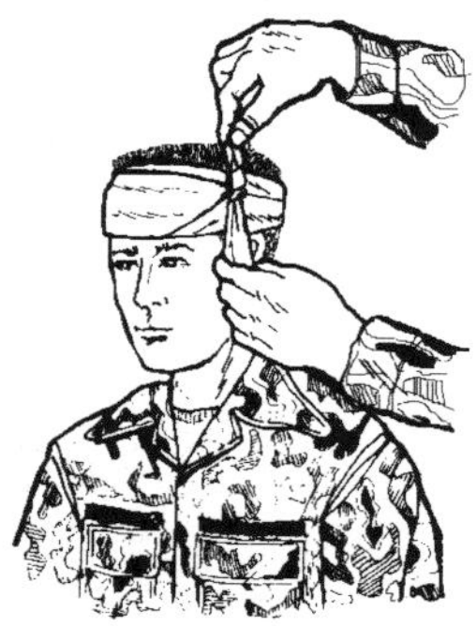

Figure 3-18. Tails tied in square knot at side of head.

(4) *Apply a dressing to a wound on top of the head.* To apply a dressing to a wound on top of the head—

(*a*) Remove the dressing from the wrapper.

(*b*) Grasp the tails of the dressing in both hands.

(*c*) Hold it (white side down) directly over the wound. **DO NOT** touch the white (sterile) side of the dressing or allow anything except the wound to come in contact with it.

(*d*) Place it over the wound (Figure 3-19).

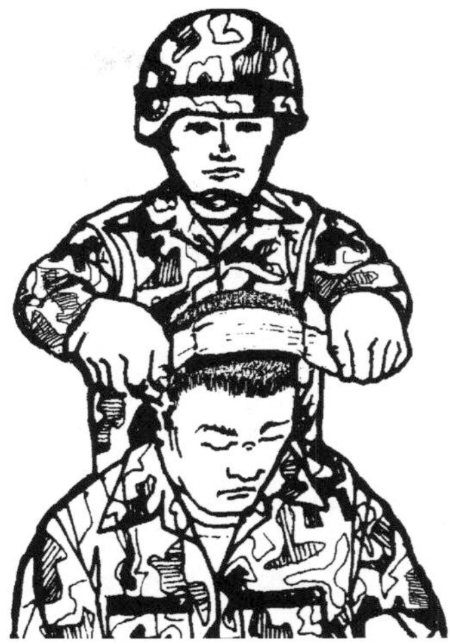

Figure 3-19. Dressing placed over wound.

(*e*) Hold it in place with one hand. If the casualty is able, he may assist.

(*f*) Wrap one tail down under the chin (Figure 3-20), up in front of the ear, over the dressing, and in front of the other ear.

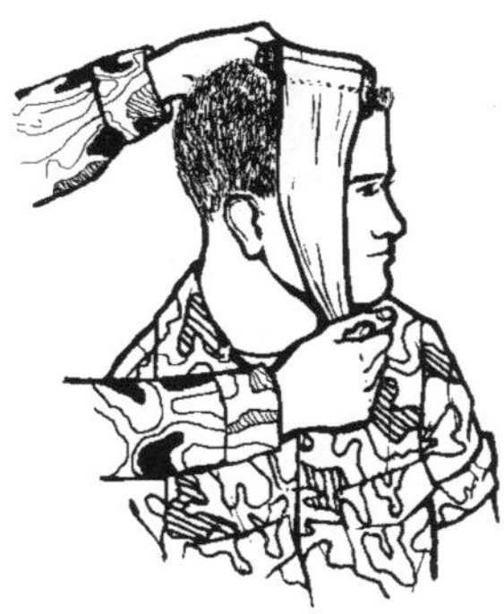

Figure 3-20. One tail of dressing wrapped under chin.

WARNING

Ensure the tails remain wide and close to the front of the chin to avoid choking the casualty.

(*g*) Wrap the remaining tail under the chin in the opposite direction and up the side of the face to meet the first tail (Figure 3-21).

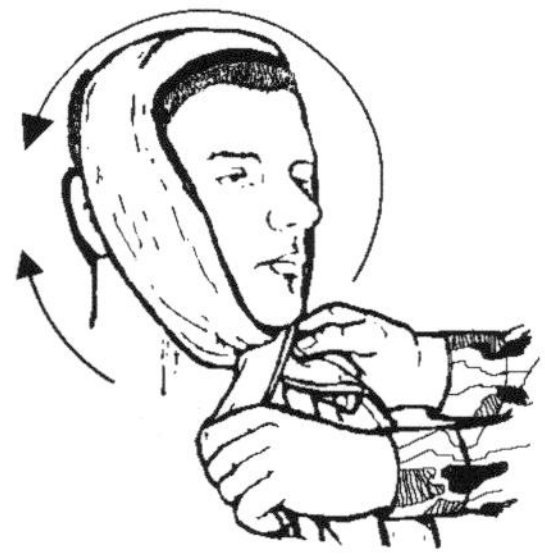

Figure 3-21. Remaining tail wrapped under chin in opposite direction.

(*h*) Cross the tails (Figure 3-22), bringing one around the forehead (above the eyebrows) and the other around the back of the head (at the base of the skull) to a point just above and in front of the opposite ear, and tie them using a square knot (Figure 3-23).

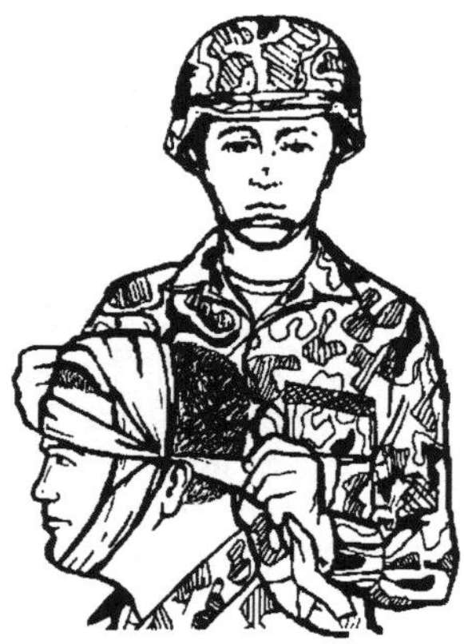

Figure 3-22. Tails of dressing crossed with one around forehead.

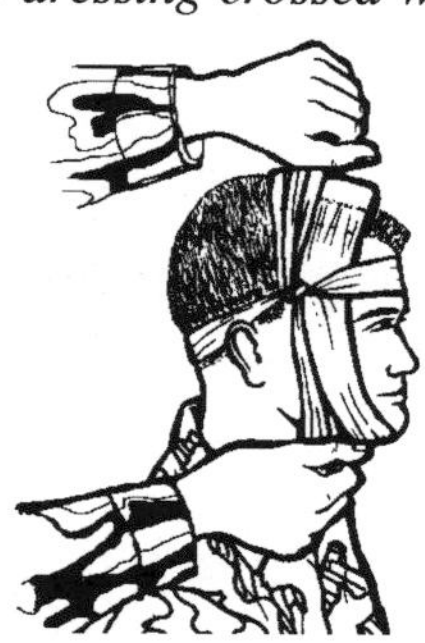

Figure 3-23. Tails tied in square knot (in front of and above ear).

(5) *Apply a triangular bandage to the head.* To apply a triangular bandage to the head—

(*a*) Turn the base (longest side) of the bandage up and center its base on the center of the forehead, letting the point (apex) fall on the back of the neck (Figure 3-24A).

(*b*) Take the ends behind the head and cross the ends over the apex.

(*c*) Take them over the forehead and tie them (Figure 3-24B).

(*d*) Tuck the apex behind the crossed part of the bandage or secure it with a safety pin, if available (Figure 3-24C).

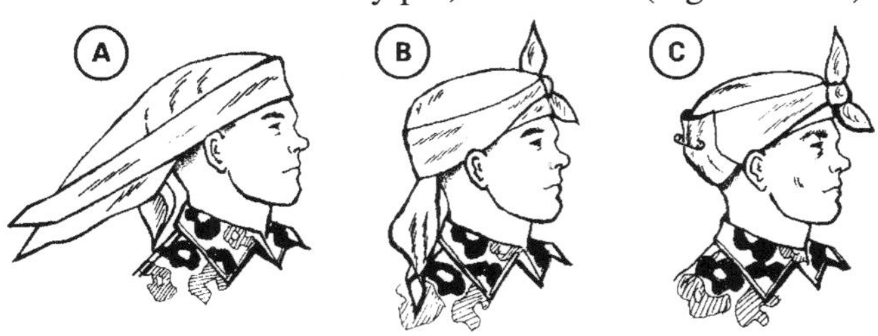

Figure 3-24. Triangular bandage applied to head (Illustrated A—C)

(6) *Apply a cravat bandage to the head.* To apply a cravat bandage to the head—

(*a*) Place the middle of the bandage over the dressing (Figure 3-25A).

(*b*) Cross the two ends of the bandage in opposite directions completely around the head (Figure 3-25B).

(*c*) Tie the ends over the dressing (Figure 3-25C).

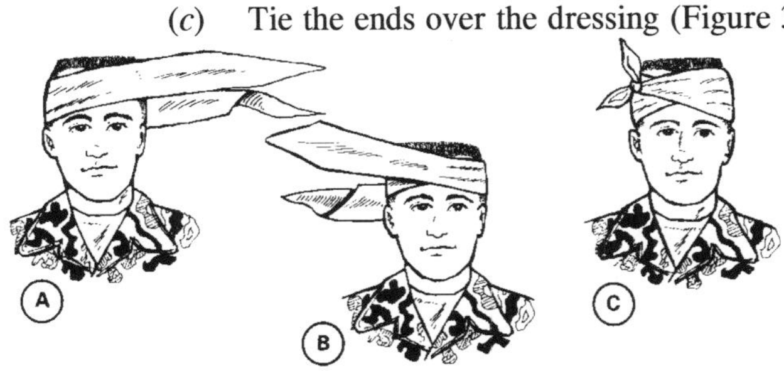

Figure 3-25. Cravat bandage applied to head (Illustrated A—C).

b. Eye Injuries. The eye is a vital sensory organ, and blindness is a severe physical handicap. Timely first aid of the eye may relieve pain and may also help to prevent shock, permanent eye injury, and possible loss of vision. Because the eye is very sensitive, any injury can be easily aggravated if it is improperly handled. Injuries of the eye may be quite severe. Cuts of the eyelids can appear to be very serious, but if the eyeball is not involved, a person's vision usually will not be damaged. However, lacerations (cuts) of the eyeball can cause permanent damage or loss of sight.

(1) *Lacerated/torn eyelids*. Lacerated eyelids may bleed heavily, but bleeding usually stops quickly. Cover the injured eye with a sterile dressing. **DO NOT** put pressure on the wound because you may injure the eyeball. Handle torn eyelids very carefully to prevent further injury. Place any detached pieces of the eyelid on a clean bandage or dressing and immediately send them with the casualty to the medical facility.

(2) *Lacerated eyeball (injury to the globe)*. Lacerations or cuts to the eyeball may cause serious and permanent eye damage. Cover the injury with a loose sterile dressing. **DO NOT** put pressure on the eyeball because additional damage may occur. An important point to remember is that when one eyeball is injured, you should immobilize both eyes. This is done by applying a bandage to both eyes. Because the eyes move together, covering both will lessen the chances of further damage to the injured eye. (However, in hazardous surroundings, leave uninjured eye uncovered to enable casualty to see.)

CAUTION

DO NOT apply pressure when there is a possible laceration of the eyeball. The eyeball contains fluid. Pressure applied over the eye will force the fluid out, resulting in permanent injury. **APPLY PROTECTIVE DRESSING WITHOUT ADDED PRESSURE**.

(3) *Extruded eyeballs*. Service members may encounter casualties with severe eye injuries that include an extruded eyeball (eyeball out-of-socket). In such instances you should gently cover the extruded eye with a loose moistened dressing and also cover the unaffected eye. **DO NOT** bind or exert pressure on the injured eye while applying the dressing. Keep the casualty quiet, place him on his back, treat for shock, and evacuate him immediately.

(4) *Burns of the eyes*. Chemical burns, thermal (heat) burns, and light burns can affect the eyes.

(*a*) *Chemical burns*. Injuries from chemical burns require immediate first aid. Mainly acids or alkalies cause chemical burns. The first aid measures consist of flushing the eyes immediately with large amounts of water for at least 5 to 20 minutes, or as long as necessary to flush out the chemical and, once flushed, bandaging the eyes. If the burn is an acid burn, you should flush the eye for at least 5 to 10 minutes. If the burn is an alkali burn, you should flush the eye for at least 20 minutes. After the eye has been flushed evacuate the casualty immediately.

(*b*) *Thermal burns*. When an individual suffers burns of the face from a fire, the eyes will close quickly due to extreme heat. This reaction is a natural reflex to protect the eyeballs; however, the eyelids remain exposed and are frequently burned. If a casualty receives burns of the eyelids or face—

- **DO NOT** apply a dressing.
- **DO NOT** touch.
- **SEEK** medical assistance immediately.

(*c*) *Light burns*. Exposure to intense light can burn an individual. Infrared rays, eclipse light (if the casualty has looked directly at the sun), or laser burns cause injuries of the exposed eyeball. Ultraviolet rays from arc welding can cause a superficial burn to the surface of the eye. These injuries are generally not painful but may cause permanent damage to the eyes. Immediate first aid is usually not required. Loosely bandaging the eyes may make the casualty more comfortable and protect his eyes from further injury caused by exposure to other bright lights or sunlight.

CAUTION

With impaled objects or significant sized foreign bodies, both eyes are usually bandaged to help secure the foreign body in the injured eye. In a battlefield environment, leave the uninjured eye uncovered so that the casualty can see.

c. *Side-of-Head or Cheek Wound*. Facial injuries to the side of the head or the cheek may bleed profusely (Figure 3-26). Prompt action is necessary to ensure that the airway remains open and also to control the bleeding. It may be necessary to apply a dressing. To apply a dressing—

(1) Remove the dressing from its wrapper.

(2) Grasp the tails in both hands.

(3) Hold the dressing directly over the wound with the white side down and place it directly on the wound (Figure 3-27A). **DO NOT** touch the white (sterile) side of the dressing or allow anything except the wound to come in contact with it.

(4) Hold the dressing in place with one hand (the casualty may assist if able). Wrap the top tail over the top of the head and bring it down in front of the ear (on the side opposite the wound), under the chin (Figure 3-27B) and up over the dressing to a point just above the ear (on the wound side).

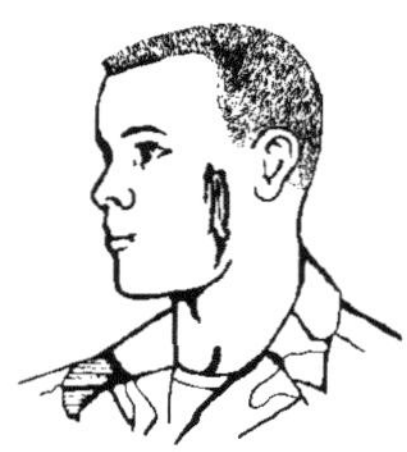

Figure 3-26. Side of head or cheek wound.

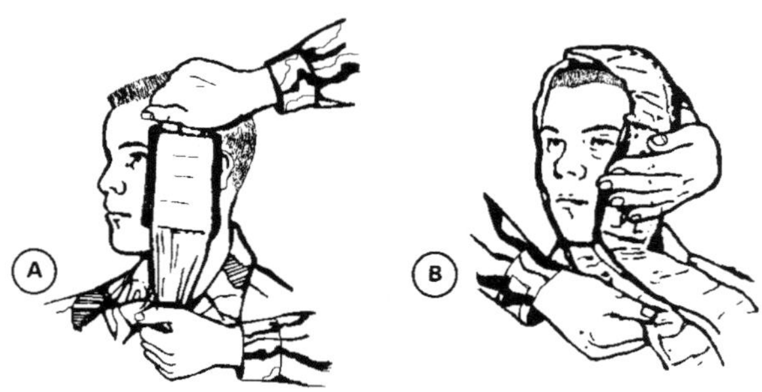

Figure 3-27. Dressing placed directly on wound. Top tail wrapped over top of head, down in front of ear, and under chin (Illustrated A—B).

NOTE

When possible, avoid covering the casualty's ear with the dressing, as this will decrease his ability to hear.

(5) Bring the second tail under the chin, up in front of the ear (on the side opposite the wound), and over the head to meet the other tail (on the wounded side) (Figure 3-28).

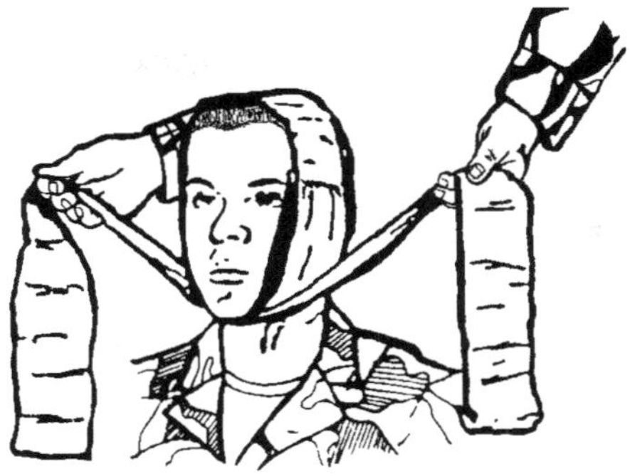

Figure 3-28. Bringing second tail under the chin.

(6) Cross the two tails (on the wound side) (Figure 3-29) and bring one end across the forehead (above the eyebrows) to a point just in front of the opposite ear (on the uninjured side).

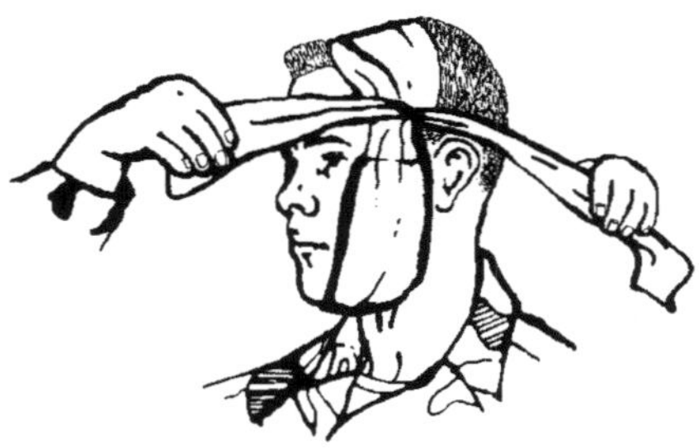

Figure 3-29. Crossing the tails on the side of the wound.

(7) Wrap the other tail around the back of the head (at the base of the skull), and tie the two ends just in front of the ear on the uninjured side with a square knot (Figure 3-30).

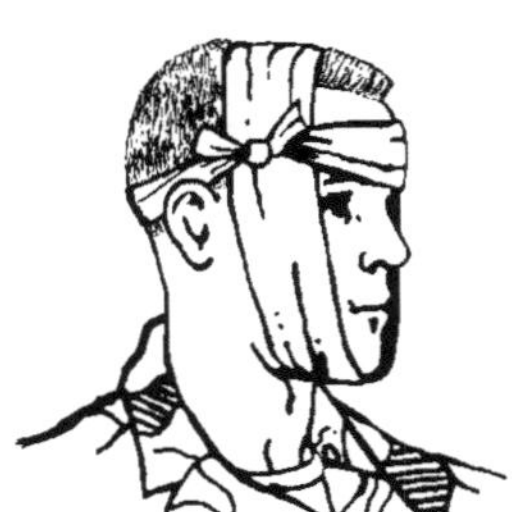

Figure 3-30. Tying the tails of the dressing in a square knot.

d. Ear Injuries. Lacerated (cut) or avulsed (torn) ear tissue may not, in itself, be a serious injury. Bleeding, or the drainage of fluids from the ear canal, however, may be a sign of a head injury, such as a skull fracture. **DO NOT** attempt to stop the flow from the inner ear canal nor put anything into the ear canal to block it. Instead, you should cover the ear lightly with a dressing. For minor cuts or wounds to the external ear, apply a cravat bandage as follows:

(1) Place the middle of the bandage over the ear (Figure 3-31A).

(2) Cross the ends, wrap them in opposite directions around the head, and tie them (Figures 3-31B and 3-31C).

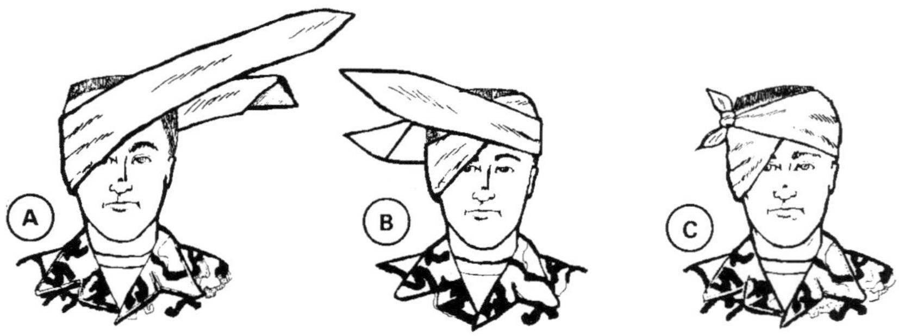

Figure 3-31. Applying cravat bandage to ear (Illustrated A—C).

(3) If possible, place some dressing material between the back of the ear and the side of the head to avoid crushing the ear against the head with the bandage.

e. Nose Injuries. Nose injuries generally produce bleeding. The bleeding may be controlled by placing an ice pack (if available) over the nose, or pinching the nostrils together. The bleeding may also be controlled by placing torn gauze (rolled) between the upper teeth and the lip.

CAUTION

DO NOT attempt to remove objects inhaled into the nose. An untrained person who removes such an object could worsen the casualty's condition and cause permanent injury.

f. Jaw Injuries. Before applying a bandage to a casualty's jaw, remove all loose or free-floating foreign material from the casualty's mouth.

If the casualty is unconscious, check for obstructions in the airway and remove if possible. If there is profuse bleeding in the oral cavity, the cavity may require loose packing with soft bandaging material (for example: Kerlix™ gauze) prior to applying a bandage. Care should be taken to avoid occluding the airway. When applying the bandage, allow the jaw enough freedom to permit passage of air and drainage from the mouth.

(1) *Apply bandages attached to field first aid dressing to the jaw.* After dressing the wound, apply the bandages using the same technique illustrated in Figure 3-32A—C.

NOTE

The dressing and bandaging procedure outlined for the jaw serves a twofold purpose. In addition to stopping the bleeding and protecting the wound, it also immobilizes a fractured jaw.

(2) *Apply a cravat bandage to the jaw.*

(*a*) Place the bandage under the chin and pull its ends upward. Adjust the bandage to make one end longer than the other (Figure 3-32A).

(*b*) Take the longer end over the top of the head to meet the short end at the temple and cross the ends over (Figure 3-32B).

(*c*) Take the ends in opposite directions to the other side of the head and tie them over the part of the bandage that was applied first (Figure 3-32C).

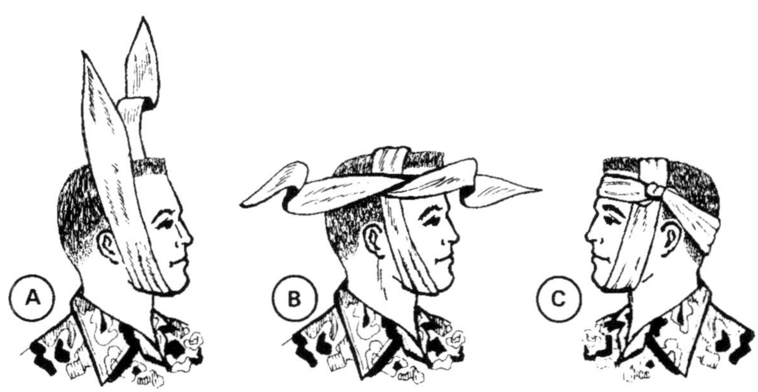

Figure 3-32. Applying a cravat bandage to jaw (Illustrated A—C).

NOTE

The cravat bandage technique is used to immobilize a fractured jaw or to maintain a sterile dressing that does not have tail bandages attached.

3-11. Shoulder Bandage

a. To apply bandages attached to the field first aid dressing—

(1) Take one bandage across the chest and the other across the back and under the arm opposite the injured shoulder.

(2) Tie the ends with a square knot (Figure 3-33).

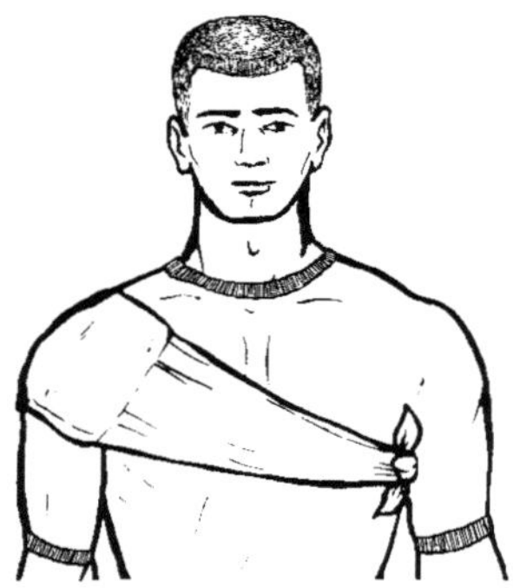

Figure 3-33. Shoulder bandage.

b. To apply a cravat bandage to the shoulder or armpit—

(1) Make an extended cravat bandage by using two triangular bandages (Figure 3-34A); place the end of the first triangular bandage along the base of the second one (Figure 3-34B).

(2) Fold the two bandages into a single extended bandage (Figure 3-34C).

(3) Fold the extended bandage into a single cravat bandage (Figure 3-34D). After folding, secure the thicker part (overlap) with two or more safety pins (Figure 3-34E).

(4) Place the middle of the cravat bandage under the armpit so that the front end is longer than the back end and safety pins are on the outside (Figure 3-34F).

(5) Cross the ends on top of the shoulder (Figure 3-34G).

(6) Take one of the bandage ends across the back and under the arm on the opposite side and the other end across the chest. Tie the ends (Figure 3-34H).

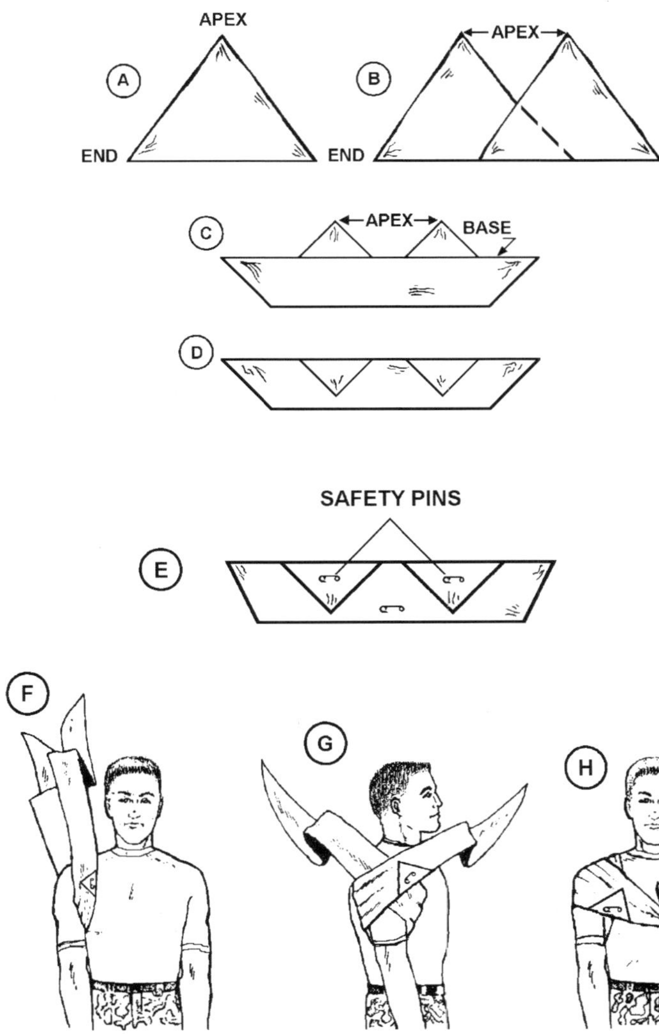

Figure 3-34. Extended cravat bandage applied to shoulder or armpit (Illustrated A—H).

Be sure to place sufficient wadding in the armpit. **DO NOT** tie the cravat bandage too tightly. Avoid compressing the major blood vessels in the armpit.

3-12. Elbow Bandage

To apply a cravat bandage to the elbow—

a. Bend the arm at the elbow and place the middle of the cravat at the point of the elbow bringing the ends upward (Figure 3-35A).

b. Bring the ends across, extending both downward (Figure 3-35B).

c. Take both ends around the arm and tie them with a square knot at the front of the elbow (Figure 3-35C).

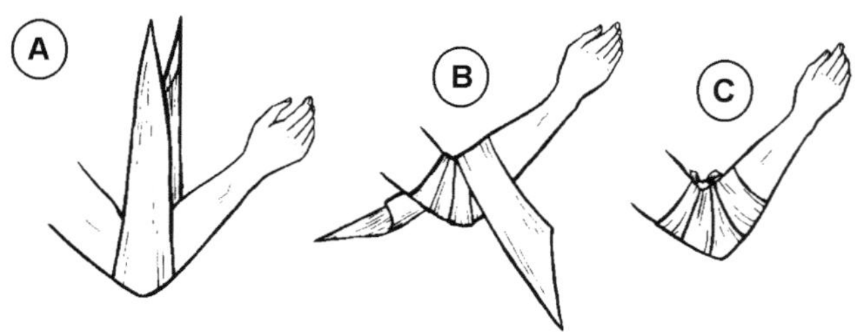

Figure 3-35. Elbow bandage (Illustrated A—C).

> **CAUTION**
>
> If an elbow fracture is suspected, **DO NOT** bend the elbow; bandage it in the position found.

3-13. Hand Bandage

a. To apply a triangular bandage to the hand—

(1) Place the hand in the middle of the triangular bandage with the wrist at the base of the bandage (Figure 3-36A). Ensure that the fingers are separated with absorbent material to prevent chafing and irritation of the skin.

(2) Place the apex over the fingers and tuck any excess material into the pleats on each side of the hand (Figure 3-36B).

(3) Cross the ends on top of the hand, take them around the wrist, and tie them (Figures 3-36C—E) with a square knot.

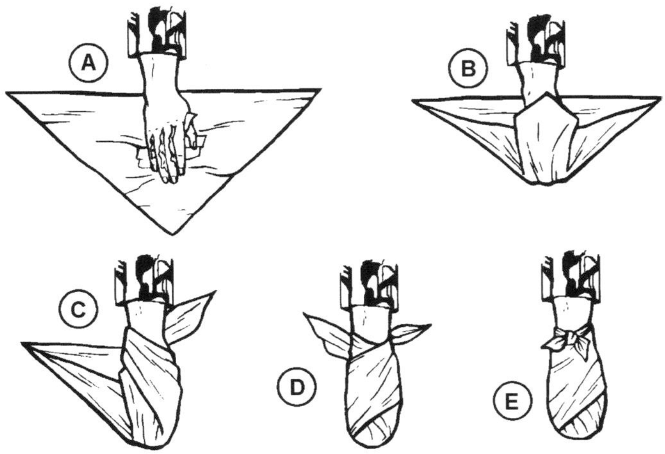

Figure 3-36. Triangular bandage applied to hand (Illustrated A—E).

b. To apply a cravat bandage to the palm of the hand—

(1) Lay the middle of the cravat over the palm of the hand with the ends hanging down on each side (Figure 3-37A).

(2) Take the end of the cravat at the little finger across the back of the hand, extending it upward over the base of the thumb; then bring it downward across the palm (Figure 3-37B).

(3) Take the thumb end across the back of the hand, over the palm, and through the hollow between the thumb and palm (Figure 3-37C).

(4) Take the ends to the back of the hand and cross them; then bring them up over the wrist and cross them again (Figure 3-37D).

(5) Bring both ends down and tie them with a square knot on top of the wrist (Figure 3-37E—F).

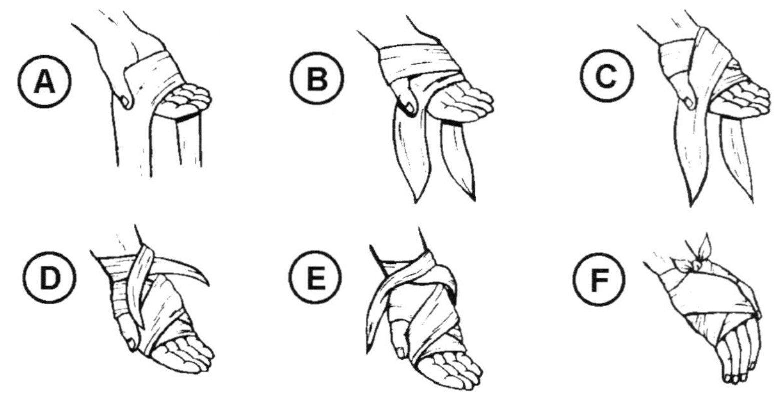

Figure 3-37. Cravat bandage applied to palm of hand (Illustrated A—F).

3-14. Leg (Upper and Lower) Bandage

To apply a cravat bandage to the leg—

a. Place the center of the cravat over the dressing (Figure 3-38A).

b. Take one end around and up the leg in a spiral motion and the other end around and down the leg in a spiral motion, overlapping part of each preceding turn (Figure 3-38B).

c. Bring both ends together and tie them (Figure 3-38C) with a square knot.

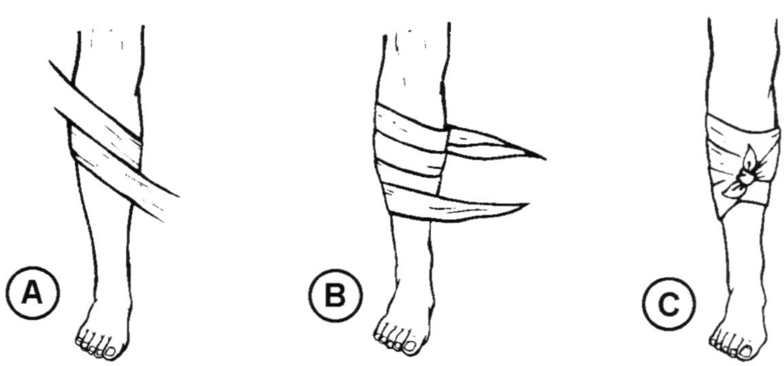

Figure 3-38. Cravat bandage applied to leg (Illustrated A—C).

3-15. Knee Bandage

To apply a cravat bandage to the knee as illustrated in Figure 3-39, use the same technique applied in bandaging the elbow.

> **CAUTION**
>
> If a fracture of the kneecap is suspected, **DO NOT** bend the knee; bandage it in the position found.

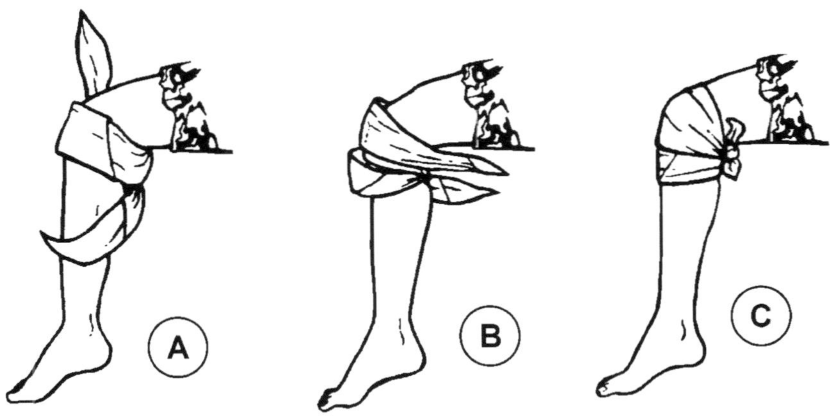

Figure 3-39. Cravat bandage applied to knee (Illustrated A—C).

3-16. Foot Bandage

To apply a triangular bandage to the foot—

a. Place the foot in the middle of the triangular bandage with the heel well forward of the base (Figure 3-40A). Ensure that the toes are separated by absorbent material to prevent chafing and irritation of the skin.

b. Place the apex over the top of the foot and tuck any excess material into the pleats on each side of the foot (Figure 3-40B).

c. Cross the ends on top of the foot, take them around the ankle, and tie them at the front of the ankle (Figure 3-40C—E).

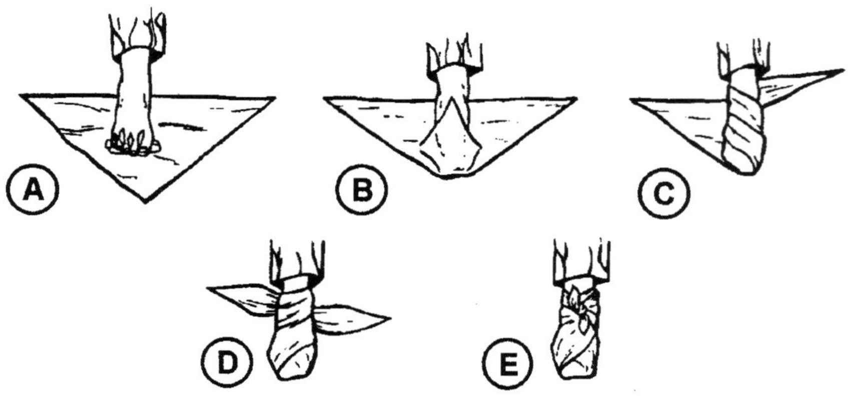

Figure 3-40. Triangular bandage applied to foot (Illustrated A—E).

CHAPTER 4

FIRST AID FOR FRACTURES

4-1. General

A fracture is any break in the continuity of a bone. Fractures can cause total disability or in some cases death by severing vital organs and/or arteries. On the other hand, they can most often be treated so there is a complete recovery. The potential for recovery depends greatly upon the first aid the individual receives before he is moved. First aid includes immobilizing the fractured part in addition to applying lifesaving measures when necessary. The basic splinting principle is to immobilize the joints above and below the fracture.

4-2. Kinds of Fractures

Figure 4-1 depicts types of fractures.

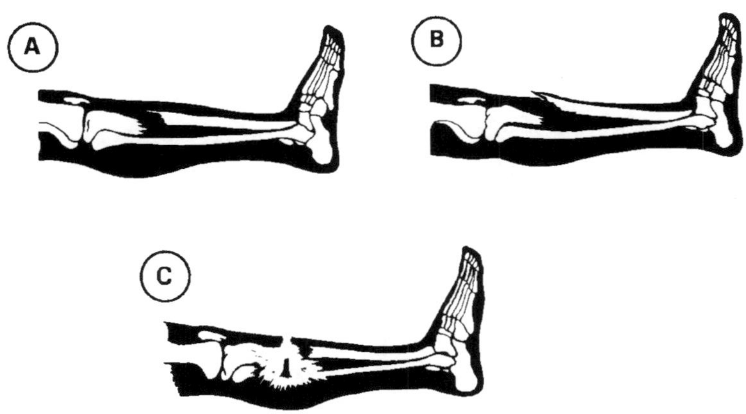

Figure 4-1. Types of fractures (Illustrated A—C).

a. Closed Fracture (Figure 4-1A). A closed fracture is a broken bone that does not break the overlying skin. The tissue beneath the skin may be damaged. A *dislocation* is when a joint, such as a knee, ankle, or shoulder, is not in the proper position. A *sprain* is when the connecting tissues of the joints have been torn. Dislocations and sprains (swelling, possible deformity, and discoloration) should be treated as closed fractures.

b. Open Fracture (Figure 4-1B and 4-1C). An open fracture is a broken bone that breaks (pierces) the overlying skin. The broken bone may come through the skin or a missile such as a bullet or shell fragment may go through the flesh and break the bone.

NOTE

An open fracture is contaminated and subject to infection.

4-3. Signs and Symptoms of Fractures

Indications of a fracture are deformity, tenderness, swelling, pain, inability to move the injured part, protruding bone, bleeding, or discolored skin at the injury site. A sharp pain when the service member attempts to move the part is also a sign of a fracture.

WARNING

DO NOT encourage the casualty to move the injured part in order to identify a fracture since such movement could cause further damage to surrounding tissues and promote shock. If you are not sure whether a bone is fractured, care for the injury as a fracture. At the site of the fracture, the bone ends are sharp and could cause vessel (artery and/or vein) damage.

4-4. Purposes of Immobilizing Fractures

A fracture is immobilized to prevent the sharp edges of the bone from moving and cutting tissue, muscle, blood vessels, and nerves. This reduces pain and helps prevent or control shock. In a closed fracture, immobilization keeps bone fragments from causing an open wound, which can become contaminated and subject to infection.

4-5. Splints, Padding, Bandages, Slings, and Swathes

a. Splints. Splints may be improvised from such items as boards, poles, sticks, tree limbs, or cardboard. If nothing is available for a splint, the chest wall can be used to immobilize a fractured arm and the uninjured leg can be used to immobilize (to some extent) the fractured leg.

b. Padding. Padding may be improvised from such items as a jacket, blanket, poncho, shelter half, or leafy vegetation.

c. *Bandages*. Bandages may be improvised from belts, rifle slings, kerchiefs, or strips torn from clothing or blankets. Narrow materials such as wire or cord should not be used to secure a splint in place. The application of wire and/or narrow material to an extremity could cause tissue damage and a tourniquet effect.

d. *Slings*. A sling is a bandage suspended from the neck to support an upper extremity. If a bandage is not available, a sling can be improvised by using the tail of a coat or shirt or pieces of cloth torn from such items as clothing and blankets. The triangular bandage is ideal for this purpose. Remember that the casualty's hand should be higher than his elbow, and the fingers should be showing at all times. The sling should be applied so that the supporting pressure is on the uninjured side.

e. *Swathes*. Swathes are any bands (pieces of cloth or load bearing equipment [LBE]) that are used to further immobilize a splinted fracture. Triangular and cravat bandages are often used and are called *swathe bandages*. The purpose of the swathe is to immobilize; therefore, the swathe bandage is placed above and/or below the fracture—not over it.

4-6. Procedures for Splinting Suspected Fractures

Before beginning first aid procedures for a fracture, gather whatever splinting materials are available. Ensure that splints are long enough to immobilize the joint above and below the suspected fracture. If possible, use at least four ties (two above and two below the fracture) to secure the splints. The ties should be square knots and should be tied away from the body on the splint. Distal pulses of the affected extremity should be checked before and after the application of the splint.

a. *Evaluate the Casualty*. Be prepared to perform any necessary lifesaving measures. Monitor the casualty for development of conditions that may require you to perform necessary lifesaving measures.

WARNING

Unless there is immediate life-threatening danger, such as a fire or an explosion, DO NOT move the casualty with a suspected back or neck injury. Improper movement may cause permanent paralysis or death.

WARNING

In a chemical environment, DO NOT remove any protective clothing. Apply the dressings and splints over the garments.

b. Locate the Site of the Suspected Fracture.

(1) Ask the casualty for the location of the injury.

- Does he have any pain?
- Where is it tender?
- Can he move the extremity?

NOTE

With the presence of an obvious deformity, do not make the casualty move extremity.

(2) Look for an unnatural position of the extremity.

(3) Look for a bone sticking out (protruding).

c. Prepare the Casualty for Splinting the Suspected Fracture.

(1) Reassure the casualty. Tell him that you will be providing first aid for him and that medical help is on the way.

(2) Loosen any tight or binding clothing.

(3) Remove all jewelry from the injured part and place it in the casualty's pocket. Tell the casualty you are doing this because if the jewelry is not removed and swelling occurs later, he may not be able to get it off and further bodily injury could result.

(4) Boots should not be removed from the casualty unless they are needed to stabilize a neck injury or there is actual bleeding from the foot.

d. Gather Splinting Materials. If standard splinting materials (splints, padding, and cravats) are not available, gather improvised materials. If splinting material is not available and the suspected fracture **CANNOT** be splinted, then swathes, or a combination of swathes and slings can be used to immobilize the extremity.

e. *Pad the Splints*. Pad the splints where they touch any bony part of the body, such as the elbow, wrist, knee, ankle, crotch, or armpit areas. Padding prevents excessive pressure on the area, which could lead to circulation problems.

f. *Check the Circulation Below the Site of the Injury*.

(1) Note any pale, white, or bluish-gray color of the skin, which may indicate impaired circulation. Circulation can also be checked by depressing the toe or fingernail beds and observing how quickly the color returns. A slower return of color to the injured side when compared with the uninjured side indicates a problem with circulation. The fingernail bed is the method to use to check the circulation in a dark-skinned casualty.

(2) Check the temperature of the injured extremity. Use your hand to compare the temperature of the injured side with the uninjured side. The body area below the injury may be colder to the touch indicating poor circulation.

(3) Question the casualty about the presence of numbness, tightness, cold, or tingling sensations.

WARNING

Casualties with fractures of the extremities may show impaired circulation, such as numbness, tingling, cold or pale to bluish skin tone. These casualties should be evacuated by medical personnel and treated as soon as possible. Prompt medical treatment may prevent possible loss of the limb.

WARNING

If it is an open fracture and the bone is protruding from the skin, *DO NOT ATTEMPT TO PUSH THE BONE BACK UNDER THE SKIN.* Apply a field dressing over the wound to protect the area.

g. Apply the Splint in Place.

(1) Splint the fracture in the position found. **DO NOT** attempt to reposition or straighten the injury. If it is an open fracture, stop the bleeding and protect the wound. Cover all wounds with field dressings before applying a splint. Remember to use the casualty's field dressing, not your own.

(2) Place one splint on each side of the fracture. Make sure that the splints reach, if possible, beyond the joints above and below the fracture.

(3) Tie the splints. Secure each splint in place above and below the fracture site with improvised (or actual) cravats. Improvised cravats, such as strips of cloth, belts, or whatever else you have, may be used. With minimal motion to the injured areas, place and tie the splints with the bandages. Push cravats through and under the natural body curvatures, and then gently position improvised cravats and tie in place. Use square knots. Tie all knots on the splint away from the casualty (Figure 4-2). **DO NOT** tie cravats directly over the suspected fracture site.

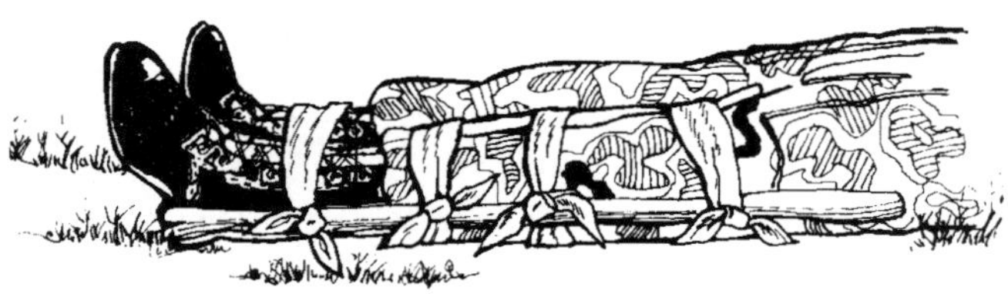

Figure 4-2. Square knots tied away from casualty.

h. Check the Splint for Tightness.

(1) **CHECK** to be sure that bandages are tight enough to securely hold splinting materials in place, but not so tight that circulation is impaired.

(2) **RECHECK** the circulation after application of the splint. Check the skin color and temperature. This is to ensure that the bandages holding the splint in place have not been tied too tightly. A fingertip check can be made by inserting the tip of the finger between the bandaged knot and the skin.

(3) **MAKE** any necessary adjustment without allowing the splint to become ineffective.

i. Apply a Sling. An improvised sling may be made from any available nonstretching piece of cloth, such as a battle dress uniform (BDU) shirt or trousers, poncho, or shelter half. Slings may also be improvised using the tail of a coat, belt, or a piece of cloth. Figure 4-3 depicts a shirttail used for support. A trousers belt or LBE may also be used for support (Figure 4-4). A sling should place the supporting pressure on the casualty's uninjured side. The supported arm should have the hand positioned slightly higher than the elbow showing the fingers.

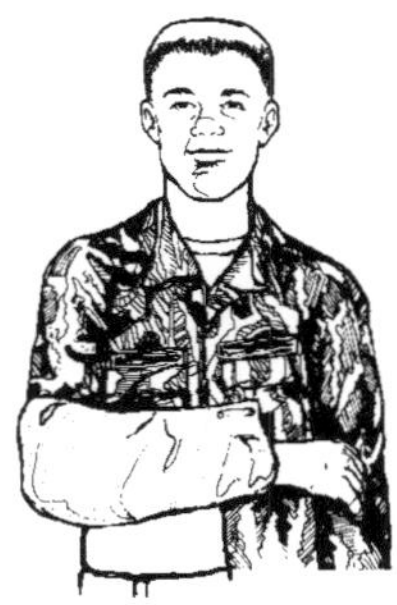

Figure 4-3. Shirttail used for support.

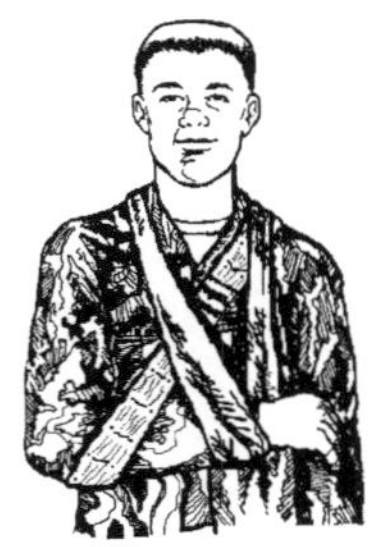

Figure 4-4. Belt used for support.

(1) Insert the splinted arm in the center of the sling (Figure 4-5).

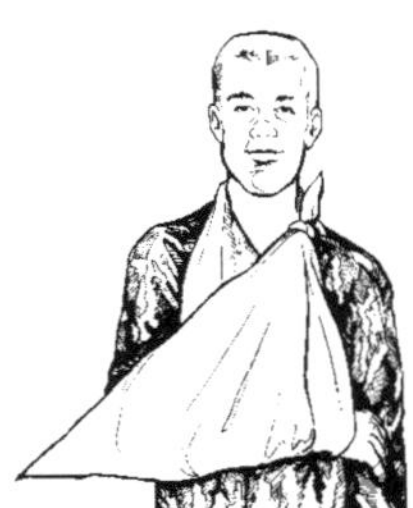

Figure 4-5. Arm inserted in center of improvised sling.

(2) Bring the ends of the sling up and tie them at the side (or hollow) of the neck on the uninjured side (Figure 4-6).

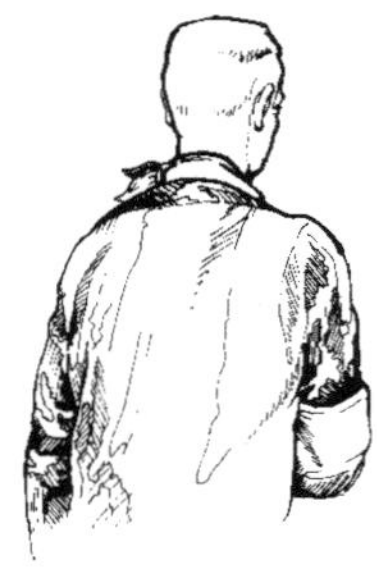

Figure 4-6. Ends of improvised sling tied to side of neck.

(3) Twist and tuck the corner of the sling at the elbow (Figure 4-7).

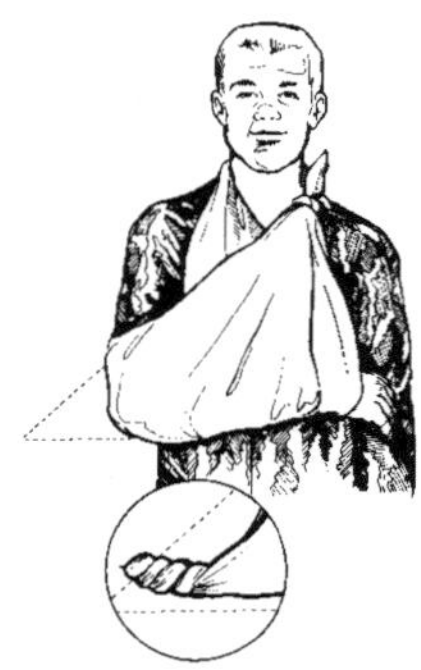

Figure 4-7. Corner of sling twisted and tucked at elbow.

j. Apply a Swathe. You may use any large piece of cloth, service member's belt, or pistol belt, to improvise a swathe.

WARNING

The swathe should not be placed directly on top of the injury, but positioned either above or below the fracture site.

(1) Apply swathes to the injured arm by wrapping the swathe over the injured arm, around the casualty's back, and under the arm on the uninjured side. Tie the ends on the uninjured side (Figure 4-8).

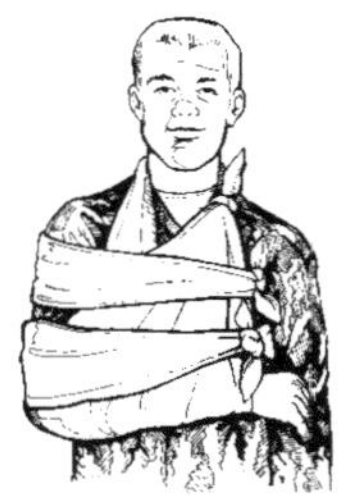

Figure 4-8. Arm immobilized with strip of clothing.

(2) A swathe is applied to an injured leg by wrapping the swathe around both legs and securing it on the uninjured side.

k. Seek Medical Assistance. Notify medical personnel, watch closely for development of life-threatening conditions and/or impaired circulation to the injured extremity. (Refer to Chapter 1 for additional information on life-threatening conditions.)

4-7. Upper Extremity Fractures

Figures 4-9 through 4-17 show how to apply slings, splints, and cravats (swathes) to immobilize and support fractures of the upper extremities. *Although the padding is not visible in some of the illustrations, it is always preferable to apply padding along the injured part for the length of the splint and especially where it touches any bony parts of the body.*

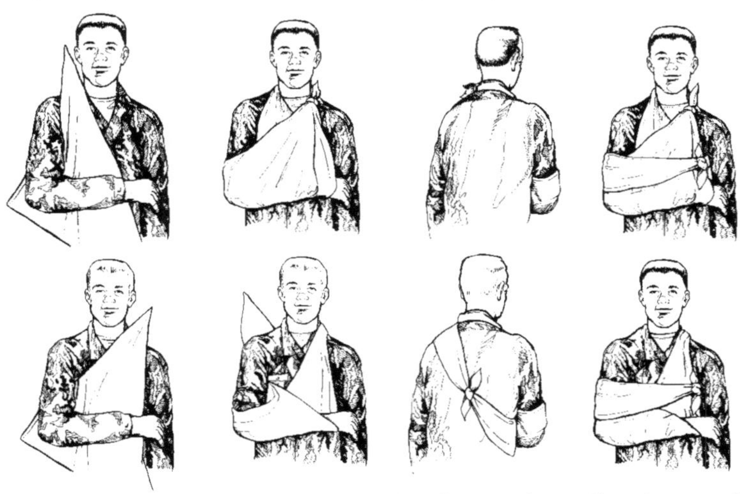

Figure 4-9. Application of triangular bandage to form sling (two methods).

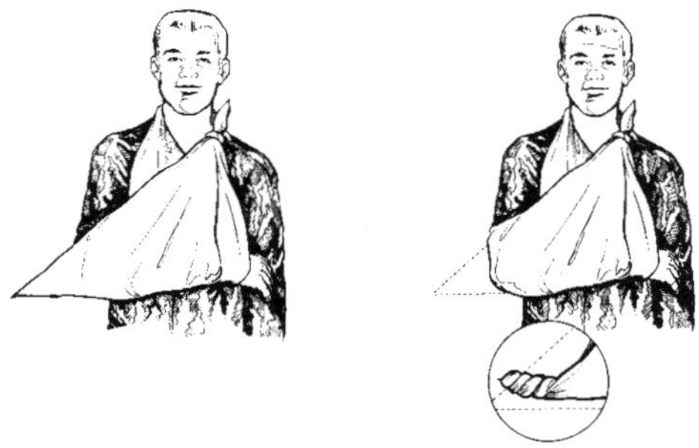

Figure 4-10. Completing sling sequence by twisting and tucking the corner of the sling at the elbow.

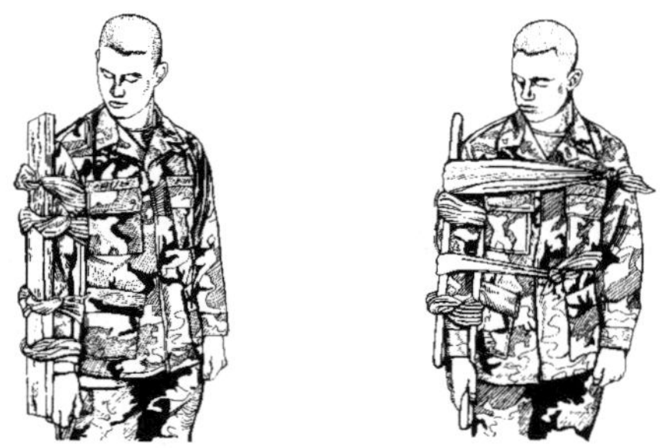

Figure 4-11. Board splints applied to fractured elbow when elbow is not bent (two methods).

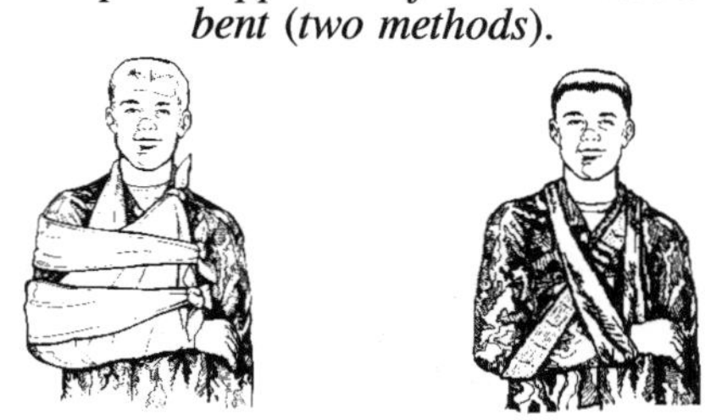

Figure 4-12. Chest wall used as splint for upper arm fracture when no splint is available.

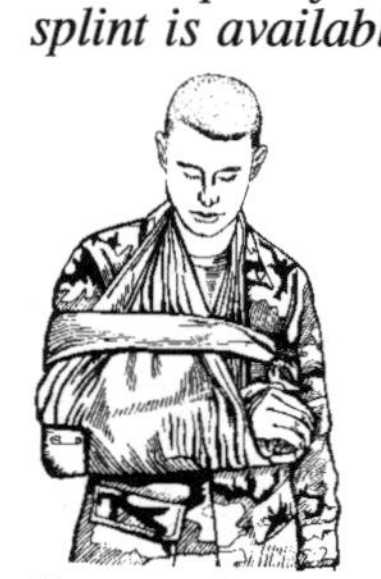

Figure 4-13. Chest wall, sling, and cravat used to immobilize fractured elbow when elbow is bent.

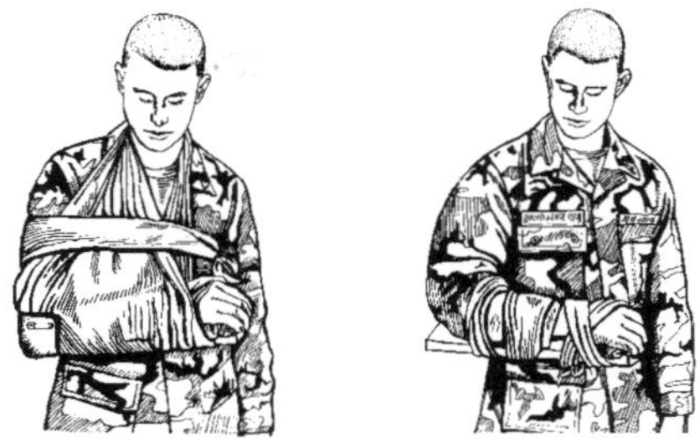

Figure 4-14. Board splint applied to fractured forearm.

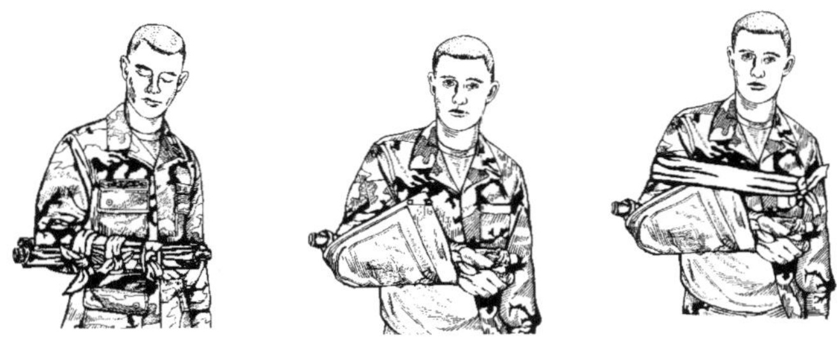

Figure 4-15. Fractured forearm or wrist splinted with sticks and supported with tail of shirt and strips of material.

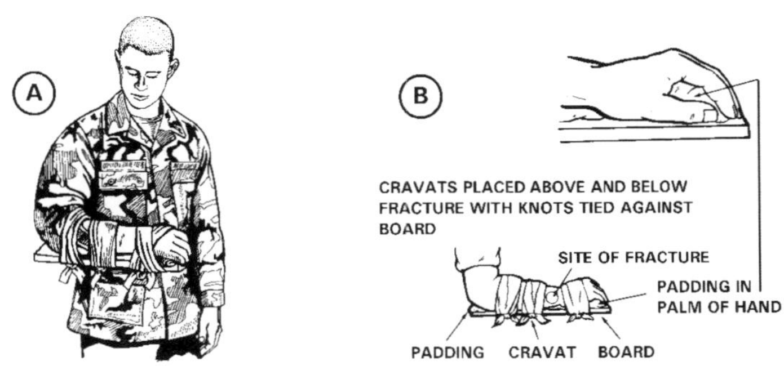

Figure 4-16. Board splint applied to fractured wrist and hand (Illustrated A—B).

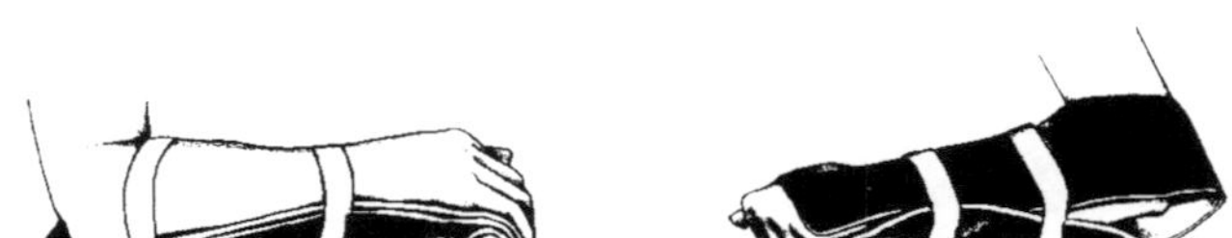

Figure 4-17. SAM® splint applied to fractured wrist or forearm.

4-8. Lower Extremity Fractures

Figures 4-18 through 4-24 show how to apply splints to immobilize fractures of the lower extremities. *Although padding is not visible in some of the illustrations, it is always preferable to apply padding along the injured part for the length of the splint and especially where it touches any bony parts of the body.*

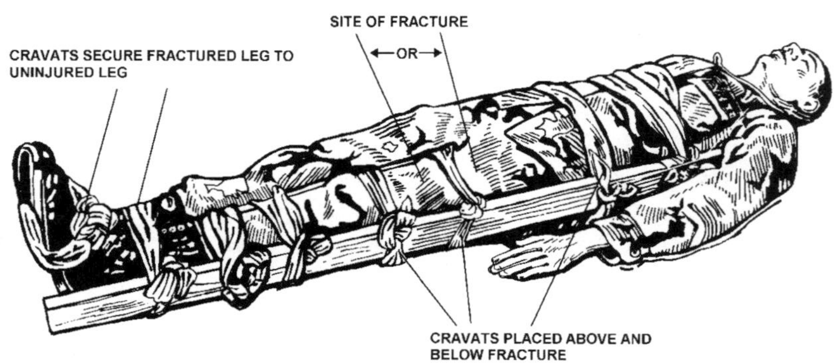

Figure 4-18. Board splints applied to fractured hip or thigh.

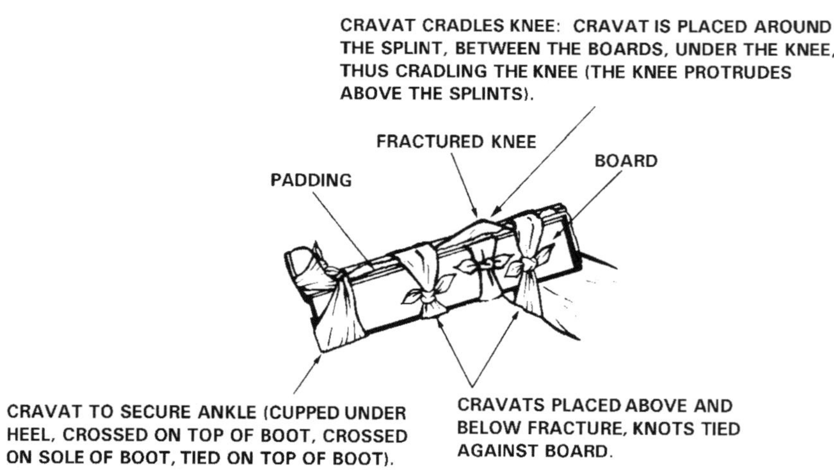

Figure 4-19. Board splint applied to fractured or dislocated knee.

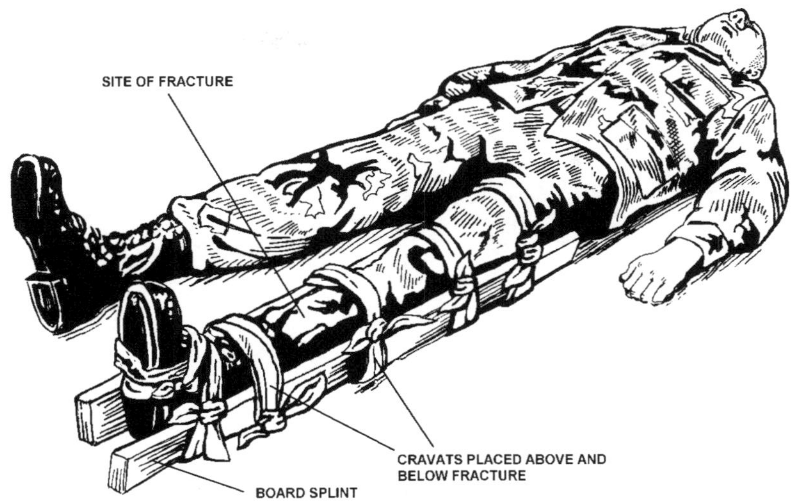

Figure 4-20. Board splints applied to fractured lower leg or ankle.

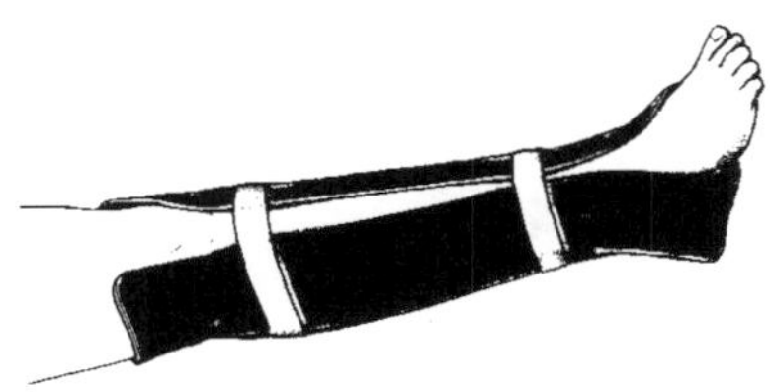

Figure 4-21. SAM® splint applied to fractured lower leg or ankle.

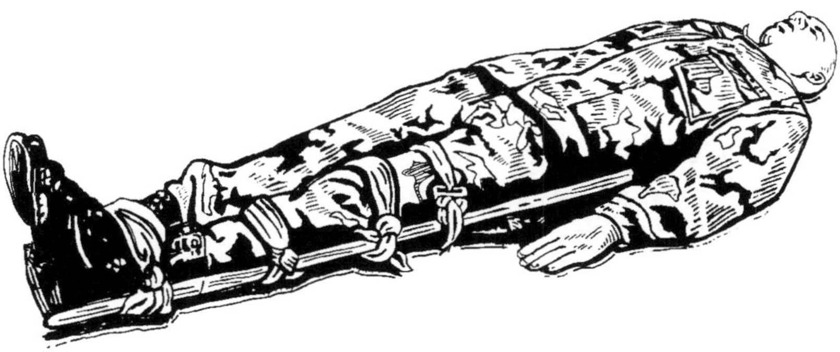

Figure 4-22. Improvised splints applied to fractured lower leg or ankle.

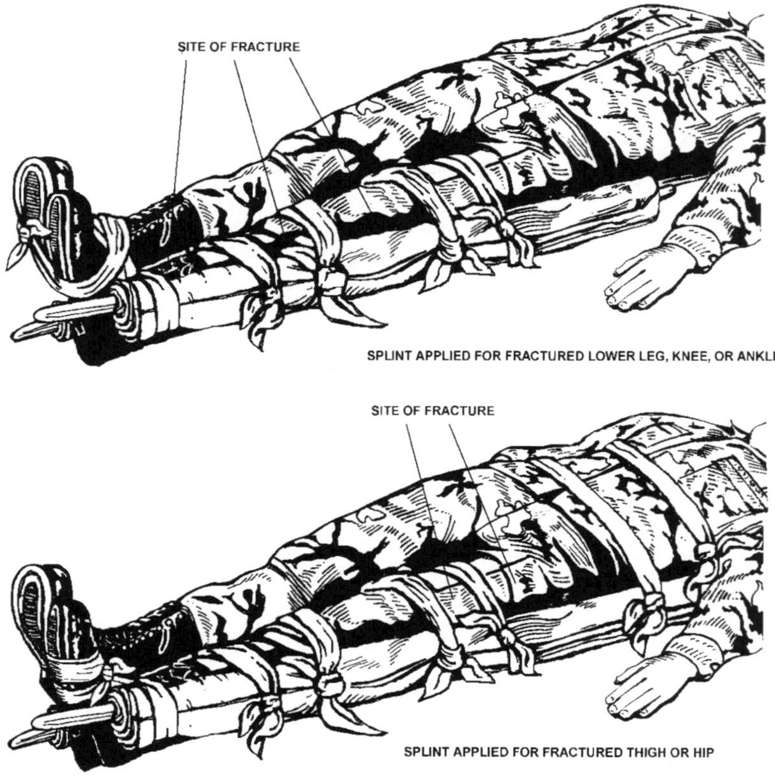

Figure 4-23. Poles rolled in a blanket and used as splints applied to fractured lower extremity.

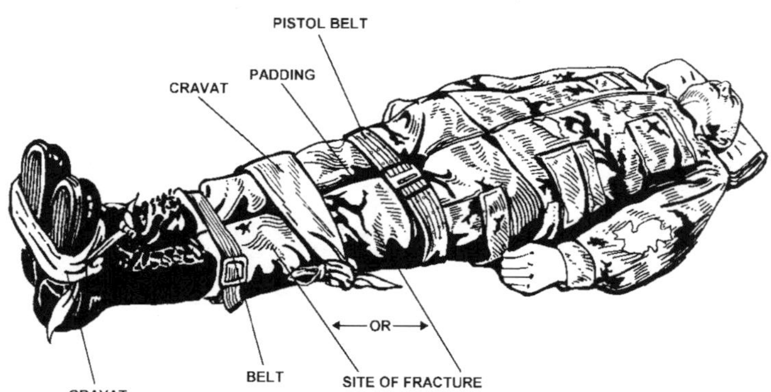

Figure 4-24. Uninjured leg used as splint for fractured leg (anatomical splint).

4-9. Jaw, Collarbone, and Shoulder Fractures

a. Apply a cravat to immobilize a fractured jaw as illustrated in Figure 4-25. Direct all bandaging support to the top of the casualty's head, not to the back of his neck. If incorrectly placed, the bandage will pull the casualty's jaw back and interfere with his breathing.

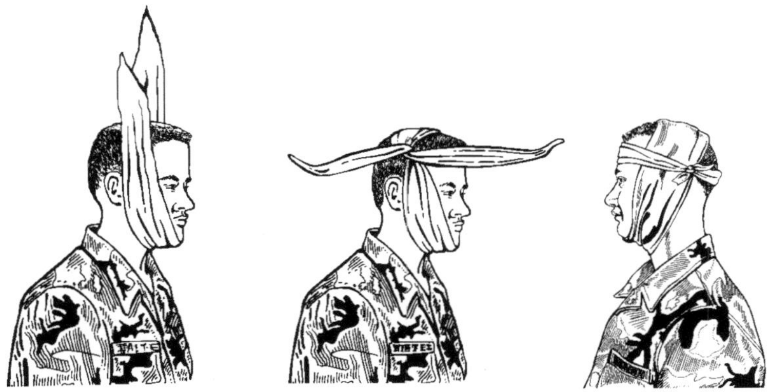

Figure 4-25. Fractured jaw immobilized.

> **WARNING**
>
> **Casualties with lower jaw (mandible) fractures cannot be laid flat on their backs because facial muscles will relax and may cause an airway obstruction.**

b. Apply two belts, a sling, and a cravat to immobilize a fractured collarbone, as illustrated in Figure 4-26.

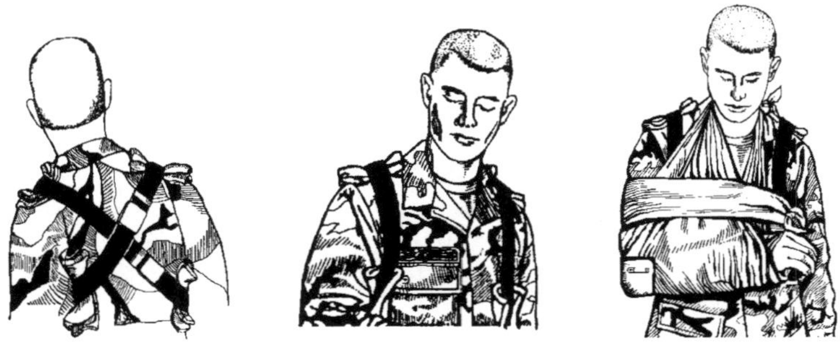

Figure 4-26. Application of belts, sling, and cravat to immobilize a fractured collarbone.

c. Apply a sling and a cravat to immobilize a fractured or dislocated shoulder, using the technique illustrated in Figure 4-27.

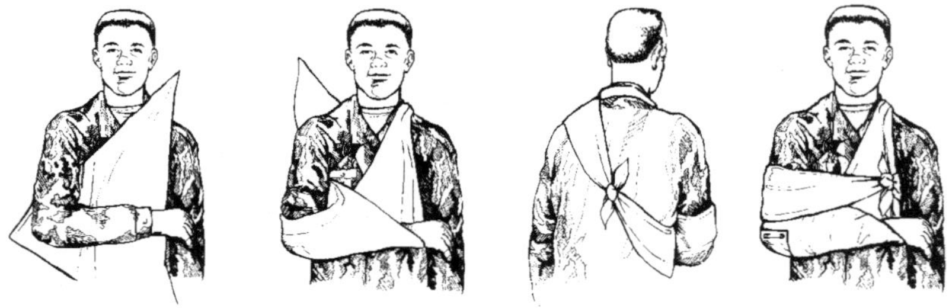

Figure 4-27. Application of sling and cravat to immobilize a fractured or dislocated shoulder.

4-10. Spinal Column Fractures

It is often impossible to be sure a casualty has a fractured spinal column. Be suspicious of any back injury, especially if the casualty has fallen or if his back has been sharply struck or bent. If a casualty has received such an injury and does not have feeling in his legs or cannot move them, you can be reasonably sure that he has a severe back injury, which should be managed as a fracture. Remember, that the possibility of a neck fracture or injury to the back should always be suspected, and it is often impossible to be sure if a casualty has a fractured spinal column. If the spine is fractured, bending it can cause the sharp bone fragments to bruise or cut the spinal cord and result in permanent paralysis or death (Figure 4-28A). The spinal column must maintain normal spinal position at the lower back (lumbar region) to help remove pressure from the spinal cord.

a. If the casualty is not to be transported until medical personnel arrive—

- Caution him not to move. Ask him if he is in pain or if he is unable to move any part of his body.

- Leave him in the position in which he is found. **DO NOT** move any part of his body, unless he is in imminent danger.

- If the casualty is lying face up, slip a blanket or other supporting material under the arch of his lower back to help support the spine in a normal position (Figure 4-28B). Take care not to place so much bulky padding as to cause potential damage by causing undo pressure on the spine. If he is lying face down, **DO NOT** put anything under any part of his body.

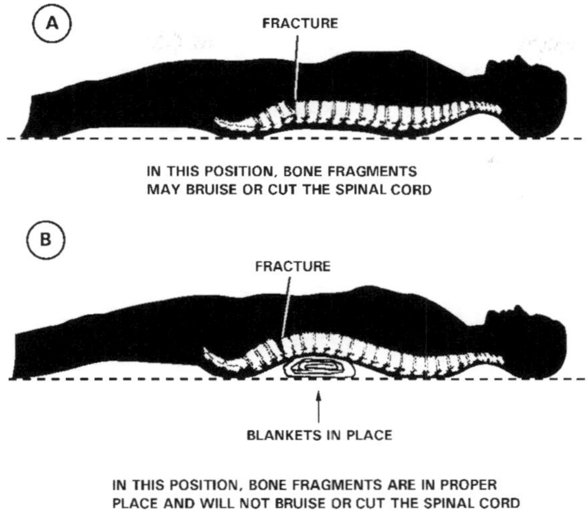

Figure 4-28. Spinal column must maintain a normal spine position.

b. If the casualty must be transported to a safe location before medical personnel arrive and if the casualty is in a—

- Face-up position, transport him by litter or use a firm substitute, such as a wide board or a door longer than his height. Loosely tie the casualty's wrists together over his waistline, using a cravat or a strip of cloth. Tie his feet together to prevent the accidental dropping or shifting of his legs. Lay a folded blanket across the litter where the arch of his back is to be placed. Using a four-man team (Figure 4-29), place the casualty on the litter without bending his spinal column or his neck.

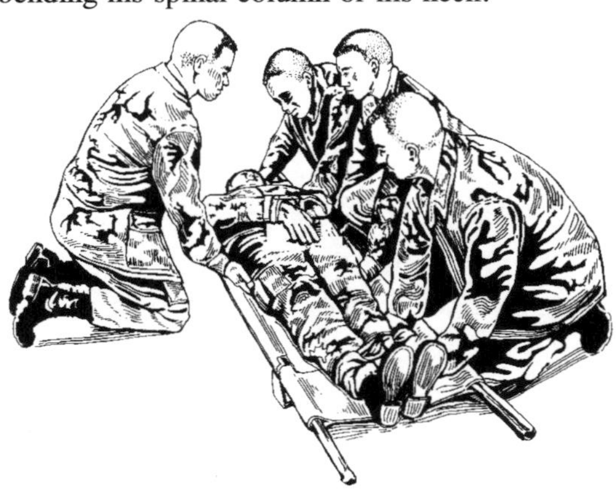

Figure 4-29. Placing face-up casualty with fractured back onto litter.

- The number two man positions himself at the casualty's head. His responsibility is to provide manual in-line (neutral) stabilization of the head and neck. The number three, and four men position themselves on one side of the casualty; all kneel on one knee along the side of the casualty. The number one man positions himself to the opposite side of the casualty (or can be on the same side of number three and four). The numbers two, three, and four men gently place their hands under the casualty. The number one man on the opposite side places his hands under the injured part to assist.

- When all four men are in position to lift, the number two man commands, "**PREPARE TO LIFT**" and then, "**LIFT**." All men, in unison, gently lift the casualty about 8 inches. Once the casualty is lifted, the number one man recovers and slides the litter under the casualty, ensuring that the blanket is in proper position. The number one man then returns to his original lift position (Figure 4-29).

- When the number two man commands, "**LOWER CASUALTY**," all men, in unison, gently lower the casualty onto the litter.

- Facedown position, he must be transported in this same position. The four-man team lifts him onto a regular or improvised litter, keeping the spinal column in a normal spinal position. If a regular litter is used, first place a folded blanket on the litter at the point where the chest will be placed.

4-11. Neck Fractures

A fractured neck is extremely dangerous. Bone fragments may bruise or cut the spinal cord just as they might in a fractured back.

a. If the casualty is not to be transported until medical personnel arrive—

- Caution him not to move. Moving may cause permanent injury or death.

- Leave the casualty in the position in which he is found. If his neck and head (cervical spine) are in an abnormal position, immediately immobilize the neck and head.

- Keep his head still, if the casualty is lying face up, raise his shoulders slightly, and slip a roll of cloth that has the bulk of a bath towel under his neck (Figure 4-31). The roll should be thick enough to arch his neck only slightly, leaving the back of his head on the ground. **DO NOT** bend his neck or head forward. **DO NOT** raise or twist his head. Immobilize the casualty's head (Figure 4-32). Do this by padding heavy objects (such as rocks or his boots filled with dirt, sand, gravel, or rock) and placing them on each side of his head. If it is necessary to use boots, after filling them, tie the top tightly or stuff with pieces of cloth to secure the contents.)

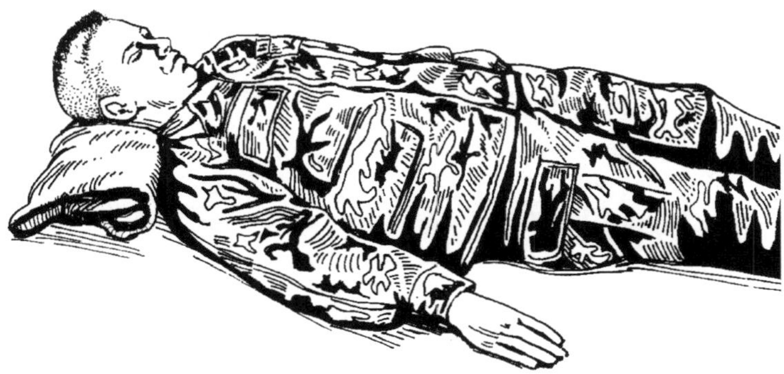

Figure 4-30. Casualty with roll of cloth (bulk) under neck.

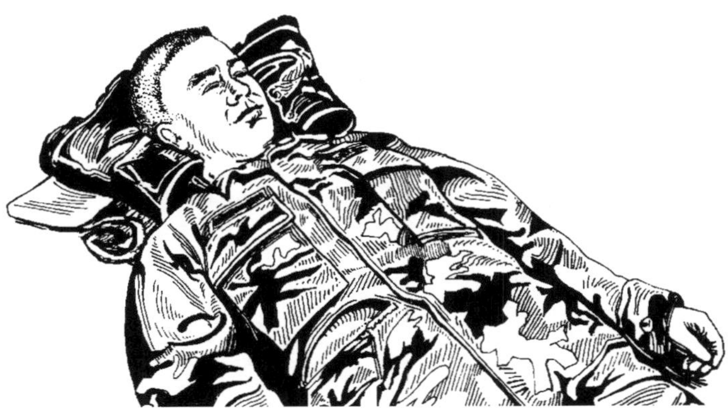

Figure 4-31. Immobilization of fractured neck.

- **DO NOT** move him if the casualty is lying face down. Immobilize the head and neck by padding heavy objects and placing them on each side of his head. DO NOT put a roll of cloth under the neck. **DO NOT** bend the neck or head, nor roll the casualty onto his back.

b. If the casualty must be prepared for transportation before medical personnel arrive—

- If the casualty has a fractured neck, at least two persons are needed because the casualty's head and trunk must be moved in unison. The two persons must work in close coordination (Figure 4-32) to avoid bending of the neck.

- A wide board is placed lengthwise beside the casualty. It should extend at least 4 inches beyond the casualty's head and feet (Figure 4-32A).

- If the casualty is lying face up, the number one man steadies the casualty's head and neck between his hands. At the same time, the number two man positions one foot and one knee against the board to prevent it from slipping. He then grasps the casualty underneath his shoulder and hip and gently slides him onto the board (Figure 4-32B).

- If the casualty is lying face down, the number one man steadies the casualty's head and neck between his hands, while the number two man gently rolls the casualty over onto the board (Figure 4-32C).

- The number one man continues to steady the casualty's head and neck. The number two man simultaneously raises the casualty's shoulders slightly, places padding under his neck, and immobilizes the casualty's head (Figures 4-32D—E).

- Any improvised supports are secured in position with a cravat or strip of cloth extended across the casualty's forehead and under the board (Figure 4-32D).

- The board is lifted onto a litter or blanket in order to transport the casualty (Figure 4-32E).

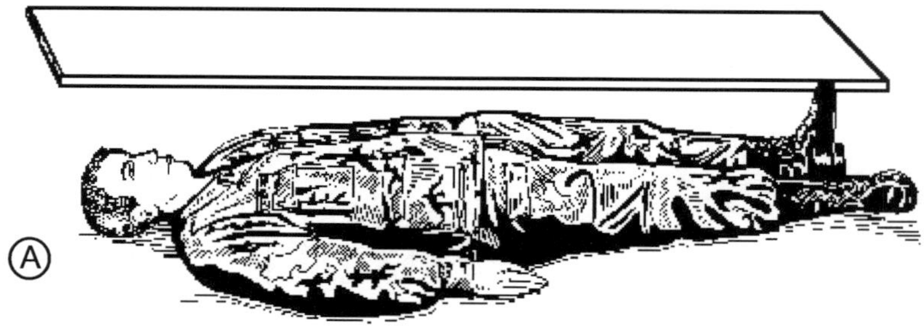

Figure 4-32. Preparing casualty with fractured neck for transportation (Illustrated A—E).

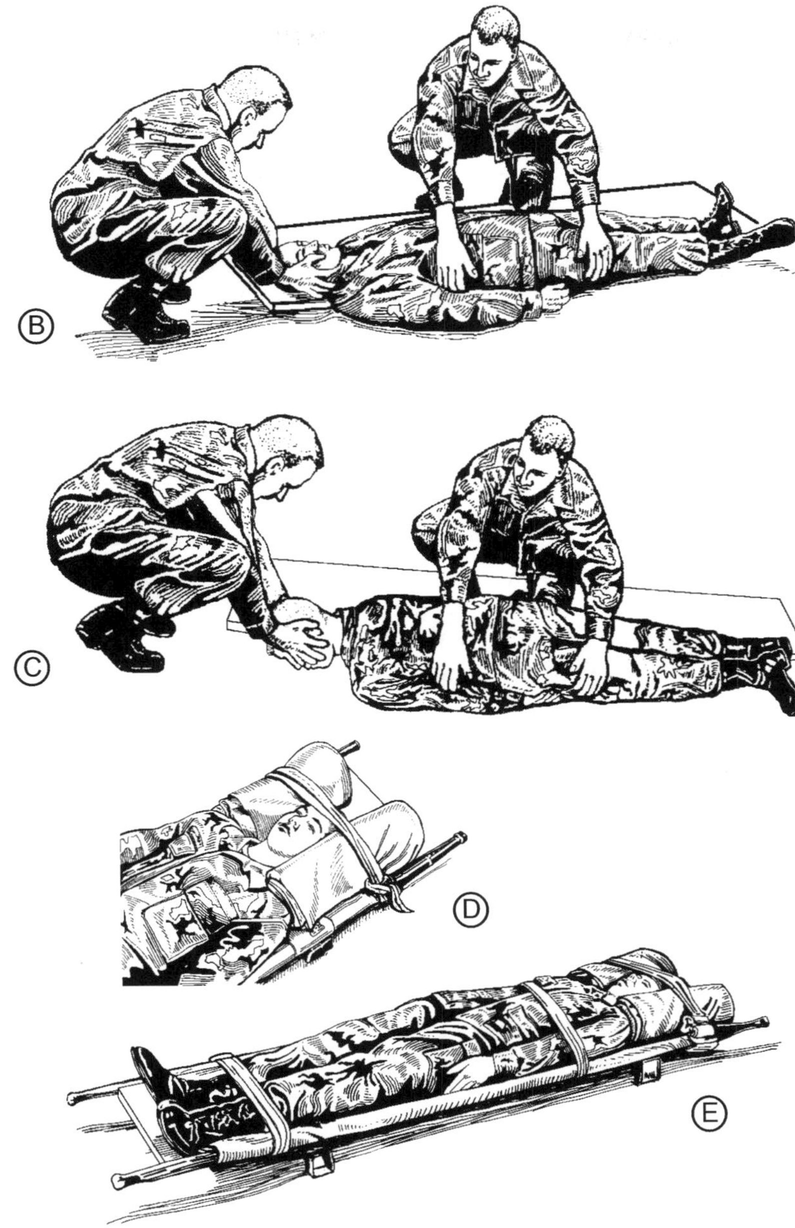

Figure 4-32. Preparing casualty with fractured neck for transportation (Illustrated A—E) (Continued).

CHAPTER 5

FIRST AID FOR CLIMATIC INJURIES

5-1. General

a. It is desirable, but not always possible, for an individual's body to become adjusted (acclimated) to an environment.

(1) The service members physical condition determines the amount of time their bodies need to adjust to the environment. Even those individuals in good physical condition need time before working or training in extremes of hot or cold weather. Climate-related injuries are usually preventable; prevention is both an individual and leadership responsibility.

(2) Several factors contribute to health and well-being in any environment—

- Diet.
- Sleep and rest.
- Exercise.
- Suitable clothing.

(3) Diet should be suited to an individual's needs in a particular climate. A special diet started for any purpose (such as weight reduction) should be done with appropriate medical supervision.

WARNING

Service members should use extreme caution when starting fad diets or taking over-the-counter herbal supplements. Medical records revealed that deaths and severe injuries occurred in individuals using dietary/ herbal supplements without medical monitoring.

NOTE

Weight loss and the use of weight loss supplements should be supervised by a trained health care provider.

(4) Specialized clothing and equipment (such as cold weather gear) for a specific environment should be obtained and used properly.

b. For information on the prevention of heat and cold injuries, refer to FM 21-10/Marine Corps Reference Publication (MCRP) 4-11.1D.

5-2. Heat Injuries

a. Heat injuries are environmental injuries. They may result when a service member—

- Is exposed to extreme heat, such as from the sun or from high temperatures.
- Does not wear proper clothing.
- Is in MOPP gear.
- Is inside closed spaces, such as inside an armored vehicle.
- Wears body armor.

b. Heat injury can be divided into three categories: heat cramps, heat exhaustion, and heatstroke.

c. Each service member must be able to recognize and give first aid for heat injuries.

WARNING

The heat casualty should be continually monitored for development of conditions which may require the performance of necessary basic lifesaving measures.

CAUTION

Do not use salt solutions in first aid procedures for heat injuries.

(1) Check the casualty for signs and symptoms of *cramping*.

- *Signs and symptoms.* Cramping is caused by an imbalance of chemicals (called electrolytes) in the body as a result of excessive sweating. This condition causes the casualty to exhibit:

- Cramping in the extremities (arms and legs).
- Abdominal (stomach) cramps.
- Excessive sweating.

NOTE

Thirst may or may not occur. Cramping can occur without the service member being thirsty.

- *First aid measures.*

  - Move the casualty to a cool, shady area or improvise shade if none is available.

  - Loosen his clothing (if not in a chemical environment).

NOTE

In a chemical environment, transport the heat casualty to a noncontaminated area as soon as the mission permits.

  - Have him slowly drink at least one canteen full of water. (The body absorbs cool water faster than warm or cold water; therefore, cool water is preferred if it is available.)

  - Seek medical assistance should cramps continue.

(2) Check the casualty for signs and symptoms of *heat exhaustion*.

- *Signs and symptoms.* Heat exhaustion is caused by loss of body fluids (dehydration) through sweating without adequate fluid replacement. It can occur in an otherwise fit individual who is involved in physical exertion in any hot environment especially if the service member is not acclimatized to that environment. These signs and symptoms are—

  - Excessive sweating with pale, moist, cool skin.
  - Headache.
  - Weakness.

- Dizziness.
- Loss of appetite.
- Cramping.
- Nausea (with or without vomiting).
- Urge to defecate.
- Chills (gooseflesh).
- Rapid breathing.
- Tingling of hands and/or feet.
- Confusion.

- *First aid measures.*

- Move the casualty to a cool, shady area or improvise shade if none is available.

- Loosen or remove his clothing and boots (unless in a chemical environment); pour water on him and fan him.

- Have him slowly drink at least one canteen of water.

- Elevate his legs.

- If possible, the casualty should not participate in strenuous activity for the remainder of the day.

- Monitor the casualty until the symptoms are gone, or medical assistance arrives.

(3) Check the casualty for signs and symptoms of *heatstroke*.

WARNING

Heatstroke is a medical emergency which may result in death if care is delayed.

- *Signs and symptoms.* A service member suffering from heatstroke has been exposed to high temperatures (such as direct sunlight) or been dressed in protective overgarments, which causes the body temperature to rise. Heatstroke occurs more rapidly in service members who are engaged in work or other physical activity in a high heat environment. Heatstroke is caused by a failure of the body's cooling mechanism which includes a decrease in the body's ability to produce sweat. The casualty's skin is red (flushed), hot, and dry. He may experience weakness, dizziness, confusion, headaches, seizures, nausea, stomach pains or cramps, and his respiration and pulse may be rapid and weak. Unconsciousness and collapse may occur suddenly.

- *First aid measures.* Cool casualty immediately by—

  - Moving him to a cool, shady area or improvising shade if none is available.

  - Loosening or removing his clothing (except in a chemical environment).

  - Spraying or pouring water on him; fanning him to permit the coolant effect of evaporation.

  - Massaging his extremities and skin, which increases the blood flow to those body areas, thus aiding the cooling process.

  - Elevating his legs.

  - Having him slowly drink at least one canteen full of water if he is conscious.

NOTE

Start cooling casualty immediately. Continue cooling while awaiting transportation and during transport to an MTF.

- *Medical assistance.* Seek medical assistance because the casualty should be transported to an MTF as soon as possible. Do not interrupt the cooling process or lifesaving measures to seek help; if someone else is present send them for help. The casualty should be continually monitored for development of conditions that may require the performance of necessary basic lifesaving measures.

d. *Table.* See Table 5-1 for further information.

Table 5-1. Heat Injuries

INJURIES	SIGNS AND SYMPTOMS	FIRST AID[1]
HEAT CRAMPS	THE CASUALTY EXPERIENCES MUSCLE CRAMPS OF THE ARMS, LEGS, AND/OR STOMACH. THE CASUALTY MAY ALSO HAVE EXCESSIVE SWEATING.	1. MOVE THE CASUALTY TO A COOL SHADY AREA OR IMPROVISE SHADE AND LOOSEN CLOTHING.[2] 2. HAVE HIM SLOWLY DRINK AT LEAST ONE CANTEEN FULL OF COOL WATER SLOWLY. 3. MONITOR THE CASUALTY AND GIVE HIM MORE WATER AS TOLERATED.
HEAT EXHAUSTION	THE CASUALTY EXPERIENCES HEAVY SWEATING WITH PALE, MOIST, COOL SKIN; HEADACHE, WEAKNESS, DIZZINESS, AND/OR LOSS OF APPETITE, HEAT CRAMPS, NAUSEA (WITH OR WITHOUT VOMITING), URGE TO DEFECATE, CHILLS (GOOSE-FLESH), RAPID BREATHING, CONFUSION, AND TINGLING OF THE HANDS AND/OR FEET.	1. MOVE THE CASUALTY TO A COOL, SHADY AREA OR IMPROVISE SHADE AND LOOSEN OR REMOVE HIS CLOTHING.[2] 2. POUR WATER ON HIM AND FAN HIM TO PERMIT THE COOLANT EFFECT OF EVAPORATION. 3. HAVE HIM SLOWLY DRINK AT LEAST ONE CANTEEN FULL OF COOL WATER. 4. ELEVATE THE CASUALTY'S LEGS. 5. SEEK MEDICAL ASSISTANCE IF SYMPTOMS CONTINUE; MONITOR UNTIL SYMPTOMS ARE GONE OR MEDICAL ASSISTANCE ARRIVES.
HEATSTROKE[3] (SUNSTROKE)	THE CASUALTY STOPS SWEATING (RED [FLUSHED] HOT, DRY SKIN). HE FIRST MAY EXPERIENCE HEADACHE, DIZZINESS, NAUSEA, FAST PULSE AND RESPIRATION, SEIZURES, AND MENTAL CONFUSION. HE MAY COLLAPSE	1. MOVE THE CASUALTY TO A COOL, SHADY AREA OR IMPROVISE SHADE AND LOOSEN OR REMOVE HIS CLOTHING, REMOVE THE OUTER GARMENTS AND PROTECTIVE

Table 5-1. Heat Injuries (Continued)

INJURIES	SIGNS AND SYMPTOMS	FIRST AID[1]
	AND SUDDENLY BECOME UNCONSCIOUS. **THIS IS A MEDICAL EMERGENCY.**	CLOTHING IF THE SITUATION PERMITS.[2] 2. START COOLING THE CASUALTY IMMEDIATELY. SPRAY OR POUR WATER ON HIM. FAN HIM. MASSAGE HIS EXTREMITIES AND SKIN. 3. ELEVATE HIS LEGS. 4. IF CONSCIOUS, HAVE HIM SLOWLY DRINK AT LEAST ONE CANTEEN FULL OF COOL WATER. 5. SEEK MEDICAL AID. CONTINUE COOLING WHILE AWAITING TRANSPORT AND CONTINUE FIRST AID WHILE EN ROUTE.

LEGEND:

1 THE FIRST AID PROCEDURE FOR HEAT RELATED INJURIES CAUSED BY WEARING INDIVIDUAL PROTECTIVE EQUIPMENT (IPE) IS TO MOVE THE CASUALTY TO A CLEAN AREA AND GIVE HIM WATER TO DRINK.
2 WHEN IN A CHEMICAL ENVIRONMENT, DO NOT LOOSEN OR REMOVE THE CASUALTY'S CLOTHING.
3 CAN BE FATAL IF NOT PROVIDED FIRST AID AND MEDICAL TREATMENT PROMPTLY.

5-3. Cold Injuries

Cold injuries are most likely to occur when conditions are moderately cold, but accompanied by wet or windy conditions. Cold injuries can usually be prevented. Well-disciplined and well-trained service members can be protected even in the most adverse circumstances. They and their leaders must know the hazards of exposure to the cold. They must know the importance of personal hygiene, exercise, care of the feet and hands, and the use of protective clothing.

a. Contributing Factors.

(1) Temperature, humidity, precipitation, and wind greatly increase likelihood of cold injuries, and the service members with wet clothing are at great risk of cold injuries. Riverine operations (river, swamp, and stream crossings) increase likelihood of cold injuries. Low temperatures and low relative humidity (dry cold) promote frostbite. Higher temperatures, together with moisture, promote immersion syndrome. Windchill accelerates the loss of body heat and may aggravate cold injuries.

(2) Relatively stationary activities such as being in an observation post or on guard duty increase the service member's vulnerability to cold injury. Also, a service member is more likely to receive a cold injury if he is—

- In contact with the ground (such as marching, performing guard duty, or engaging in other outside activities).
- Immobile for long periods (such as while riding in an unheated or open vehicle).
- Standing in water, such as in a foxhole.
- Out in the cold for days without being warmed.
- Deprived of an adequate diet and rest.
- Not able to take care of his personal hygiene.

(3) Physical fatigue contributes to apathy, which leads to inactivity, personal neglect, carelessness, and reduced heat production. In turn, these increase the risk of cold injury. Service members with prior cold injuries have a higher-than-normal risk of subsequent cold injury; not necessarily involving the body part previously injured.

(4) Depressed or unresponsive service members are also vulnerable because they are less active. These service members tend to be careless about precautionary measures, especially warming activities, when cold injury is a threat.

(5) Excessive use of alcohol or drugs leading to faulty judgment or unconsciousness in a cold environment increases the risk of becoming a cold injury casualty.

b. *Signs and Symptoms*. Once a service member becomes familiar with the factors that contribute to cold injury, he must learn to recognize cold injury signs and symptoms.

(1) Many service members suffer cold injury without realizing what is happening to them. They may be cold and generally uncomfortable. These service members often do not notice the injured part because it is already numb from the cold.

(2) Superficial cold injury usually can be detected by numbness or tingling sensations. These signs and symptoms often can be relieved simply by loosening boots or other clothing and by exercising to improve circulation. In more advanced cases involving deep cold injury, the service member often is not aware that there is a problem until the affected part feels like a stump or block of wood.

(3) Outward signs of cold injury include discoloration of the skin at the site of injury. In light-skinned persons, the skin first reddens and then becomes pale or waxy white. In dark-skinned persons, grayness in the skin is usually evident. An injured foot or hand feels cold to the touch. Swelling may be an indication of deep injury. Also note that blisters may occur after rewarming the affected parts. Service members should work in pairs (buddy teams) to check each other for signs of discoloration and other symptoms.

c. First Aid Measures. First aid for cold injuries depends on whether they are superficial or deep. Rewarming the affected part using body heat can adequately treat cases of superficial cold injury. (For example, this can be done by covering cheeks with hands, putting fingertips in armpits, or placing the casualty's feet under the clothing of a buddy [next to his belly].) The injured part should **NOT** be massaged, exposed to a fire or stove, rubbed with snow, slapped, chafed, or soaked in cold water. Walking on injured feet should be avoided. Deep cold injury (frostbite) is very serious and requires prompt first aid to avoid or to minimize the loss of parts or all of the fingers, toes, hands, or feet. The sequence for treating cold injuries depends on whether the condition is life-threatening. The first priority in managing cold injuries is to remove the casualty from the cold environment (such as building an improvised shelter). Other injuries the casualty may have are provided first aid simultaneously while waiting for transportation or evacuation. If the casualty is to be transported in a nonmedical vehicle, first aid measures should be continued en route to the MTF.

d. Conditions Caused by Cold. Conditions caused by cold include chilblain, immersion syndrome (immersion foot and trench foot), frostbite, snow blindness, dehydration, and hypothermia.

(1) *Chilblain.*

- *Signs and symptoms.* Chilblain is caused by repeated prolonged exposure of bare skin at temperatures from 60° Fahrenheit (F) to

32°F, or 20°F for acclimated, dry, unwashed skin. The area may be acutely swollen, red, tender, and hot with itchy skin. There may be no loss of skin tissue in untreated cases but continued exposure may lead to infected, ulcerated, or bleeding lesions.

- *First aid measures*. Within minutes, the area usually responds to locally applied body heat. Rewarm the affected part by applying firm steady pressure with your hands, or placing the affected part under your arms or against the stomach of a buddy. **DO NOT** rub or massage affected areas.

NOTE

Medical personnel should evaluate the injury, because signs and symptoms of tissue damage may be slow to appear.

(2) *Immersion syndrome (immersion foot and trench foot)*. Immersion foot and trench foot are injuries that result from fairly long exposure of the feet to wet conditions at temperatures from approximately 32°F to 50°F. Inactive feet in damp or wet socks and boots, or tightly laced boots which impair circulation, are even more susceptible to injury. This injury can be very serious; it can lead to loss of toes or parts of the feet. If exposure of the feet has been prolonged and severe, the feet may swell so much that pressure closes the blood vessels and cuts off circulation. Should an immersion injury occur, dry the feet thoroughly and transport the casualty to an MTF by the fastest means possible.

- *Signs and symptoms*. At first, the parts of the affected foot are cold and painless, the pulse is weak, and numbness may be present. Second, the parts may feel hot, and burning and shooting pains may begin. In later stages, the skin is pale with a bluish cast and the pulse decreases. Other signs and symptoms that may follow are blistering, swelling, redness, heat, hemorrhaging (bleeding), and gangrene.

- *First aid measures*. First aid measures are required for all stages of immersion syndrome injury. Rewarm the injured part gradually by exposing it to warm air. Protect it from trauma and secondary infections. Dry, loose clothing or several layers of warm coverings are preferable to extreme heat. Under no circumstances should the injured part be exposed to an open fire. Elevate the injured part to relieve the swelling. Transport the casualty to an MTF as soon as possible. When the part is rewarmed, the casualty often feels a burning sensation and pain. Symptoms may persist for days or weeks even after rewarming.

NOTE

When providing first aid for immersion foot and trench foot— **DO NOT** massage the injured part. **DO NOT** moisten the skin. **DO NOT** apply heat or ice.

(3) *Frostbite*. Frostbite is the injury of tissue caused from exposure to cold, usually below 32°F depending on the windchill factor, duration of exposure, and adequacy of protection. Individuals with a history of cold injury are likely to suffer an additional cold injury. The body parts most easily frostbitten are the cheeks, nose, ears, chin, forehead, wrists, hands, and feet. Frostbite may involve only the skin (superficial), or it may extend to a depth below the skin (deep). Deep frostbite is very serious and requires prompt first aid to avoid or to minimize the loss of parts or all of the fingers, toes, hands, or feet.

- *Signs and symptoms*.
    - Loss of sensation (numb feeling) in any part of the body.
    - Sudden blanching (whitening) of the skin of the affected part, followed by a momentary tingling sensation.
    - Redness of skin in light-skinned service members; grayish coloring in dark-skinned service members.
    - Blisters.
    - Swelling or tender areas.
    - Loss of previous sensation of pain in affected area.
    - Pale, yellowish, waxy-looking skin.
    - Frozen tissue that feels solid (or wooden) to the touch.

CAUTION

Deep frostbite is a very serious injury and requires immediate first aid and subsequent medical treatment to avoid or minimize loss of body parts.

- *First aid measures.*

  - *Face, ears, and nose.* Cover the casualty's affected area with his and/or your bare hands until sensation and color return.

  - *Hands.* Open the casualty's field jacket and shirt. (In a chemical environment, do not loosen or remove the clothing and protective overgarments.) Place the affected hands under the casualty's armpits. Close the field jacket and shirt to prevent additional exposure.

  - *Feet.* Remove the casualty's boots and socks if he does not need to walk any further to receive additional treatment. (Thawing the casualty's feet and forcing him to walk on them will cause additional pain and injury.) Place the affected feet under clothing and against the body of another service member.

WARNING

DO NOT attempt to thaw the casualty's feet or other frozen areas if he will be required to walk or travel to an MTF for additional medical treatment. The possibility of additional injury from walking is less when the feet are frozen than when they are thawed. (However, if possible avoid walking.) Thawing in the field increases the possibilities of infection, gangrene, or other injury.

NOTE

Thawing may occur spontaneously during transportation to the MTF; this cannot be avoided since the body in general must be kept warm.

In all of the above areas, ensure that the casualty is kept warm and that he is covered (to avoid further injury). Seek medical treatment as soon as possible. Reassure the casualty, protect the affected area from further injury by covering it lightly with a blanket or any dry clothing, and seek shelter out of the wind. Remove or loosen constricting clothing (except in a contaminated environment) and increase insulation. Ensure the casualty exercises as much as possible, avoiding trauma to the injured part, and is prepared for pain when thawing occurs. Protect the frostbitten part from additional injury. **DO NOT—**

- Rub the injured part with snow or apply cold water soaks.

- Warm the part by massage or exposure to open fire because the frozen part may be burned due to the lack of feeling.

- Use ointments or other salves.

- Manipulate the part in any way to increase circulation.

- Use alcohol or tobacco because this reduces the body's resistance to cold.

NOTE

Remember, when freezing extends to a depth below the skin, it is a much more serious injury. Extra care is required to reduce or avoid the chances of losing all or part of the toes or feet. This also applies to the fingers and hands.

(4) *Snow blindness.* Snow blindness is the effect that glare from an ice field or snowfield has on the eyes. It is more likely to occur in hazy, cloudy weather than when the sun is shining. Glare from the sun will cause an individual to instinctively protect his eyes. However, in cloudy weather, he may be overconfident and expose his eyes longer than when the threat is more obvious. He may also neglect precautions such as the use of protective eyewear. Waiting until discomfort (pain) is felt before using protective eyewear is dangerous because a deep burn of the eyes may already have occurred.

- *Signs and symptoms.* Symptoms of snow blindness are a sensation of grit in the eyes with pain in and over the eyes, made worse by moving the eyeball. Other signs and symptoms are watering, redness, headache, and increased pain on exposure to light.

- *First aid measures.* First aid measures consist of blindfolding or covering the eyes with a dark cloth which stops painful eye movement. Complete rest is desirable. If further exposure to light is not preventable, the eyes should be protected with dark bandages or the darkest glasses available. Once unprotected exposure to sunlight stops, the condition usually heals in a few days without permanent damage. The casualty should be evacuated to the nearest MTF.

(5) *Dehydration.* Dehydration occurs when the body loses too much fluid. A certain amount of body fluid is lost through normal body processes. A normal daily intake of liquids replaces these losses. When individuals are engaged in any strenuous exercises or activities, fluid is lost

through sweating and this loss creates an imbalance of fluids in the body, and if not matched by rehydration it can contribute to dehydration. The danger of dehydration is as prevalent in cold regions as it is in hot regions. In hot weather, the individual is aware of his body losing fluids through sweat. In cold weather, however, it is extremely difficult to realize that this condition exists since sweating is not as apparent as in a hot environment. The danger of dehydration in cold weather operations is a serious problem. In cold climates, sweat evaporates so rapidly or is absorbed so thoroughly by layers of heavy clothing that it is rarely visible on the skin. Dehydration also occurs during cold weather operations because drinking is inconvenient. Dehydration will weaken or incapacitate a casualty for a few hours, or sometimes, several days. Because rest is an important part of the recovery process, casualties must take care that limited movement during their recuperative period does not enhance the risk of becoming a cold injury casualty.

- *Signs and symptoms*. The symptoms of cold weather dehydration are similar to those encountered in heat exhaustion. The mouth, tongue, and throat become parched and dry, and swallowing becomes difficult. The casualty may have nausea (with or without vomiting) along with extreme dizziness and fainting. The casualty may also feel generally tired and weak and may experience muscle cramps. Focusing the eyes may also become difficult.

- *First aid measures*. The casualty should be kept warm and his clothes should be loosened (if not in a chemical environment) to allow proper circulation. Shelter from wind and cold must be provided. Fluid replacement should begin immediately and the service member transported to an MTF as soon as possible.

(6) *Hypothermia (general cooling)*. When exposed to prolonged cold weather a service member may become both mentally and physically numb, thus neglecting essential tasks or requiring more time and effort to achieve them. Under some conditions (particularly cold water immersion), even a service member in excellent physical condition may die in a matter of minutes. The destructive influence of cold on the body is called *hypothermia*. This means bodies lose heat faster than they can produce it. Hypothermia can occur from exposure to temperatures either above or below freezing, especially from immersion in cold water, wet-cold conditions, or from the effect of wind. Physical exhaustion and insufficient food intake may also increase the risk of hypothermia. General cooling of the entire body to a temperature below 95°F is caused by continued exposure to low or rapidly dropping temperatures, cold moisture, snow, or ice. Fatigue, poor physical condition, dehydration, faulty blood circulation, alcohol or other drug use, trauma, and immersion can cause hypothermia. Remember, cold

may affect the body systems slowly and almost without notice. Service members exposed to low temperatures for extended periods may suffer ill effects even if they are well protected by clothing.

- *Signs and symptoms*. As the body cools, there are several stages of progressive discomfort and impairment. A sign that is noticed immediately is shivering. Shivering is an attempt by the body to generate heat. The pulse is faint or very difficult to detect. People with temperatures around 90°F may be drowsy and mentally slow. Their ability to move may be hampered, stiff, and uncoordinated, but they may be able to function minimally. Their speech may be slurred. As the body temperature drops further, shock becomes evident as the person's eyes assume a glassy state, breathing becomes slow and shallow, and the pulse becomes weaker or absent. The person becomes very stiff and uncoordinated. Unconsciousness may follow quickly. As the body temperature drops even lower, the extremities freeze, and a deep (or core) body temperature (below 85°F) increases the risk of irregular heart action. This irregular heart action or heart standstill can result in sudden death.

- *First aid measures*. Except in cases of the most severe hypothermia (marked by coma or unconsciousness and a weak pulse), first aid measures for hypothermia are directed towards protecting the casualty from further loss of body heat. For the casualty who is conscious, first aid measures are directed at rewarming the body evenly and without delay. Provide heat by using a hot water bottle or field expedient or another service member's body heat.

CAUTION

DO NOT expose the casualty to an open fire, as he may become burned.

NOTE

When using a hot water bottle or field expedient (canteen filled with warm water), the bottle or canteen must be wrapped in cloth prior to placing it next to the casualty. This will reduce the chance of burning the casualty's skin.

Always call or send for help as soon as possible and protect the casualty immediately with dry clothing or a sleeping bag. Then, move him to a warm place. Evaluate other injuries and provide first aid as required. First aid measures can be performed while the casualty is waiting transportation or while he is en route. In the case of an accidental breakthrough into ice water, or other hypothermic accident, strip the casualty of wet clothing immediately and bundle him into a sleeping bag. Rescue breathing should be started at once if the casualty's breathing has stopped or is irregular or shallow. Warm liquids (**NOT HOT**) may be given gradually if the casualty is conscious. **DO NOT** force liquids on an unconscious or semiconscious casualty because he may choke. The casualty should be transported on a litter because the exertion of walking may aggravate circulation problems. Medical personnel should immediately treat any hypothermia casualty. Hypothermia is life threatening until normal body temperature has been restored. The first aid measures for a casualty with severe hypothermia are based upon the following principles: attempt to avoid further heat loss, handle the casualty gently, and transport the casualty as soon as possible to the nearest MTF. If at all possible, the casualty should be evacuated by medical personnel.

WARNING

Rewarming a severely hypothermic casualty is extremely dangerous in the field due to the possibility of such complications as rewarming, shock and disturbances in the rhythm of the heartbeat. These conditions require treatment by medical personnel.

NOTE

Resuscitation of casualties with hypothermic complications is difficult if not impossible to do outside of an MTF setting.

CAUTION

The casualty is unable to generate his own body heat. Therefore, merely placing him in a blanket or sleeping bag is not sufficient.

e. *Table.* See Table 5-2 for further information.

Table 5-2. Injuries Caused by Cold and Wet Conditions

INJURIES	SIGNS/SYMPTOMS	FIRST AID
CHILBLAIN	RED SWOLLEN, HOT, TENDER, ITCHING SKIN. CONTINUED EXPOSURE MAY LEAD TO INFECTED (ULCERATED OR BLEEDING) SKIN LESIONS.	1. AREA USUALLY RESPONDS TO LOCALLY APPLIED REWARMING (BODY HEAT). 2. DO NOT RUB OR MASSAGE AREA. 3. SEEK MEDICAL AID.
IMMERSION SYNDROME (IMMERSION FOOT/TRENCH FOOT)	AFFECTED PARTS ARE COLD, NUMB, AND PAINLESS. PARTS MAY THEN BE HOT, WITH BURNING AND SHOOTING PAINS. ADVANCED STAGE: SKIN PALE WITH BLUISH CAST; PULSE DECREASES; BLISTERING, SWELLING, HEAT, HEMORRHAGING, AND GANGRENE MAY FOLLOW.	1. GRADUAL REWARMING BY EXPOSURE TO WARM AIR. 2. DO NOT MASSAGE OR MOISTEN SKIN. 3. PROTECT AFFECTED PARTS FROM TRAUMA. 4. DRY FEET THOROUGHLY, AVOID WALKING. 5. SEEK MEDICAL AID.
FROSTBITE	LOSS OF SENSATION (NUMB FEELING) IN ANY PART OF THE BODY. SUDDEN BLANCHING (WHITENING) OF THE SKIN OF THE AFFECTED PART, FOLLOWED BY A MOMENTARY TINGLING SENSATION. REDNESS OF SKIN IN LIGHT-SKINNED SERVICE MEMBERS; GRAYISH COLORING IN DARK-SKINNED SERVICE MEMBERS. BLISTERS. SWELLING OR TENDER AREAS. LOSS OF PREVIOUS SENSATION OF PAIN IN THE AFFECTED AREA. PALE YELLOWISH, WAXY-LOOKING SKIN. FROZEN TISSUE THAT FEELS SOLID (WOODEN) TO THE TOUCH.	1. WARM THE AREA AT THE FIRST SIGN OF FROSTBITE, USING FIRM, STEADY PRESSURE OF THE HAND, UNDERARM, OR ABDOMEN. 2. FACE, EARS, NOSE: COVER AREA WITH HANDS (CASUALTY'S OWN OR BUDDY'S). 3. HANDS: OPEN FIELD JACKET AND PLACE CASUALTY'S HANDS AGAINST HIS BODY, THEN CLOSE THE JACKET TO PREVENT HEAT LOSS. 4. FEET: REMOVE THE CASUALTY'S BOOTS AND SOCKS AND PLACE HIS FEET AGAINST THE BODY OF ANOTHER SERVICE MEMBER.

Table 5-2. Injuries Caused by Cold and Wet Conditions (Continued)

INJURIES	SIGNS/SYMPTOMS	FIRST AID
		5. WARNING: DO NOT ATTEMPT TO THAW THE CASUALTY'S FEET OR OTHER FROZEN AREAS IF HE WILL BE REQUIRED TO WALK OR TRAVEL TO AN MTF FOR ADDITIONAL TREATMENT. THE POSSIBILITY OF INJURY FROM WALKING IS LESS WHEN THE FEET ARE FROZEN THAN WHEN THEY HAVE BEEN THAWED. (HOWEVER, IF POSSIBLE AVOID WALKING.) THAWING IN THE FIELD INCREASES THE POSSIBILITY OF INFECTION, GANGRENE, OR INJURY. 6. LOOSEN OR REMOVE CONSTRICTING CLOTHING AND REMOVE ANY JEWELRY. 7. INCREASE INSULATION (COVER WITH BLANKET OR OTHER DRY MATERIAL). ENSURE CASUALTY EXERCISES AS MUCH AS POSSIBLE, AVOIDING TRAUMA TO INJURED PART.
SNOW BLINDNESS	EYES MAY FEEL SCRATCHY. WATERING, REDNESS, HEADACHE, AND INCREASED PAIN WITH EXPOSURE TO LIGHT CAN OCCUR.	1. COVER THE EYES WITH A DARK CLOTH. 2. SEEK MEDICAL AID.
DEHYDRATION	SIMILAR TO HEAT EXHAUSTION (REFER TO TABLE 5-1).	1. KEEP WARM. 2. CASUALTY NEEDS FLUID REPLACEMENT, REST, AND PROMPT MEDICAL AID.
HYPOTHERMIA	CASUALTY IS COLD. SHIVERING. CORE TEMPERATURE IS LOW. CONSCIOUSNESS MAY BE	**MILD HYPOTHERMIA** 1. REWARM BODY

Table 5-2. Injuries Caused by Cold and Wet Conditions (Continued)

INJURIES	SIGNS/SYMPTOMS	FIRST AID
	ALTERED. UNCOORDINATED MOVEMENTS MAY OCCUR. SHOCK AND COMA MAY RESULT AS BODY TEMPERATURE DROPS.	EVENLY AND WITHOUT DELAY. (NEED TO PROVIDE HEAT SOURCE; CASUALTY'S BODY UNABLE TO GENERATE HEAT.) 2. KEEP DRY, PROTECT FROM THE ELEMENTS. 3. WARM (NOT HOT) LIQUIDS MAY BE GIVEN GRADUALLY (TO CONSCIOUS CASUALTIES ONLY). 4. BE PREPARED TO START BASIC LIFE SUPPORT MEASURES FOR THE CASUALTY. 5. SEEK MEDICAL TREATMENT IMMEDIATELY. **SEVERE HYPOTHERMIA** 1. STABILIZE THE TEMPERATURE. 2. ATTEMPT TO AVOID FURTHER HEAT LOSS. 3. HANDLE THE CASUALTY GENTLY. 4. EVACUATE TO THE NEAREST MTF AS SOON AS POSSIBLE. **5. WARNING: HYPOTHERMIA IS A MEDICAL EMERGENCY. PROMPT MEDICAL ATTENTION IS NECESSARY.**

CHAPTER 6

FIRST AID FOR BITES AND STINGS

6-1. General

Snakebites, insect bites, or stings can cause intense pain and/or swelling. If not treated promptly and correctly, they can cause serious illness or death. The severity of a snakebite depends upon: whether the snake is poisonous or nonpoisonous, the type of snake, the location of the bite, and the amount of venom injected. Bites from humans and other animals, such as dogs, cats, bats, raccoons, and rats, can cause severe bruises and infection and tears or lacerations of tissue. Awareness of the potential sources of injuries can reduce or prevent them from occurring. Knowledge and prompt application of first-aid measures can lessen the severity of injuries from bites and stings and keep the service member from becoming a serious casualty.

6-2. Types of Snakes

a. Nonpoisonous Snakes. There are approximately 130 different varieties of nonpoisonous snakes in the United States. They have oval-shaped heads and round eyes. Unlike poisonous snakes, discussed below, nonpoisonous snakes do not have fangs with which to inject venom. Figure 6-1 depicts the characteristics of a nonpoisonous snake.

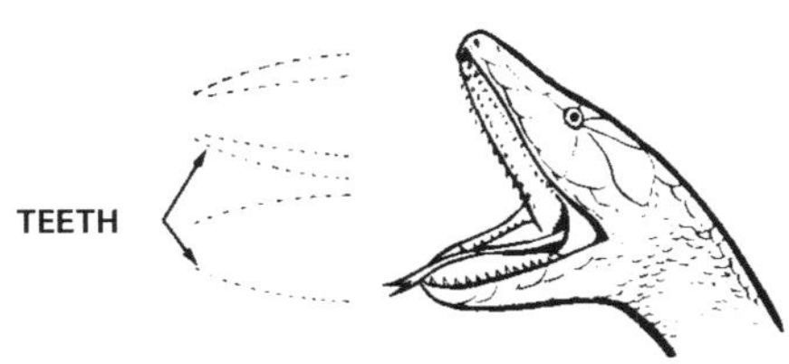

Figure 6-1. Characteristics of nonpoisonous snake.

b. Poisonous Snakes. Poisonous snakes are found throughout the world, primarily in tropical to moderate climates. Within the United States, there are four kinds: rattlesnakes, copperheads, water moccasins (cottonmouth), and coral snakes. Poisonous snakes in other parts of the world include sea snakes, the fer-de-lance, the bushmaster, and the tropical rattlesnake in tropical Central America; the Malayan pit viper in the tropical Far East; the cobra in Africa and Asia; the mamba (or black mamba) in central and southern Africa; and the krait in India and Southeast Asia. Refer to Figure 6-2 for characteristics of a poisonous pit viper.

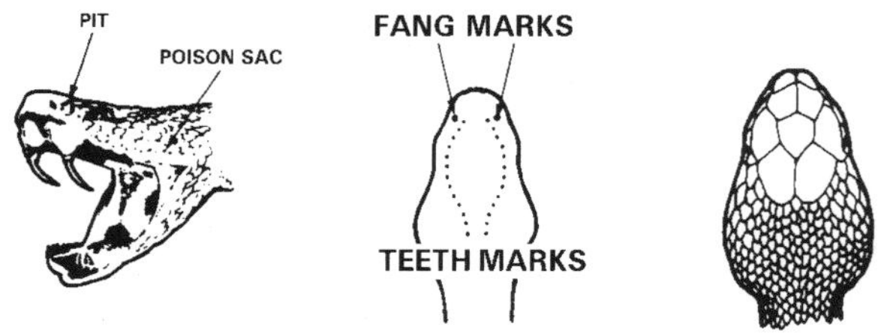

Figure 6-2. Characteristics of poisonous pit viper.

c. Pit Vipers (Poisonous). Figure 6-3 depicts a variety of poisonous snakes.

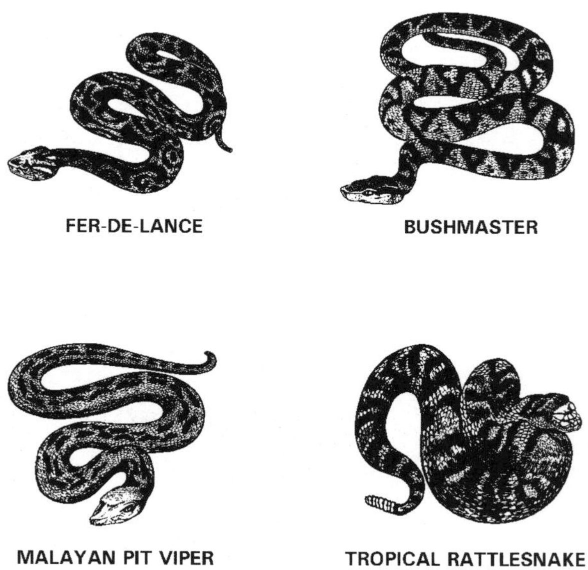

Figure 6-3. Poisonous snakes.

(1) Rattlesnakes, bushmasters, copperheads, fer-de-lance, Malayan pit vipers, and water moccasins (cottonmouth) are called pit vipers because of the small, deep pits between the nostrils and eyes on each side of the head (Figure 6-2). In addition to their long, hollow fangs, these snakes have other identifying features: thick bodies, slit-like pupils of the eyes, and flat, almost triangular-shaped heads. Color markings and other identifying characteristics, such as rattles or a noticeable white interior of the mouth (cottonmouth), also help distinguish these poisonous snakes. Further

identification is provided by examining the bite pattern of the wound for signs of fang entry. Occasionally there will be only one fang mark, as in the case of a bite on a finger or toe where there is no room for both fangs, or when the snake has broken off a fang.

(2) The casualty's condition provides the best information about the seriousness of the situation, or how much time has passed since the bite occurred. Pit viper bites are characterized by severe burning pain. Discoloration and swelling around the fang marks usually begins within 5 to 10 minutes after the bite. If only minimal swelling occurs within 30 minutes, the bite will almost certainly have been from a nonpoisonous snake or possibly from a poisonous snake which did not inject venom. The venom destroys blood cells, causing a general discoloration of the skin. Blisters and numbness in the affected area follow this reaction. Other signs, which can occur, are weakness, rapid pulse, nausea, shortness of breath, vomiting, and shock.

d. Corals, Cobras, Kraits, and Mambas. Corals (Figure 6-4), cobras (Figure 6-5), kraits, and mambas all belong to the same group even though they are found in different parts of the world. All four inject their venom through short, grooved fangs, leaving a characteristic bite pattern.

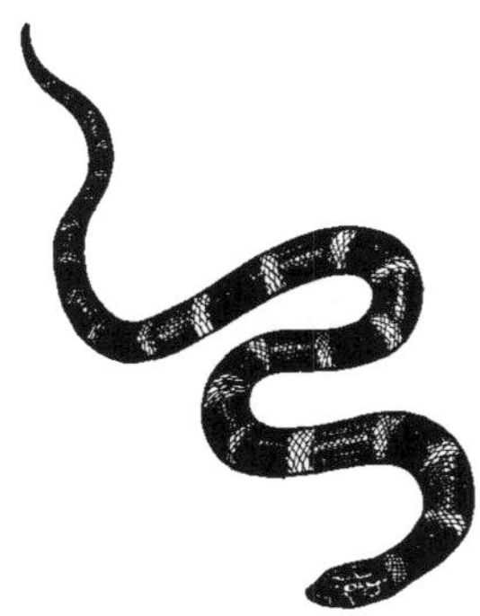

Figure 6-4. Coral snake.

(1) The small coral snake, found in the Southeastern US, is brightly colored with bands of red, yellow (or almost white), and black completely encircling the body. Other nonpoisonous snakes have the same coloring, but on the coral snake found in the US, the red ring always touches the yellow ring. To know the difference between a harmless snake and the coral snake found in the United States, remember the following:

"Red on yellow will kill a fellow,
Red on black, venom will lack."

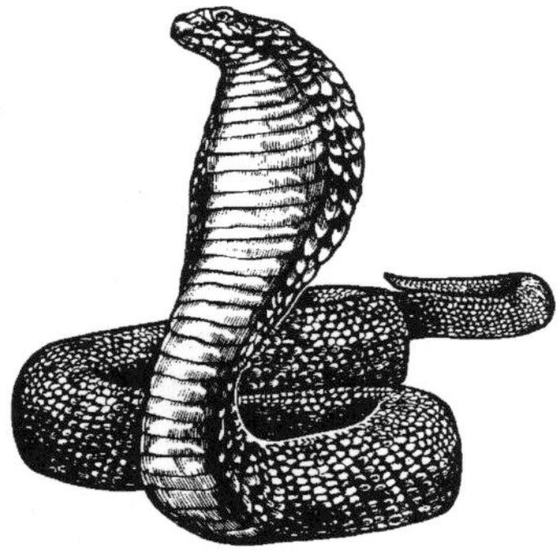

Figure 6-5. Cobra snake.

(2) The venom of corals, cobras, kraits, and mambas produces symptoms different from those of pit vipers. Because there is only minimal pain and swelling, many people believe that the bite is not serious. Delayed reactions in the nervous system normally occur between 1 to 7 hours after the bite. Symptoms include blurred vision, drooping eyelids, slurred speech, drowsiness, and increased salivation and sweating. Nausea, vomiting, shock, respiratory difficulty, paralysis, convulsions, and coma will usually develop if the bite is not treated promptly.

e. *Sea Snakes*. Sea snakes (Figure 6-6) are found in the warm water areas of the Pacific and Indian oceans, along the coasts, and at the mouths of some larger rivers. Their venom is **VERY** poisonous, but their fangs are only 1/4 inch long. The first aid outlined for land snakes also applies to sea snakes.

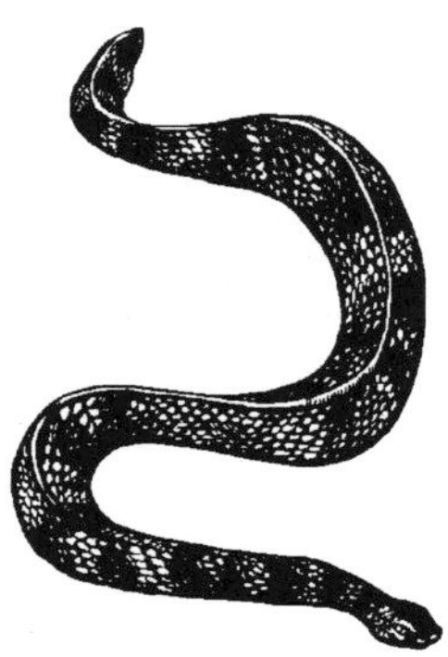

Figure 6-6. Sea snake.

6-3. Snakebites

a. Poisonous snakes **DO NOT** always inject venom when they bite or strike a person. However, all snakes may carry tetanus (lockjaw); anyone bitten by a snake, whether poisonous or nonpoisonous, should immediately seek medical attention.

- Poison is injected from the venom sacs through grooved or hollow fangs. Depending on the species, these fangs are either long or short. Pit vipers have long hollow fangs. These fangs are folded against the roof of the mouth and extend when the snake strikes. This allows them to strike quickly and then withdraw. Cobras, coral snakes, kraits, mambas, and sea snakes have short, grooved fangs. These snakes are less effective in their attempts to bite, since they must chew after striking to inject enough venom (poison) to be effective. Figure 6-7 depicts the characteristics of a poisonous snakebite.

- In the event you are bitten, attempt to identify and/or kill the snake. Take it to medical personnel for inspection/identification. This provides valuable information to medical personnel who deal with snakebites. **TREAT ALL SNAKEBITES AS POISONOUS.**

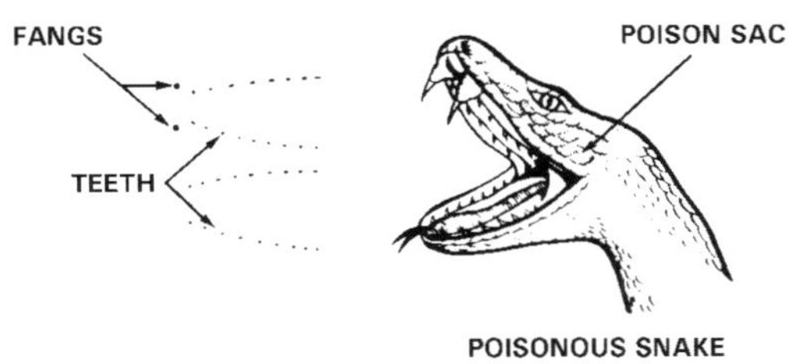

Figure 6-7. Characteristics of poisonous snakebite.

b. The venoms of different snakes cause different effects. Pit viper venom (hemotoxin [blood toxin]) destroys tissue and blood cells. Cobras, adders, and coral snakes inject powerful venom (neurotoxin [nerve toxin]) which affect the central nervous system, causing respiratory paralysis. Water moccasins and sea snakes have venom that is both hemotoxic and neurotoxic.

c. The identification of poisonous snakes is very important since medical treatment will be different for each type of venom. *Unless it can be positively identified, the snake should be killed and saved.* When this is not possible or when doing so is a serious threat to others, identification may sometimes be difficult since many venomous snakes resemble harmless varieties. When dealing with snakebite problems in foreign countries, seek advice, professional or otherwise, which may help identify species in the particular area of operations.

d. Get the casualty to an MTF as soon as possible and with minimum movement. Until evacuation or treatment is possible, have the casualty lie quietly and not move any more than necessary. If the casualty has been bitten on an extremity, **DO NOT** elevate the limb; keep the extremity level with the body. Keep the casualty comfortable and reassure him. If the casualty is alone when bitten, he should go to the medical facility himself rather than wait for someone to find him. Unless the snake has been positively identified, attempt to kill it and send it with the casualty. Be sure that retrieving the snake does not endanger anyone or delay transporting the casualty.

(1) If the bite is on an arm or leg, place a constricting band (narrow cravat [swathe], or narrow gauze bandage) one to two fingerbreadths above and below the bite (Figure 6-8). If the bite is on the hand or foot, place a single band above the wrist or ankle. The band should be tight enough to stop the flow of blood near the skin, but not tight enough to interfere with circulation. In other words, it should not have a tourniquet-like affect. If no swelling is seen, place the bands about 1 inch from either side of the bite. If swelling is present, put the bands on the unswollen part at the edge of the swelling. If the swelling extends beyond the band, move the band to the new edge of the swelling. (If possible, leave the old band on, place a new one at the new edge of the swelling, and then remove and save the old one in case the process has to be repeated.)

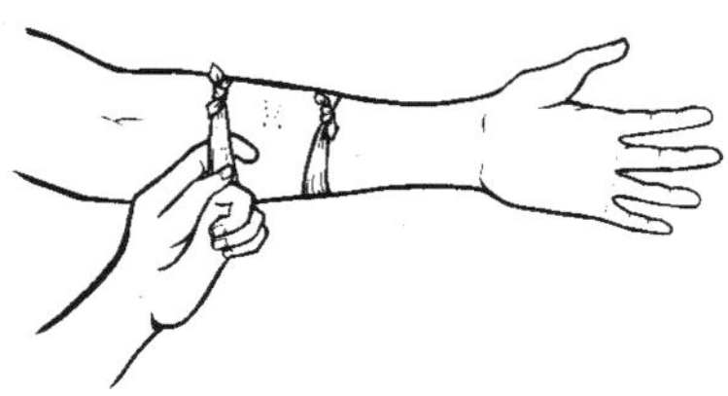

Figure 6-8. Constricting band.

CAUTION

DO NOT attempt to cut open the bite nor suck out the venom. If the venom should seep through any damaged or lacerated tissues in your mouth, you could immediately lose consciousness or even die.

(2) If the bite is located on an arm or leg, immobilize it at a level below the heart. **DO NOT** elevate an arm or leg even with or above the level of the heart.

CAUTION

When a splint is used to immobilize the arm or leg, take **EXTREME** care to ensure the splinting is done properly and does not bind. Watch it closely and adjust it if any changes in swelling occur.

(3) When possible, clean the area of the bite with soap and water. **DO NOT** use ointments of any kind.

(4) **NEVER** give the casualty food, alcohol, stimulants (coffee or tea), drugs, or tobacco.

(5) Remove rings, watches, or other jewelry from the affected limb.

6-4. Human or Animal Bites

Human or other land animal bites may cause lacerations or bruises. In addition to damaging tissue, bites always present the possibility of infection.

a. Human Bites. Human bites that break the skin may become seriously infected since the mouth is heavily contaminated with bacteria. Medical personnel **MUST** treat all human bites.

b. Animal Bites. Land animal bites can result in both infection and disease. Tetanus, rabies, and various types of fevers can follow an untreated animal bite. Because of these possible complications, the animal causing the bite should, if possible, be captured or killed (without damaging its head) so that it can be tested for disease.

c. First Aid.

(1) Cleanse the wound thoroughly with soap.

(2) Flush it well with water.

(3) Cover it with a sterile dressing.

(4) Immobilize the injured arm or leg, if appropriate.

(5) Transport the casualty immediately to an MTF.

NOTE

If unable to capture or kill the animal, provide medical personnel with any information that will help identify it.

6-5. Marine (Sea) Animals

With the exception of sharks and barracuda, most marine animals will not deliberately attack. The most frequent injuries from marine animals are wounds by biting, stinging, or puncturing. Wounds inflicted by marine animals can be very painful, but are rarely fatal.

a. Sharks, Barracuda, and Alligators. Wounds from these marine animals can involve major trauma as a result of bites and lacerations. Bites from large marine animals are potentially the most life threatening of all injuries from marine animals. Major wounds from these animals can be treated by controlling the bleeding, preventing shock, giving basic life support, splinting the injury, and by securing prompt medical aid.

b. Turtles, Moray Eels, and Corals. These animals normally inflict minor wounds. Treat by cleansing the wound(s) thoroughly and by splinting if necessary.

c. Jellyfish, Portuguese Man-of-War, Anemones, and Others. This group of marine animals inflict injury by means of stinging cells in their tentacles. Contact with the tentacles produces burning pain with a rash and small hemorrhages on the skin. Shock, muscular cramping, nausea, vomiting, and respiratory distress may also occur. Gently remove the clinging tentacles with a towel and wash or treat the area. Use diluted ammonia or alcohol, meat tenderizer, and talcum powder. If symptoms become severe or persist, seek medical assistance.

d. Spiny Fish, Urchins, Stingrays, and Cone Shells. These animals inject their venom by puncturing the skin with their spines. General signs and symptoms include swelling, nausea, vomiting, generalized cramps, diarrhea, muscular paralysis, and shock. Deaths are rare. Treatment consists of soaking the wounds in hot water (when available) for 30 to 60 minutes. This inactivates the heat sensitive toxin. In addition, further first aid measures (controlling bleeding, applying a dressing, and so forth) should be carried out as necessary.

CAUTION

Be careful not to scald the casualty with water that is too hot because the pain of the wound will mask the normal reaction to heat.

6-6. Insect (Arthropod) Bites and Stings

An insect bite or sting can cause great pain, allergic reaction, inflammation, and infection. If not treated correctly, some bites/stings may cause serious illness or even death. When an allergic reaction is not involved, first aid is a simple process. In any case, medical personnel should examine the casualty at the earliest possible time. It is important to properly identify the spider, bee, or creature that caused the bite/sting, especially in cases of allergic reaction.

a. *Types of Insects*. The insects found throughout the world that can produce a bite or sting are too numerous to mention in detail. Commonly encountered stinging or biting insects include brown recluse spiders (Figure 6-9), black widow spiders (Figure 6-10), tarantulas (Figure 6-11), scorpions (Figure 6-12), urticating caterpillars, bees, wasps, centipedes, conenose beetles (kissing bugs), ants, and wheel bugs. Upon being reassigned, especially to overseas areas, take the time to become acquainted with the types of insects to avoid.

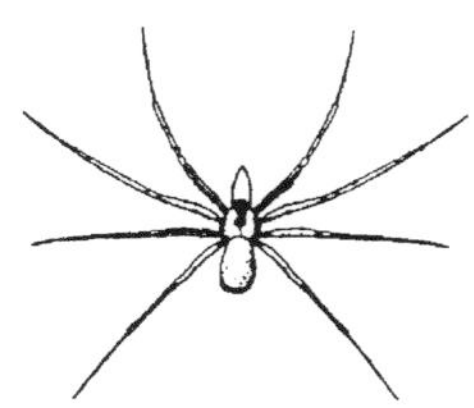

Figure 6-9. Brown recluse spider.

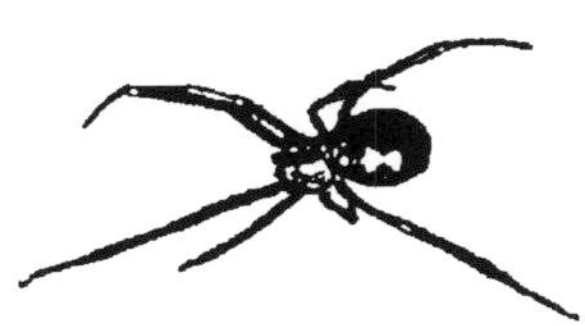

Figure 6-10. Black widow spider.

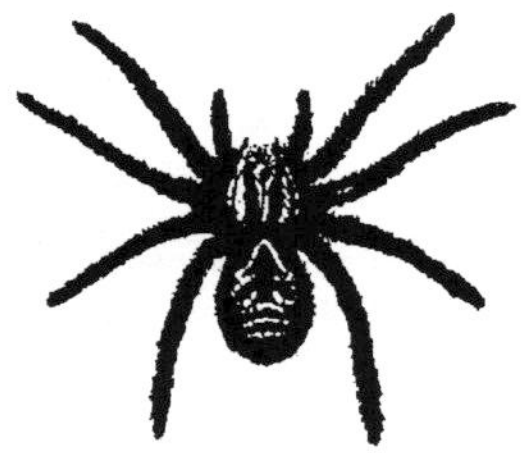

Figure 6-11. Tarantula.

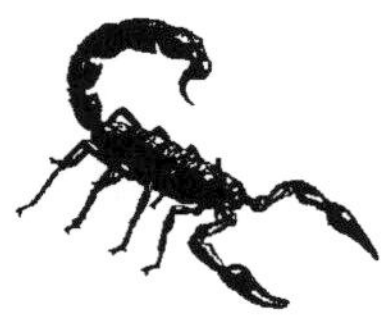

Figure 6-12. Scorpion.

b. Signs and Symptoms. Discussed in paragraphs (1) and (2) below are the most common effects of insect bites/stings. They can occur alone or in combination with the others.

(1) *Less serious.* Commonly seen signs/symptoms are pain, irritation, swelling, heat, redness, and itching. Hives or wheals (raised areas of the skin that itch) may occur. These are the least severe of the allergic reactions that commonly occur from insect bites/stings. They are usually dangerous only if they affect the air passages (mouth, throat, nose, and so forth), which could interfere with breathing. The bites/stings of bees, wasps, ants, mosquitoes, fleas, and ticks are usually not serious and normally produce mild and localized symptoms. A tarantula's bite is usually no worse than that of a bee sting. Scorpions are rare and their stings (except for a specific species found only in the Southwest desert) are painful but usually not dangerous.

(2) *Serious.* Emergency allergic or hypersensitive reactions sometimes result from the stings of bees, wasps, and ants. Many people are allergic to the venom of these particular insects. Bites or stings from these insects may produce more serious reactions, to include generalized itching and hives, weakness, anxiety, headache, breathing difficulties, nausea, vomiting, and diarrhea. Very serious allergic reactions (called *anaphylactic shock*) can lead to complete collapse, shock, and even death. Spider bites (particularly from the black widow and brown recluse spiders) can also be

serious. Venom from the black widow spider affects the nervous system. This venom can cause muscle cramps, a rigid, nontender abdomen, breathing difficulties, sweating, nausea, and vomiting. The brown recluse spider generally produces local rather than system-wide problems; however, local tissue damage around the bite can be severe and can lead to an ulcer and even gangrene.

c. First Aid. There are certain principles that apply regardless of what caused the bite/sting. Some of these are—

- If there is a stinger present (for example, from a bee), remove the stinger by scraping the skin's surface with a fingernail or knife. **DO NOT** squeeze the sac attached to the stinger because it may inject more venom.

- Wash the area of the bite/sting with soap and water (alcohol or an antiseptic may also be used) to help reduce the chances of an infection and remove traces of venom.

- Remove jewelry from bitten extremities because swelling may occur.

- In most cases of insect bites the reaction will be mild and localized; use ice or cold compresses (if available) on the site of the bite/sting. This will help reduce swelling, ease the pain, and slow the absorption of venom. Meat tenderizer (to neutralize the venom) or calamine lotion (to reduce itching) may be applied locally. If necessary, seek medical assistance.

- In more serious reactions (severe and rapid swelling, allergic symptoms, and so forth) treat the bite/sting like you would treat a snakebite; that is, apply constricting bands above and below the site.

- Be prepared to perform basic life-support measures, such as rescue breathing.

- Reassure the casualty and keep him calm.

- In serious reactions, attempt to capture the insect for positive identification; however, be careful not to become a casualty yourself.

- If the reaction to the bite/sting appears serious, seek medical assistance.

WARNING

Insect bites/stings may cause *anaphylactic shock* (a shock caused by a severe allergic reaction). This is a life-threatening event and a TRUE MEDICAL EMERGENCY. Be prepared to perform the basic life-support measures and to immediately transport the casualty to an MTF.

NOTE

Be aware that some allergic or hypersensitive individuals may carry identification or emergency insect bite treatment kits. If the casualty is having an allergic reaction and has such a kit, administer the medication in the kit according to the instructions which accompany the kit.

d. Supplemental Information. For additional information concerning biting insects, see FM 21-10.

6-7. First Aid for Bites and Stings

See the table below for information on bites and stings.

Table 6-1. First Aid Measures for Bites and Stings

TYPES	FIRST AID MEASURES
SNAKEBITE	1. MOVE CASUALTY AWAY FROM THE SNAKE. 2. REMOVE JEWELRY FROM THE AFFECTED AREA, IF APPLICABLE. 3. REASSURE CASUALTY AND KEEP HIM QUIET. 4. APPLY CONSTRICTING BAND, 1-2 FINGERBREADTHS FROM THE BITE. YOU SHOULD BE ABLE TO INSERT A FINGER BETWEEN THE BAND AND THE SKIN. *a. ARM OR LEG BITE.* PLACE ONE BAND ABOVE AND ONE BAND BELOW THE BITE SITE. *b. HAND OR FOOT BITE.* PLACE ONE BAND ABOVE THE WRIST OR ANKLE.

Table 6-1. First Aid Measures for Bites and Stings

TYPES	FIRST AID MEASURES
	5. IMMOBILIZE THE AFFECTED PART IN A POSITION BELOW THE LEVEL OF THE HEART. 6. KILL THE SNAKE (IF POSSIBLE, WITHOUT DAMAGING ITS HEAD OR ENDANGERING YOURSELF) AND SEND IT WITH THE CASUALTY. 7. SEEK MEDICAL ASSISTANCE IMMEDIATELY.
BROWN RECLUSE SPIDER OR BLACK WIDOW SPIDER BITE	1. KEEP CASUALTY QUIET. 2. REMOVE ALL JEWELRY FROM AFFECTED PART, IF APPLICABLE. 3. WASH THE AREA. 4. APPLY ICE OR FREEZE PACK, IF AVAILABLE. 5. SEEK MEDICAL ASSISTANCE.
TARANTULA BITE OR SCORPION STING OR ANT BITE	1. WASH THE AREA. 2. REMOVE ALL JEWELRY FROM AFFECTED PART, IF APPLICABLE. 3. APPLY ICE OR FREEZE PACK, IF AVAILABLE. 4. APPLY BAKING SODA, CALAMINE LOTION, OR MEAT TENDERIZER (IF AVAILABLE) TO BITE SITE TO RELIEVE PAIN AND ITCHING. 5. IF THE SITE OF THE BITE IS ON THE FACE, NECK (POSSIBLE AIRWAY PROBLEMS), OR GENITAL AREA, OR IF LOCAL REACTION SEEMS SEVERE, OR IF THE STING IS BY THE DANGEROUS TYPE OF SCORPION FOUND IN THE SOUTHWEST UNITED STATES DESERT, KEEP THE CASUALTY AS QUIET AS POSSIBLE. SEEK MEDICAL ASSISTANCE.
BEE STING	1. IF THE STINGER IS PRESENT, REMOVE BY SCRAPING WITH A KNIFE OR FINGERNAIL. DO NOT SQUEEZE VENOM SAC ON STINGER; MORE VENOM MAY BE INJECTED. 2. REMOVE ALL JEWELRY FROM AFFECTED PART, IF APPLICABLE.

Table 6-1. First Aid Measures for Bites and Stings

TYPES	FIRST AID MEASURES
	3. WASH THE AREA. 4. APPLY ICE OR FREEZE PACK, IF AVAILABLE. 5. IF ALLERGIC SIGNS OR SYMPTOMS APPEAR, BE PREPARED TO PERFORM BASIC LIFE SUPPORT MEASURES. SEEK IMMEDIATE MEDICAL ASSISTANCE.

CHAPTER 7

FIRST AID IN A NUCLEAR, BIOLOGICAL, AND CHEMICAL ENVIRONMENT

7-1. General

American forces have not been exposed to NBC weapons/agents on the battlefield since World War I. In future conflicts and wars we can expect the use of such agents. Nuclear, biological, and chemical weapons will rapidly degrade unit effectiveness by forcing troops to wear protective clothing and by creating confusion and fear. Through training in protective procedures and first aid, units can maintain their effectiveness on the integrated battlefield.

7-2. First Aid Materials

You may be issued the following materials to protect, decontaminate, and use as first aid for NBC exposure. You must know how to use the items; some items are described in *a* through *d* below. It is equally important that you know when to use them.

a. Nerve Agent Pyridostigmine Pretreatment (*NAPP*). You may be issued a blister pack of pretreatment tablets when your commander directs. The NAPP is a pretreatment; it is not an antidote. It improves the effectiveness of the nerve agent antidote. When ordered to take the pretreatment you must take one tablet every 8 hours, mission permitting. This must be taken prior to exposure to nerve agents, since it may take several hours to develop adequate blood levels.

NOTE

Commanders must follow investigational new drug protocols for use of the NAPP.

b. M291 Skin Decontaminating Kit. The M291 Skin Decontaminating Kit (Figure 7-1) contains six packets of XE-555 decontaminant resin.

WARNING

For external use only. May be slightly irritating to the eyes. Keep decontaminating powder out of eyes. Use water to wash toxic agent out of eyes.

c. *Nerve Agent Antidote Kit, MARK I.* Each service member is issued three MARK Is for use in first aid for nerve agent poisoning (Figure 7-2 and paragraph 7-6).

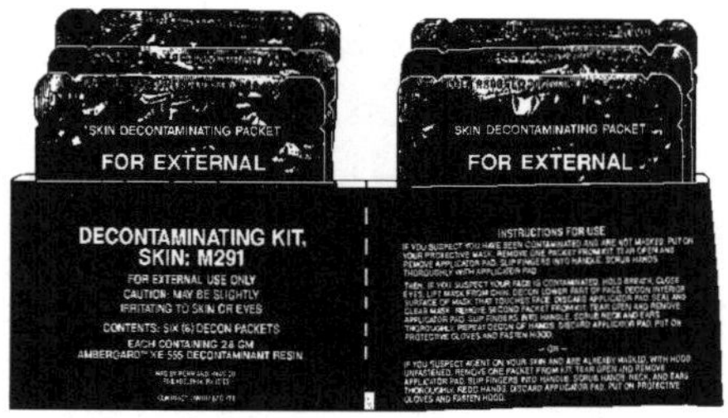

Figure 7-1. M291 Skin Decontamination Kit.

d. *Antidote Treatment, Nerve Agent, Autoinjector.* A new nerve agent antidote injection device, Antidote Treatment, Nerve Agent, Autoinjector (ATNAA) is currently under development that will replace the MARK I. The ATNAA is a multichambered device with the atropine and pralidoxime chloride in separate chambers. Both antidotes will be administered through a single needle.

7-3. Classification of Chemical and Biological Agents

a. Chemical agents are classified according to the primary physiological effects they produce, such as blistering, choking, vomiting, and incapacitating agents.

b. Biological warfare agents are classified according to the effect they have on man. The effects include their ability to incapacitate and cause death. Most biological warfare agents are delivered as aerosols that effect the respiratory tract; some can be delivered by releasing infected insects, by contaminating food and water, and by injection (injecting material in individuals by terrorist, not mass exposure). These agents are found in living organisms such as fungi, bacteria, and viruses.

WARNING

Swallowing water or food contaminated with nerve, blister, and other chemical agents and with some biological agents can be fatal. NEVER consume water or food that is suspected of being contaminated until it has been tested and found safe for consumption by medical personnel.

7-4. Conditions for Masking Without Order or Alarm

a. Once an attack with a chemical or biological agent is detected or suspected, or information is available that such an agent is about to be used, you must **STOP BREATHING** and mask immediately. **DO NOT WAIT** to receive an order or alarm under the following circumstances:

- Your position is hit by artillery missiles, rockets that produce vapors, smoke, and mists, and aerial sprays.
- Smoke or vapor cloud from an unknown source is present or approaching.
- A suspicious odor, liquid, or solid is present.
- A chemical or biological warfare agent attack is occurring.
- You are entering an area known or suspected of being contaminated.
- When casualties are being received from an area where chemical or biological agents have reportedly been used.
- You have one or more of the following symptoms:
  - An unexplained runny nose.
  - A sudden unexplained headache.
  - A feeling of choking or tightness in the chest or throat.
  - Dimness of vision.
  - Irritation of the eyes.
  - Difficulty in or increased rate of breathing without obvious reasons.
  - Sudden feeling of depression.
  - Dread, anxiety, or restlessness.
  - Dizziness or light-headedness.

- Slurred speech.
- Unexplained laughter or unusual behavior is noted in others.
- Numerous unexplained ill personnel.
- Service members suddenly collapsing without evident cause.
- Animals or birds exhibiting unusual behavior or suddenly dying.

b. For further information on protection and masking procedures, refer to FM 3-4, FM 4-02.7, FM 8-284, and FM 8-285.

7-5. First Aid for a Chemical Attack

Your field protective mask gives protection against biological and chemical warfare agents as well as radiological fallout. With practice you can mask in 9 seconds or less, or put on your mask with hood within 15 seconds.

a. Stop breathing. Don your mask, seal it properly, and clear and check it; then resume breathing. Give the alarm, and continue the mission. Keep your mask on until the "all clear" signal has been given.

NOTE

Keep your mask on until the area is no longer hazardous and you are told to unmask.

b. If symptoms of nerve agent poisoning (paragraph 7-7) appear, immediately give yourself one MARK I or ATNAA.

CAUTION

Do not inject a nerve agent antidote until you are sure you need it.

c. If your eyes and face become contaminated, you must immediately try to get under cover. You need shelter to prevent further contamination while performing decontamination procedures on your face. If no overhead cover is available, put your poncho over your head before beginning the decontamination process. Then you put on the remaining protective clothing. If vomiting occurs, the mask should be lifted momentarily and drained—with your eyes closed and while holding your breath—then replaced, cleared, and sealed.

d. If nerve agents are used, mission permitting, watch for persons needing nerve agent antidotes and immediately follow procedures outlined in paragraph 7-8*b* or *c*.

e. Decontaminate your skin immediately and clothing and equipment as soon as the mission permits.

7-6. Background Information on Nerve Agents

a. Nerve agents are among the deadliest of chemical agents. Nerve agents enter the body by inhalation, by ingestion, and through the skin. Depending on the route of entry and the amount, nerve agents can produce injury or death within minutes. Nerve agents can achieve their effects with small amounts. Nerve agents are absorbed rapidly, and the effects are felt immediately upon entry into the body. You will be issued three MARK Is or three ATNAAs and one Convulsant Antidote for Nerve Agent (CANA). Each MARK I consists of one atropine autoinjector and one pralidoxime chloride (2 PAM Cl) autoinjector (Figure 7-2A). Each ATNAA consist of a multichambered autoinjector with the atropine and pralidoxime chloride in separate chambers (Figure 7-2C). The CANA is a single autoinjector with flanges (Figure 7-2B). Procedures for use of both the MARK I and ATNAA are described below. You will use either the MARK I or the ATNAA in self-aid and buddy aid as issued.

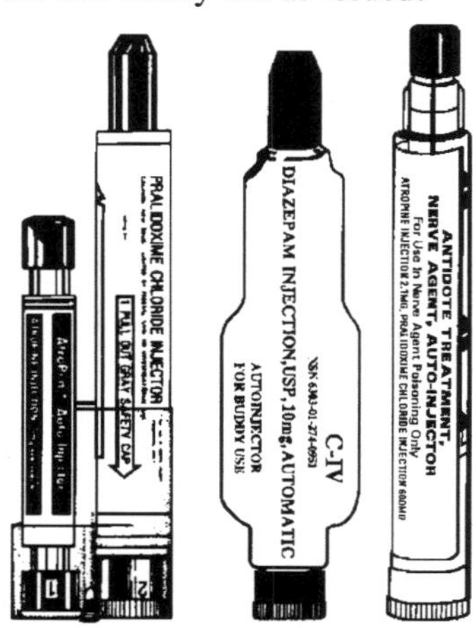

A B C

Figure 7-2. Nerve Agent Antidote Kit, MARK I, CANA, and ATNAA.

b. When you have the signs and symptoms of nerve agent poisoning, you should immediately put on the protective mask and then inject yourself with one set of the MARK I or ATNAA. Do not administer the CANA. You should inject yourself in the outer (lateral) thigh muscle (Figure 7-3) or if you are thin, in the upper outer (lateral) part of the buttocks (Figure 7-4).

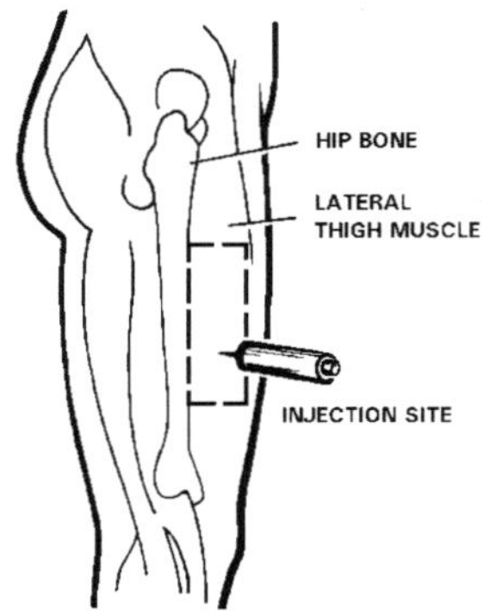

Figure 7-3. Thigh injection site.

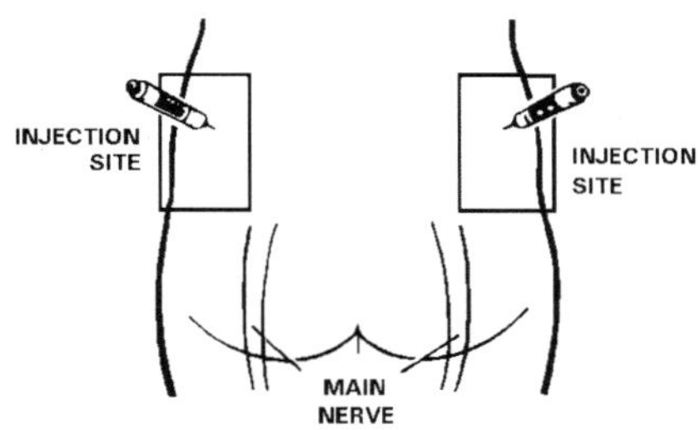

Figure 7-4. Buttocks injection site.

c. Also, you may come upon an unconscious chemical agent casualty who will be unable to care for himself and who will require first aid. You should be able to successfully—

(1) Mask him if he is unmasked.

(2) Inject him, if necessary, with all of **HIS** autoinjectors.

(3) Decontaminate his skin.

(4) Seek medical assistance.

7-7. Signs and Symptoms of Nerve Agent Poisoning

The symptoms of nerve agent poisoning are grouped as **MILD**—those that you recognize and for which you can perform self-aid, and **SEVERE**—those which require buddy aid.

a. MILD Signs and Symptoms.

- Unexplained runny nose.
- Unexplained sudden headache.
- Sudden drooling.
- Difficulty seeing (dimness of vision and miosis).
- Tightness in the chest or difficulty in breathing.
- Localized sweating and muscular twitching in the area of contaminated skin.
- Stomach cramps.
- Nausea.
- Tachycardia followed by bradycardia. (*Tachycardia* is an abnormally rapid heartbeat with a heart rate of over 100 beats per minute. *Bradycardia* is a slow heart rate of less than 60 beats per minute.)

b. SEVERE Signs and Symptoms.

- Strange or confused behavior.
- Wheezing, dyspnea (difficulty in breathing), and coughing.
- Severely pinpointed pupils.
- Red eyes with tearing.
- Vomiting.
- Severe muscular twitching and general weakness.
- Involuntary urination and defecation.

- Convulsions.
- Unconsciousness.
- Respiratory failure.
- Bradycardia.

7-8. First Aid for Nerve Agent Poisoning

First aid for nerve agent poisoning consists of administering the MARK I or ATNAA and CANA.

a. *Injection Site.* The injection site for administering the antidotes is normally in the outer thigh muscle. The thigh injection site is the area about a hand's width above the knee to a hand's width below the hip joint (Figure 7-3). It is important that the injection be given into a large muscle area. If the individual is thinly built, then the injections should be administered into the upper outer quarter (quadrant) of the buttock (Figure 7-4). Injecting in the buttocks of a thinly built individual avoids injury to the thighbone.

b. *Self-Administer MARK I.* If you experience any or all of the nerve agent **MILD** symptoms (paragraph 7-7*a*), you must **IMMEDIATELY** put on your protective mask and self-administer one MARK I (Figure 7-2A). Follow the procedure given in Table 7-1. The MARK I is carried in your protective mask carrier, pocket of the MOPP overgarment, or other location as specified in your unit tactical standing operating procedure (TSOP). (In cold weather, the MARK I should be stored in an inside pocket of your clothing to protect the antidote from freezing. A frozen MARK I cannot be immediately used to provide you with antidote, when needed. (However, the MARK I can still be used after complete thawing.)

Table 7-1. Self Aid for Nerve Agent Poisoning

MARK I*	ATNAA*
STEP 1. OBTAIN ONE MARK I.**	STEP 1. OBTAIN ONE ATNAA.**
STEP 2. CHECK INJECTION SITE.	STEP 2. CHECK INJECTION SITE.
STEP 3. HOLD MARK I AT EYE LEVEL WITH NONDOMINANT HAND WITH THE LARGE INJECTOR ON TOP (FIGURE 7-5A).	STEP 3. HOLD ATNAA WITH DOMINANT HAND (FIGURE 7-12A).

Table 7-1. Self Aid for Nerve Agent Poisoning (Continued)

MARK I*	ATNAA*
STEP 4. GRASP SMALL INJECTOR (ATROPINE) (FIGURE 7-5B) AND REMOVE FROM CLIP (FIGURE 7-5C).	STEP 4. GRASP SAFETY CAP WITH NONDOMINANT HAND AND REMOVE FROM INJECTOR (FIGURE 7-12B).
STEP 5. CLEAR HARD OBJECTS FROM INJECTION SITE.	STEP 5. CLEAR HARD OBJECTS FROM INJECTION SITE.
STEP 6. INJECT ATROPINE AT INJECTION SITE APPLYING EVEN PRESSURE TO THE INJECTOR (FIGURE 7-6 OR 7-7). HOLD IN PLACE FOR 10 SECONDS.	STEP 6. INJECT ATNAA AT INJECTION SITE APPLYING EVEN PRESSURE TO THE INJECTOR (FIGURE 7-14 OR 7-15). HOLD IN PLACE FOR 10 SECONDS.
STEP 7. HOLD USED INJECTOR WITH NONDOMINANT HAND.	STEP 7. BEND NEEDLE OF USED INJECTOR BY PRESSING ON A HARD SURFACE TO FORM A HOOK.
STEP 8. GRASP THE LARGE (2 PAM Cl) INJECTOR (FIGURE 7-8B) AND PULL IT FROM CLIP (FIGURE 7-8C). DROP CLIP TO GROUND.	STEP 8. ATTACH USED INJECTOR TO BLOUSE POCKET FLAP OF BDO/JSLIST (FIGURE 7-16).
STEP 9. INJECT 2 PAM Cl AT INJECTION SITE APPLYING EVEN PRESSURE TO THE INJECTOR (FIGURE 7-6 OR 7-7). HOLD IN PLACE FOR 10 SECONDS.	STEP 9. MASSAGE INJECTION SITE, MISSION PERMITTING.
STEP 10. BEND THE NEEDLES OF ALL USED INJECTORS BY PRESSING ON A HARD SURFACE TO FORM A HOOK.	
STEP 11. ATTACH ALL USED INJECTORS TO BLOUSE POCKET FLAP OF BDO/JSLIST (FIGURE 7-9).	
STEP 12. MASSAGE INJECTION SITE, MISSION PERMITTING.	

* USE STEPS LISTED FOR TYPE OF ANTIDOTE DEVICE ISSUED.

** ONLY ADMINISTER ONE MARK I OR ATNAA AS SELF-AID. DO NOT SELF-ADMINISTER CANA.

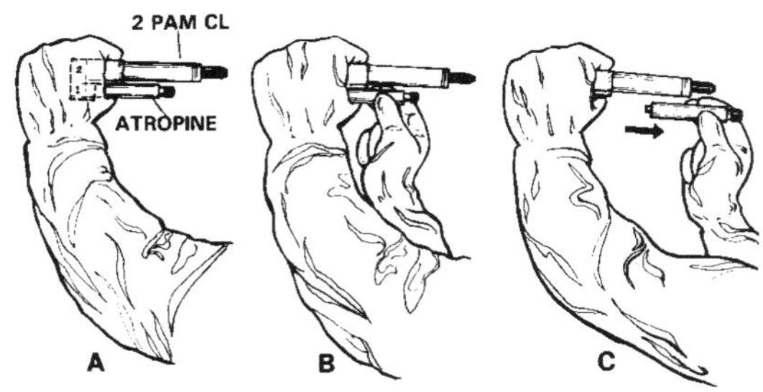

Figure 7-5. Removing the atropine autoinjector from the MARK I clip.

CAUTION

DO NOT cover or hold the needle end with your hand, thumb, or fingers—you might accidentally inject yourself. An accidental injection into the hand **WILL NOT** deliver an effective dose of the antidote, especially if the needle goes through the hand.

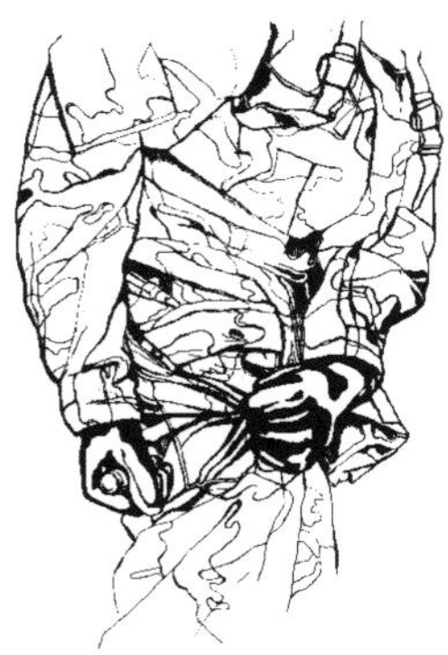

Figure 7-6. Thigh injection site for self-aid.

NOTE

If you are thinly built, inject yourself into the upper outer quadrant of the buttock (Figure 7-7). There is a nerve that crosses the buttocks; hitting this nerve can cause paralysis. Therefore, you must only inject into the *upper outer quadrant* of the buttock.

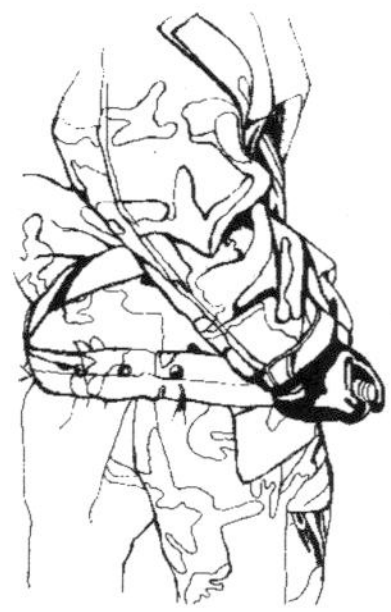

Figure 7-7. Buttocks injection site for self-aid.

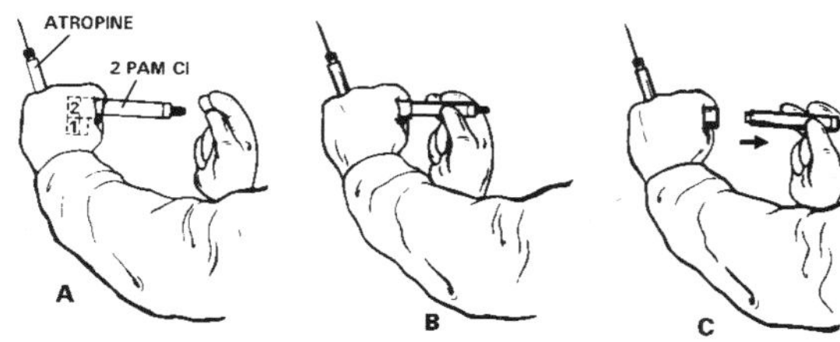

Figure 7-8. Removing the 2 PAM Cl autoinjector from the MARK I clip.

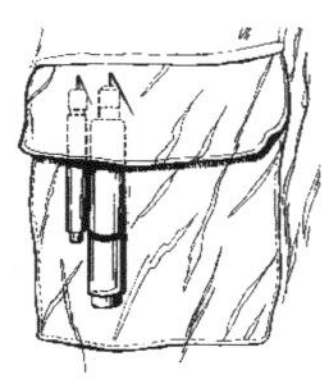

Figure 7-9. One set of used MARK I autoinjectors attached to pocket flap.

NOTES

1. **DO NOT** give yourself another set of injections. If you are able to walk without assistance, know who you are, and where you are, you **WILL NOT** need the second set of injections. (If not needed, giving yourself a second set of MARK I injections or ATNAA may create a nerve agent antidote overdose, which could cause incapacitation [inability to perform mission or defend yourself].)

2. If you continue to have symptoms of nerve agent poisoning, seek someone else (a buddy) to check your symptoms and administer the additional sets of injections, if required.

c. Buddy Evaluation and Buddy Aid. Service members may seek assistance after self-aid (self-administering one MARK I or ATNAA) or may become incapacitated after self-aid. A buddy must evaluate the individual to determine if additional antidotes are required to counter the effects of the nerve agent. Also, service members may experience **SEVERE** symptoms of nerve agent poisoning (paragraph 7-7*b*); they will not be able to treat themselves. In either case, other service members must perform buddy aid as quickly as possible. Before initiating buddy aid, determine if one set of MARK I autoinjectors has already been used so that no more than three sets of the antidote are administered. Buddy aid also includes administering the CANA with the third MARK I or ATNAA to prevent convulsions. Follow the procedures indicated in Table 7-2.

WARNING

Squat, DO NOT kneel, when masking the casualty or administering the nerve agent antidote to the casualty. Kneeling may force the chemical agent into or through your protective clothing.

CAUTION

DO NOT use your own MARK I, ATNAA, or CANA on a casualty. If you use your own, you may not have any antidote if needed for self-aid.

WARNING

DO NOT inject into areas close to the hip, knee, or thigh-bone.

Table 7-2. Buddy Aid/Combat Lifesaver Aid for Nerve Agent Casualty.

MARK I*	ATNAA*	CANA**
STEP 1. MASK THE CASUALTY AND POSITION HIM ON HIS SIDE (SWIMMER'S POSITION).	STEP 1. MASK THE CASUALTY AND POSITION HIM ON HIS SIDE (SWIMMER'S POSITION).	STEP 1. OBTAIN BUDDY'S CANA.
STEP 2. POSITION YOURSELF NEAR THE CASUALTY'S THIGH.	STEP 2. POSITION YOURSELF NEAR THE CASUALTY'S THIGH.	STEP 2. CHECK INJECTION SITE.

Table 7-2. Buddy Aid/Combat Lifesaver Aid for Nerve Agent Casualty (Continued).

MARK I*	ATNAA*	CANA**
STEP 3. OBTAIN BUDDY'S THREE OR REMAINING MARK Is.	STEP 3. OBTAIN BUDDY'S THREE OR REMAINING ATNAAs.	STEP 3. HOLD CANA IN A CLOSED FIST WITH DOMINANT HAND (FIGURE 7-12A).
STEP 4. CHECK INJECTION SITE.	STEP 4. CHECK INJECTION SITE.	STEP 4. GRASP SAFETY CAP WITH NONDOMINANT HAND AND REMOVE FROM INJECTOR (FIGURE 7-12B).
STEP 5. HOLD MARK I WITH NONDOMINANT HAND (FIGURE 7-5A).	STEP 5. HOLD ATNAA IN A CLOSED FIST WITH DOMINANT HAND (FIGURE 7-12A).	STEP 5. CLEAR HARD OBJECTS FROM INJECTION SITE.
STEP 6. GRASP SMALL INJECTOR (ATROPINE) AND REMOVE FROM CLIP (FIGURE 7-5B).	STEP 6. GRASP SAFETY CAP WITH NONDOMINANT HAND AND REMOVE FROM INJECTOR (FIGURE 7-12B).	STEP 6. INJECT CANA AT INJECTION SITE BY APPLYING EVEN PRESSURE TO THE INJECTOR, NOT A JABBING MOTION (FIGURE 7-14 OR 7-15). HOLD IN PLACE FOR 10 SECONDS.
STEP 7. CLEAR HARD OBJECTS FROM INJECTION SITE.	STEP 7. CLEAR HARD OBJECTS FROM INJECTION SITE.	STEP 7. BEND NEEDLE OF INJECTOR BY PRESSING ON A HARD SURFACE TO FORM A HOOK.
STEP 8. INJECT ATROPINE AT INJECTION SITE BY APPLYING EVEN PRESSURE TO THE INJECTOR, NOT A JABBING MOTION (FIGURE 7-10 OR 7-11). HOLD IN PLACE FOR 10 SECONDS.	STEP 8. INJECT ATNAA AT INJECTION SITE BY APPLYING EVEN PRESSURE TO THE INJECTOR, NOT A JABBING MOTION (FIGURE 7-14 OR 7-15). HOLD IN PLACE FOR 10 SECONDS.	STEP 8. ATTACH USED INJECTOR TO BLOUSE POCKET FLAP OF BDO/JSLIST (FIGURE 7-16).
STEP 9. HOLD USED INJECTOR BETWEEN LITTLE FINGER AND RING FINGER OF NONDOMINANT HAND (FIGURE 7-5A).	STEP 9. BEND NEEDLE OF INJECTOR BY PRESSING ON A HARD SURFACE TO FORM A HOOK.	STEP 9. MASSAGE INJECTION SITE, MISSION PERMITTING.
STEP 10. PULL LARGE INJECTOR (2 PAM CI) FROM CLIP (FIGURE 7-5C). DROP CLIP TO GROUND.	STEP 10. ATTACH ALL USED INJECTORS TO BLOUSE POCKET FLAP OF BDO/JSLIST (FIGURE 7-16).	

Table 7-2. Buddy Aid/Combat Lifesaver Aid for Nerve Agent Casualty (Continued).

MARK I*	ATNAA*	CANA**
STEP 11. INJECT 2 PAM CI AT INJECTION SITE BY APPLYING EVEN PRESSURE TO THE INJECTOR, NOT A JAB-BING MOTION (FIGURE 7-10 OR 7-11). HOLD IN PLACE FOR 10 SECONDS.	STEP 11. MASSAGE INJECTION SITE, MISSION PERMITTING.	
STEP 12. REPEAT STEPS ABOVE FOR REMAINING MARK Is.		
STEP 13. BEND THE NEEDLES OF ALL USED INJECTORS BY PRESSING ON A HARD SURFACE TO FORM A HOOK.		
STEP 14. ATTACH ALL USED INJECTORS TO BLOUSE POCKET FLAP OF BDO/JSLIST (FIGURE 7-13).		
STEP 15. MASSAGE INJECTION SITE, MISSION PERMITTING.		

* USE STEPS LISTED FOR TYPE OF ANTIDOTE DEVICE ISSUED.
** CANA IS USED IN BUDDY AID/CLS AID ONLY. DO NOT USE IN SELF-AID.

NOTE

If the casualty is thinly built, inject the antidote into the buttock. Only inject the antidote into the upper outer portion of the casualty's buttock (Figure 7-11). This avoids hitting the nerve that crosses the buttocks (Figure 7-4). Hitting this nerve can cause paralysis.

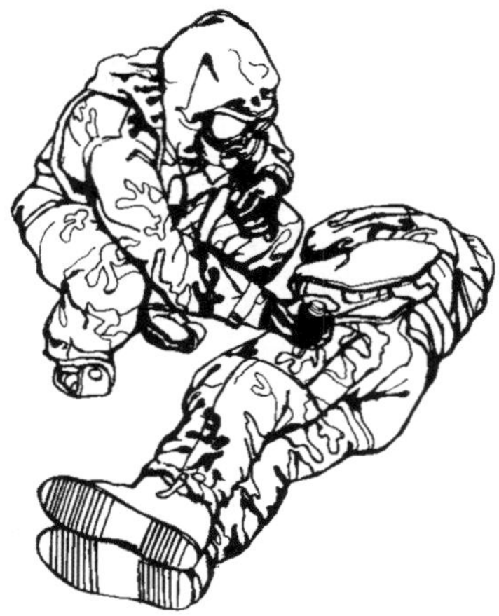

Figure 7-10. Injecting the casualty's thigh (Mark I or CANA).

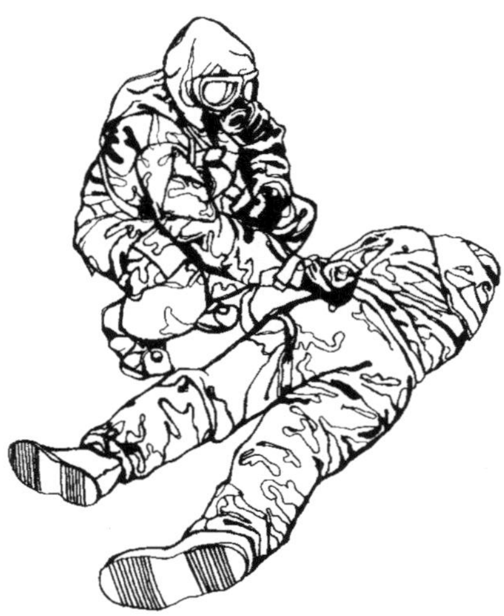

Figure 7-11. Injecting the casualty's buttocks (Mark I or CANA).

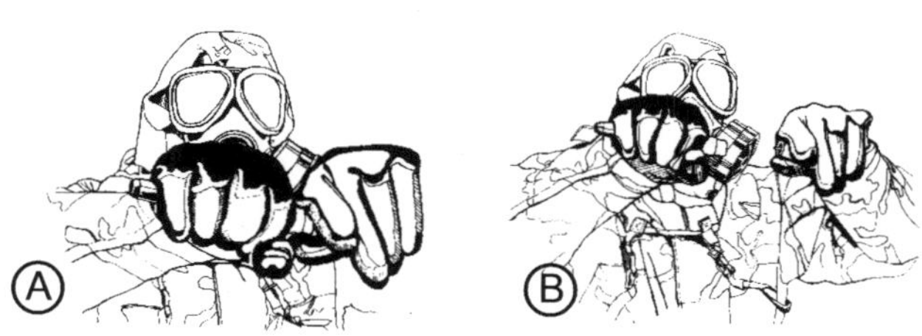

Figure 7-12. Preparing CANA or ATNAA for injection.

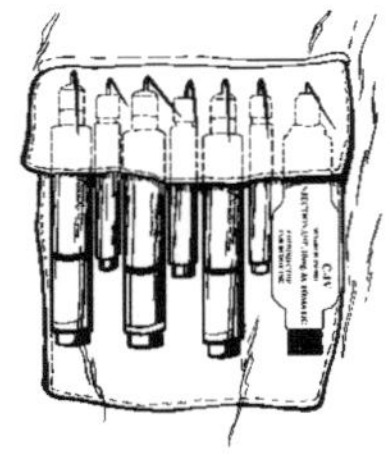

Figure 7-13. Three sets of used MARK I autoinjectors and one CANA autoinjector attached to pocket flap.

d. Self-Administer Antidote Treatment Nerve Agent Autoinjector. If you experience any or all of the nerve agent **MILD** symptoms (paragraph 7-7*b*), you must **IMMEDIATELY** self-administer one ATNAA following the procedure given Table 7-1.

NOTE

If you are thinly-built, inject yourself into the upper outer quarter (quadrant) of the buttock (Figure 7-15). There is a nerve that crosses the buttocks; hitting this nerve can cause paralysis. Therefore, you must only inject into the upper outer quarter (quadrant) of the buttocks.

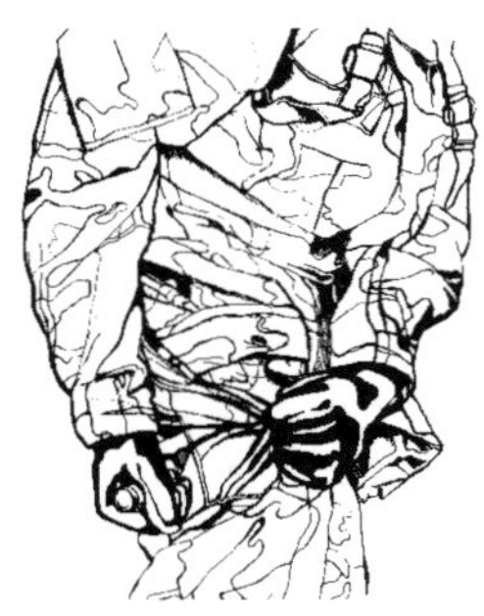

Figure 7-14. Self-administration of ATNAA (thigh).

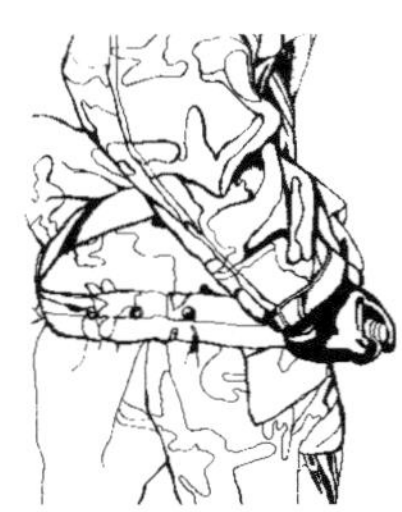

Figure 7-15. Self-administration of ATNAA (buttock).

NOTE

If you continue to have symptoms of nerve agent poisoning, seek someone else (a buddy) to check your symptoms and administer your remaining sets of injections, if required.

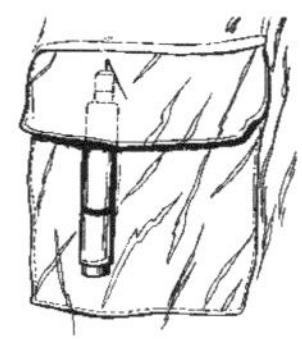

Figure 7-16. Used ATNAA attached to clothing.

e. Buddy Assistance. Service members may seek assistance after self-aid (self-administering one ATNAA) or may become incapacitated after self-aid. A buddy must evaluate the individual to determine if additional antidotes are required to counter the effects of the nerve agent. Also, service members may experience **SEVERE** symptoms of nerve agent poisoning (paragraph 7-7*b*); they will not be able to treat themselves. In either case, other service members must perform buddy aid as quickly as possible. Before initiating buddy aid, determine if one ATNAA has already been used so that no more than three ATNAA are administered. Buddy aid also includes administering the CANA with the third ATNAA to prevent convulsions. Follow the procedures indicated in Table 7-2.

WARNING

Squat, DO NOT kneel, when masking the casualty or administering the nerve agent antidotes to the casualty. Kneeling may force any chemical agent on your overgarment into or through your protective clothing.

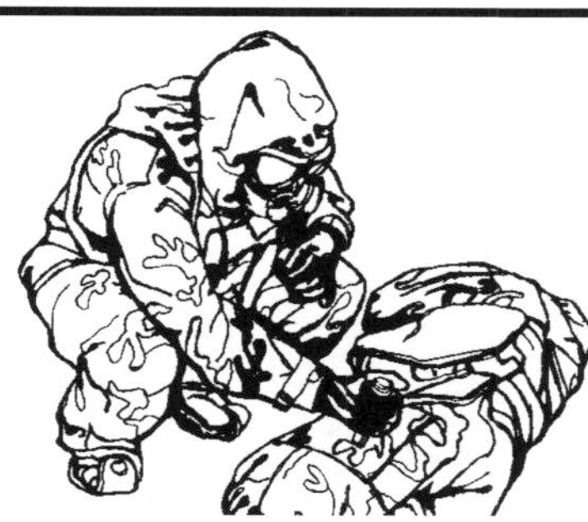

Figure 7-17. Buddy injecting casualty's outer thigh (ATNAA or CANA).

NOTE

If the casualty is thinly built, inject the antidote into the buttocks (Figure 7-18). Only inject the antidote into the upper outer portion of the casualty's buttocks. This avoids hitting the nerve that crosses the buttocks (Figure 7-4). Hitting this nerve can cause paralysis.

WARNING

DO NOT inject into areas close to the hip, knee, or thighbone.

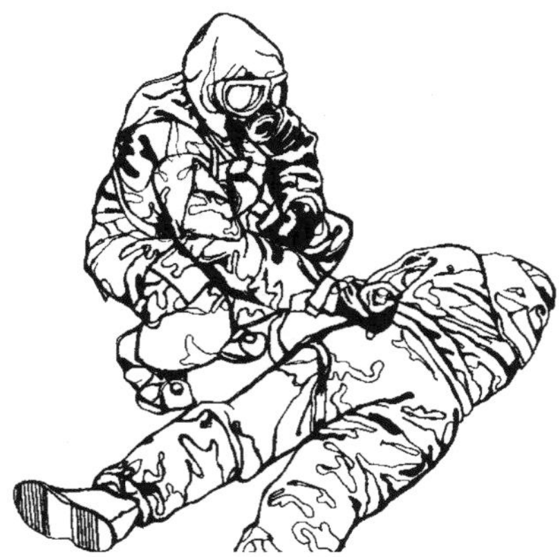

Figure 7-18. Buddy injecting casualty's buttocks (ATNAA or CANA).

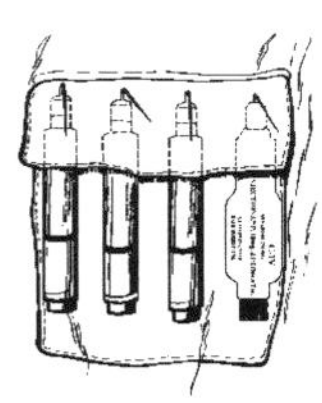

Figure 7-19. Three used ATNAAs and one CANA autoinjector attached to clothing.

f. Combat Lifesaver.

(1) The combat lifesaver must check to verify if the individual has received three sets of MARK I or ATNAAs. If not, the combat lifesaver performs first aid as described for buddy aid above. If the

individual has received the initial three sets of MARK I, then the combat lifesaver may administer additional atropine injections at approximately 15 minute intervals until atropinization is achieved (that is a heart rate above 90 beats per minute, reduced bronchial secretions, and reduced salivations). Administer additional atropine at intervals of 30 minutes to 4 hours to maintain atropinization or until the casualty is placed under the care of medical personnel. Check the heart rate by lifting the casualty's mask hood and feeling for a pulse at the carotid artery. Request medical assistance as soon as the tactical situation permits.

(2) The CLS should administer additional CANA to casualties suffering convulsions. Administer a second, and if needed, a third CANA at 5 to 10 minute intervals for a maximum of three injections (30 milligrams diazepam). Follow the steps and procedures described in buddy aid for administering the CANA. **DO NOT** give more than two additional injections for a total of three (one self-aid plus two by the CLS).

7-9. Blister Agents

Blister agents (vesicants) include mustard (H and HD), nitrogen mustards (HN), lewisite (L), and other arsenicals, mixtures of mustards and arsenicals, and phosgene oxime (CX). Blister agents may act on the eyes, mucous membranes, lungs, and skin. They burn and blister the skin or any other body parts they contact. Even relatively low doses may cause serious injury. Blister agents damage the respiratory tract (nose, sinuses, and windpipe) when inhaled and cause vomiting and diarrhea when absorbed. Lewisite and CX cause immediate pain on contact. However, mustard agents are deceptive as there is little or no pain at the time of exposure. Thus, in some cases, signs of injury may not appear for several hours after exposure.

a. Protective Measures. Your protective mask with hood and protective overgarment provide protection against blister agents. If it is known or suspected that blister agents are being used, **STOP BREATHING**, put on your mask and your protective overgarment.

CAUTION

Large drops of liquid vesicants on the protective overgarment ensemble may penetrate it if allowed to stand for an extended period. Remove large drops as soon as possible.

b. Signs and Symptoms of Blister Agent Poisoning.

(1) Immediate and intense pain upon contact with L, LH (lewisite and mustard) mixture, and CX. No initial pain upon contact with mustard.

(2) Inflammation and blisters (burns) resulting in tissue destruction. The severity of a chemical burn is directly related to the concentration of the agent and the duration of contact with the skin. The longer the agent is in contact with the tissue, the more serious the injury will be.

(3) Vomiting and diarrhea. Exposure to high concentrations of vesicants may cause vomiting or diarrhea.

(4) Death. The blister agent vapors absorbed during ordinary field exposure will probably not cause enough internal body (systemic) damage to result in death. However, death may occur from prolonged exposure to high concentrations of vapor or from extensive liquid contamination over wide areas of the skin, particularly *when decontamination is neglected or delayed.*

c. First Aid Measures.

(1) Use your M291 Skin Decontaminating Kit to decontaminate your skin and use water to flush contaminated eyes. Decontamination of vesicants must be done immediately (within 1 minute is best).

(2) If blisters form, cover them loosely with a field dressing and secure the dressing.

CAUTION

Blisters are actually burns. **DO NOT** attempt to decontaminate the skin where blisters have formed, as the agent has already been absorbed.

(3) If you receive blisters over a wide area of the body, you are considered seriously burned. Seek medical assistance immediately.

(4) If vomiting occurs, the mask should be lifted momentarily and drained—while the eyes are closed and the breath is held—and replaced, cleared, and sealed.

(5) Remember, if vomiting or diarrhea occurs after having been exposed to blister agents, seek medical assistance immediately.

7-10. Choking Agents (Lung-Damaging Agents)

Chemical agents that attack lung tissue, primarily causing fluid buildup (pulmonary edema), are classified as choking agents (lung-damaging agents). This group includes phosgene (CG), diphosgene (DP), chlorine (Cl), and chloropicrin (PS). Of these four agents, CG is the most dangerous and is more likely to be employed by the enemy in future conflict.

a. Protective Measures. Your protective mask gives adequate protection against choking agents.

b. Signs and Symptoms. During and immediately after exposure to choking agents (depending on agent concentration and length of exposure), you may experience some or all of the following signs and symptoms:

- Tears (lacrimation).
- Coughing.
- Choking.
- Tightness of chest.
- Nausea and vomiting.
- Headaches.

c. Self-Aid.

(1) The protective mask should be put on immediately when any of the conditions described in *b* above exist. Another indication of a CG attack is an odor like newly mown hay; however, **DO NOT** rely upon odor as indication of a chemical attack.

(2) If some CG is inhaled, normal combat duties should be continued unless there is difficulty in breathing, nausea, vomiting, or more than the usual shortness of breath during exertion. If any of the above symptoms occur and the mission permits, remain at quiet rest until medical evacuation is accomplished.

d. Death. With ordinary field exposure to choking agents, death will probably not occur. *However, prolonged exposure to high concentrations of the vapor and neglect or delay in masking can be fatal.*

7-11. Cyanogen (Blood) Agents

Cyanogen agents interfere with proper oxygen utilization in the body. Hydrogen cyanide (AC) and cyanogen chloride (CK) are the primary agents in this group.

a. Protective Measures. Your protective mask with a fresh filter gives adequate protection against field concentrations of cyanogen agent vapor. The protective overgarments, as well as the mask, are needed when exposed to liquid AC.

b. Signs and Symptoms. During and immediately after exposure to cyanogen agents (depending on agent concentration and length of exposure), you may experience some or all of the following signs and symptoms:

- Tearing (lacrimation).
- Eye, nose, and throat irritation.
- Sudden stimulation of breathing (unable to hold breath).
- Nausea.
- Coughing.
- Tightness of chest.
- Headache.
- Light-headedness (dizziness).
- Unconsciousness.

c. First Aid.

(1) *Hydrogen cyanide.* During any chemical attack, if you get a sudden stimulation of breath or detect an odor like bitter almonds, **PUT ON YOUR MASK IMMEDIATELY**. Speed is absolutely essential since this agent acts so rapidly that within a few seconds its effects will make it impossible for service members to put on their mask by themselves. Stop breathing until the mask is on, if at all possible. This may be very difficult since the agent strongly stimulates respiration.

(2) *Cyanogen chloride.* Put your mask on immediately if you experience any irritation of the eyes, nose, or throat. Service members

who are unable to mask should be masked by the nearest service member (buddy).

d. Medical Assistance. If you suspect that you have been exposed to blood agents, seek medical assistance immediately.

7-12. Incapacitating Agents

An incapacitating agent is a chemical agent which produces temporary, disabling conditions which persist for hours to days after exposure. Unlike riot control agents, which usually are momentary or fleeting in action, incapacitating agents have a persistent effect. It is likely that smoke-producing munitions or aerosols will disseminate such agents, thus making breathing their means of entry into the body. The protective mask is, therefore, essential.

a. There are no specific first aid measures to relieve the symptoms of incapacitating agents. Supportive first aid and physical restraint may be indicated. If the casualty is stuporous or comatose, be sure that respiration is unobstructed; then turn him on his side in case vomiting should occur. Complete cleansing of the skin with soap and water should be done as soon as possible; or, the M291 Skin Decontaminating Kit can be used if washing is impossible. Remove weapons and other potentially harmful items from service members who are suspected of having these symptoms. Harmful items include cigarettes, matches, medications, and small items that might be swallowed accidentally. Delirious (confused) persons have been known to attempt to eat items bearing only a superficial resemblance to food.

b. Incapacitating agents (anticholinergic drugs BZ type) may produce alarming dryness and coating of the lips and tongue; however, there is usually no danger of immediate dehydration. Fluids should be given sparingly, if at all, because of the danger of vomiting and because of the likelihood of temporary urinary retention due to paralysis of bladder muscles.

c. If the body temperature is elevated and mucous membranes are dry, immediate and vigorous cooling (as for heatstroke) is indicated. Methods that can be used to cool the skin are spraying with cool water and air circulation (fanning); applying alcohol soaked cloths and air circulation; and providing maximum exposure to air in a shaded area, along with maximum air circulation. Such cases are usually a result of anticholinergic poisoning. Rapid evacuation should be accomplished since medical treatment with the appropriate medication may be lifesaving.

CAUTION

DO NOT use **ice** for cooling the skin.

d. Reassurance and a firm, but friendly, attitude by individuals providing first aid will be beneficial if the casualty appears to comprehend what is being said. Conversation is a waste of time if the service member is incoherent or cannot understand what is being said. In such cases, the less said, the better it is—these casualties will benefit more from prompt and vigorous restraint and evacuation to an MTF.

7-13. Incendiaries

Incendiaries can be grouped as WP, thickened gasoline, metal, and oil and metal. You must learn to protect yourself against these incendiaries.

a. White phosphorus is used primarily as a smoke producer but can be used for its incendiary effect to ignite field expedients and combustible materials. The burns from WP are usually multiple, deep, and variable in size. When particles of WP get on the skin or clothing, they continue to burn until deprived of air. They also have a tendency to stick to a surface and must be brushed off or picked out.

(1) If burning particles of WP strike and stick to your clothing, quickly take off the contaminated clothing before the WP burns through to the skin.

(2) If burning WP strikes your skin, smother the flame with water, a wet cloth, or mud.

NOTE

Since WP is soluble in oil, **DO NOT** use grease, oily ointments, or eye ointments to smother the flame.

(3) Keep the WP particles covered with a wet material to exclude air until you can remove them or have them removed from your skin.

(4) Remove the WP particles from the skin by brushing them with a wet cloth and by picking them out with a knife, bayonet, stick, or other available object.

(5) Seek medical assistance when the mission permits.

b. Thickened fuel mixtures (napalm) have a tendency to cling to clothing and body surfaces, thereby producing prolonged exposure and severe burns. The first aid for these burns is the same as for other heat burns. The heat and irritating gases given off by these combustible mixtures may cause lung damage, which must be treated by medical personnel.

c. Metal incendiaries pose special problems. Thermite particles on the skin should be immediately cooled with water and then removed. The first aid for these burns is the same as for other heat burns. Particles of magnesium on the skin burn quickly and deeply. Like other metal incendiaries, they must be removed. Ordinarily, medical personnel should do the complete removal of these particles as soon as possible. Immediate medical treatment is required.

d. Oil and metal incendiaries have much the same effect on contact with the skin and clothing as those discussed (*b* and *c* above). First aid measures for burns are discussed in Chapter 3.

7-14. Biological Agents and First Aid

a. Biological attacks can result in combat ineffectiveness by introducing disease-causing organisms into a troop population.

b. Once a disease is identified, first aid or medical treatment is initiated, depending on the seriousness of the disease. First aid measures are concerned with observable symptoms of the disease such as diarrhea or vomiting.

7-15. Toxins

Toxins are alleged to have been used in past conflicts. Witnesses and victims have described the agent as toxic rain (or yellow rain) because it was reported to have been released from aircraft as a yellow powder or liquid that covered ground, structures, vegetation, and people.

a. *Signs and Symptoms.* The occurrence of the symptoms from toxins may appear in a period of a few minutes to several hours depending on the particular toxin, the service member's susceptibility, and the amount of toxin inhaled, ingested, or deposited on the skin. Symptoms from toxins usually involve the central nervous system but are often preceded by less prominent symptoms, such as nausea, vomiting, diarrhea, cramps, or stomach irritation and burning sensation. Typical neurological symptoms often develop rapidly in severe cases; for example, visual disturbances, inability to swallow, speech difficulty, lack of muscle coordination, and sensory abnormalities (numbness of mouth, throat, or extremities). Yellow rain (mycotoxins) also may have hemorrhagic symptoms, which could include any or all of the following:

- Dizziness.
- Severe itching or tingling of the skin.
- Formation of multiple, small, hard blisters.
- Coughing up blood.
- Shock (which could result in death).

b. *Self-Aid.* Upon recognition of an attack employing toxins, you must immediately take the following actions:

(1) Stop breathing, put on your protective mask with hood, and then resume breathing. Next, put on your protective clothing.

(2) Should severe itching of the face become unbearable, quickly—

- Loosen the cap on your canteen.
- Take and hold a deep breath and lift your mask.
- While holding your breath, close your eyes and flush your face with generous amounts of water.

CAUTION

DO NOT rub or scratch your eyes. Try not to let the water run onto your clothing or protective overgarment.

- Put your protective mask back on, seat it properly, clear it, and check it for a seal; then resume breathing.
- Decontaminate your skin by bathing with soap and water as soon as the mission permits.

- Change clothing and decontaminate your protective mask using soap and water. Replace the filters if directed.

(3) If vomiting occurs, the mask should be lifted momentarily and drained—while the eyes are closed and the breath is held—and replaced, cleared, and sealed.

c. *Medical Assistance.* If you suspect that you have been exposed to toxins, you should seek medical assistance immediately.

7-16. Nuclear Detonation

a. Three types of injuries may result from a nuclear detonation. These are thermal, blast, and radiation injuries. Many times the casualty will have a combination of these types of injuries. First aid for thermal and blast injuries is provided based on observable injuries, such as burns, hemorrhage, or fractures.

b. The signs and symptoms of radiation illness in the initial phase include the rapid onset of nausea, vomiting, and malaise (tiredness). The only first aid procedure for radiological casualties is decontamination.

CHAPTER 8

FIRST AID FOR PSYCHOLOGICAL REACTIONS

8-1. General

Psychological first aid is as natural and reasonable as physical first aid and is just as familiar. When you were hurt as a child, the understanding attitude of your parents did as much as the psychological effect of a bandage. Later, your disappointment or grief was eased by supportive words from a friend. Certainly, taking a walk and talking things out with a friend are familiar ways of dealing with an emotional crisis. The same natural feelings that make us want to help a person who is injured make us want to give a helping hand to a buddy who is upset. *Psychological first aid* really means nothing more complicated than assisting people with emotional distress whether it results from physical injury, disease, or excessive stress. Emotional distress is not always as visible as a wound or a broken bone. However, overexcitement, severe fear, excessive worry, deep depression, misdirected irritability, and anger are signs that stress has reached the point of interfering with effective coping. The more noticeable the symptoms become, the more urgent the need for you to be of help and the more important it is for you to know *how* to help.

8-2. Importance of Psychological First Aid

You must know how to give psychological first aid to be able to help yourself, your buddies, and your unit in order to keep performing the mission. Psychological first aid measures are simple and easy to understand. Your decision of what to do depends upon your ability to observe the service member and understand his needs. Making the best use of resources requires ingenuity on your part. A stress reaction resulting in poor judgment can cause injury or even death to yourself or others on the battlefield. It can be even more dangerous if other persons are affected by the judgment of an emotionally upset service member. If it is detected early enough, the affected service member stands a good chance of remaining in his unit as an effective member. If it is not detected early and if the service member becomes more emotionally upset, he may become a threat to himself and to others.

8-3. Situations Requiring Psychological First Aid

- Psychological first aid (buddy aid) is most needed at the first sign that a service member cannot perform the mission because of emotional distress. Stress is inevitable in combat, in hostage and terrorist situations, and in civilian disasters such as floods, hurricanes, or industrial accidents. Most emotional reactions to such situations are temporary, and the service member can still carry on with encouragement. Painful or disruptive symptoms may last for minutes, hours, or days. However, if the stress symptoms are seriously disabling, they may be psychologically contagious and endanger not only the emotionally upset service member but also the entire unit.

- Sometimes people continue to function well during a disastrous event, but suffer from emotional scars which impair their job performance or quality of life at a later time. Painful memories and dreams may recur for months and years and still be considered a normal reaction. However, if the memories are so painful that the person must avoid all situations which arouse them, becomes socially withdrawn, or shows symptoms of anxiety, depression, or substance abuse, he needs treatment. Experience with police, firemen, emergency medical technicians, and others who deal with disasters has proved that the routine application of psychological first aid to all the participants, including those who have functioned well, greatly reduces the likelihood of future serious post-traumatic stress disorders (PTSDs).

8-4. Interrelationship of Psychological and Physical First Aid

Psychological first aid should go hand in hand with physical first aid. The discovery of a physical injury or cause for an inability to function does not rule out the possibility of a psychological injury (or vice versa). The person suffering from pain, shock, fear of serious injury, or fear of death does not respond well to joking, indifference, or fearful-tearful attention. Fear and anxiety may take as high a toll of the service member's strength as does the loss of blood.

8-5. Goals of Psychological First Aid

The goals of psychological first aid are to—

- Be supportive; assist the service member in dealing with his stress reaction.

- Prevent, and if necessary control, behavior harmful to himself and to others.

- Return the service member to duty as soon as possible after dealing with the stress reaction.

8-6. Respect for Others' Feelings

a. Accept the service member you are trying to help without censorship or ridicule. Respect his right to his own feelings. Even though your feelings, beliefs, and behavior are different, DO NOT blame or make light of him for the way he feels or acts. Your purpose is to help him in this tough situation, not to be his critic. A person DOES NOT WANT to be upset and worried. When he seeks help, he needs and expects consideration of his fears, not abrupt dismissal or ridicule.

b. Realize that people are the products of a wide variety of factors. All people DO NOT react the same way to the same situations. Each individual has complex needs and motivations, both conscious and unconscious, that are uniquely his own. Often the one thing that finally causes the person to become overloaded by a stressful situation is not the stressor itself, but some other problem.

8-7. Emotional and Physical Disability

a. Accept emotional disability as being just as real as physical disability. If a service member's ankle is seriously sprained in a fall, no one expects him to run right away. A service member's emotions may be temporarily strained by the overwhelming stress of battle or other traumatic incident. DO NOT demand that he pull himself together immediately and carry on without a break. Some individuals can pull themselves together immediately, but others cannot. The service member whose emotional stability has been disrupted has a disability just as real as the service member who has sprained his ankle. There is an unfortunate tendency in many people to regard as real only what they can see, such as a wound or bleeding. Some people tend to assume that damage involving a person's mind and emotions is just imagined, that he is not really sick or injured, and that he could overcome his trouble by using his will power.

b. The terms *it's all in your head, snap out of it,* and *get control of yourself* are often used by people who believe they are being helpful. Actually, these terms are expressions of hostility because they show lack of understanding. They only emphasize weakness and inadequacy. Such terms are of no use in psychological first aid.

c. Every physically injured person has some emotional reaction to the fact that he is injured.

(1) It is normal for an injured person to feel upset. The more severe the injury, the more insecure and fearful he becomes, especially

if the injury is to a body part which is highly valued. For example, an injury to the eyes or the genitals, even though relatively minor, is likely to be extremely upsetting. An injury to some other part of the body may be especially disturbing to an individual for his own particular reason. For example, an injury of the hand may be a terrifying blow to a surgeon or an injury to the eye of a pilot.

(2) An injured service member always feels less secure, more anxious, and more afraid not only because of what has happened to him but because of what he imagines may happen as a result of his injury. This fear and insecurity may cause him to be irritable, uncooperative, or unreasonable. As you help him, always keep in mind that such behavior has little or nothing to do with you personally. He needs your patience, reassurance, encouragement, and support.

8-8. Combat and Other Operational Stress Reactions

Stress reaction is a temporary emotional disorder or inability to function, experienced by a previously normal service member as a reaction to the overwhelming or cumulative stress of combat. Stress reaction gets better with reassurance, rest, physical replenishment, and activities that restore confidence. All service members are likely to feel stress reaction under conditions of intense and/or prolonged stress. They may even become stress reaction casualties, unable to perform their mission for hours or days. Other combat and operational stress reactions (COSRs) may result in negative behavior, but are not termed *stress reaction,* as they need more intensive treatment. These negative COSRs may result in misconduct stress behaviors such as drug and alcohol abuse, criminal acts, looting, desertion, and self-inflicted wounds. These harmful COSRs can often be prevented by good psychological first aid. Service members who commit misconduct stress behaviors may require disciplinary action rather than medical treatment.

8-9. Reactions to Stress

Most service members react to stressful incidents after the situation has passed. All service members feel some fear. This fear may be greater than they have experienced at any other time, or they may be more aware of their fear. In such a situation, they should not be surprised if they feel shaky or become sweaty, nauseated, or confused. These reactions are normal and are not a cause for concern. However, some reactions, either short- or long-term, will cause problems if left unchecked. See paragraph 8-13 for more information.

a. Emotional Reactions.

(1) The most obvious combat stress reaction (CSR) is inefficient performance. This can be demonstrated by—

- Slow thinking (or reaction time).
- Difficulty recognizing priorities and seeing what needs to be done.
- Difficulty getting started.
- Indecisiveness and having trouble focusing attention.
- Tendency to do familiar tasks and be preoccupied with familiar details. (This can reach the point where the person is very passive, such as just sitting or wandering about not knowing what to do.)

(2) A less common reaction may be uncontrolled emotional outbursts; this can be demonstrated by crying, screaming, or laughing. Some service members will react in the opposite way. They will be very withdrawn and silent and try to isolate themselves from everyone. These service members should be encouraged to remain with their assigned unit. Uncontrolled reactions may appear by themselves or in any combination (the person may be crying uncontrollably one minute and then laughing the next). In this state, the person is restless and cannot keep still. He may run about, apparently without purpose. Inside, he feels a great rage or fear and his physical acts may show this. In his anger he may indiscriminately strike out at others.

b. Loss of Adaptability.

(1) In a desperate attempt to get away from the danger, which has overwhelmed him, a service member may panic and become confused. His mental ability may be so impaired he cannot think clearly or even follow simple commands. His judgment may be faulty and he may not be aware of his actions, such as standing up in his fighting position during an attack.

(2) In other cases, overwhelming stress may produce symptoms that are often associated with head injuries. For example, the service member may appear dazed or be found wandering around aimlessly. He may appear confused and disoriented and may seem to have a complete or partial loss of memory. In such cases, especially when no eyewitnesses can provide evidence that the service member has NOT suffered a head injury, it is necessary for him to be rapidly medically evacuated. **DO NOT** allow the

service member to expose himself to further personal danger until the cause of the problem has been determined.

c. Sleep Disturbance and Repetition of Dreams. A person who has been overwhelmed by stress often has difficulty sleeping. The service member may experience nightmares related to the stressors. Remember that nightmares, in themselves, are not considered abnormal when they occur soon after a period of intensive stress. As time passes, the nightmares usually become less frequent and less intense. In extreme cases, a service member, even when awake, may think repeatedly of the incident, feel as though it is happening again, and act out parts of his stress over and over again. For some persons, this repetitious reexperiencing of the stressful event may be necessary for eventual recovery; therefore, it should not be discouraged or viewed as abnormal. For the person reexperiencing the event, such reaction may be disruptive. The service member needs to be encouraged to *ventilate* about the incident. Ventilation is a technique where the service member is given the opportunity to talk extensively, often repetitiously about the experience.

8-10. Severe Stress or Stress Reaction

You do not need specialized training to recognize severe stress or stress reaction that will cause problems for the service member, the unit, or the mission. Reactions that are less severe, however, are more difficult to detect. To determine whether a person needs help, you must observe him to see whether he is doing something meaningful, performing his duties, taking care of himself, behaving in an unusual fashion, or acting out of character.

8-11. Application of Psychological First Aid

The emotionally disturbed service member has built a barrier against fear. He does this for his own protection, although he is probably not aware that he is doing it. If he finds that he does not have to be afraid and that there are normal, understandable things about him, he will feel safer in dropping this barrier. Persistent efforts to make him realize that you want to understand him will be reassuring, especially if you remain calm. Nothing can cause an emotionally disturbed person to become even more fearful than feeling that others are afraid of him. Try to remain calm. Familiar things, such as a cup of coffee, the use of his name, attention to a minor wound, being given a simple job to do, or the sight of familiar people and activities, will add to his ability to overcome his fear. He may not respond well if you get excited, angry, or abrupt.

a. *Ventilation.* After the service member becomes calmer, he is likely to have dreams about the stressful event. He also may think about it when he is awake or even repeat his personal reaction to the event. One benefit of this natural pattern is that it helps him master the stress by going over it just as one masters the initial fear of parachuting from an aircraft by doing it over and over again. Eventually, it is difficult to remember how frightening the event was initially. In giving first aid to the emotionally disturbed service member, you should let him follow this natural pattern. Encourage him to talk. Be a good listener. Let him tell, in his own words, what actually happened. If home front problems or worries have contributed to the stress, it will help him to talk about them. Your patient listening will prove to him that you are interested in him, and by describing his personal problem, he can work at mastering his fear. If he becomes overwhelmed in the telling, suggest a cup of coffee or a break. Whatever you do, assure him that you will listen again as soon as he is ready. Do try to help put the service member's perception of what happened back into realistic perspective; but DO NOT argue about it.

b. *Activity.*

(1) A person who is emotionally disturbed as the result of a combat action is a casualty of anxiety and fear. He is disabled because he has become temporarily overwhelmed by his anxiety. A good way to control fear is through activity. Almost all service members, for example, experience a considerable sense of anxiety and fear while they are poised, awaiting the opening of a big offensive; but this is normally relieved, and they actually feel better once they begin to move into action. They take pride in effective performance and pleasure in knowing that they are good service members, perhaps being completely unaware that overcoming their initial fear was their first major accomplishment.

(2) Useful activity is very beneficial to the emotionally disturbed service member who is not physically incapacitated. After you help a service member get over his initial fear, help him to regain some self-confidence. Make him realize his job is continuing by finding him something useful to do. Encourage him to be active. Get him to help load trucks, clean up debris, or dig fighting positions. If possible, get him back to his usual duty. Seek out his strong points and help him apply them. Avoid having him just sit around. You may have to provide direction by telling him what to do and where to do it. The instructions should be clear and simple and should be repeated. A person who has panicked is likely to argue. Respect his feelings, but point out more immediate, obtainable, and demanding needs. Channel his excessive energy and, above all, DO NOT argue. If you cannot get him interested in doing more profitable work, it may be necessary to enlist aid in controlling his overactivity before it spreads to the group and

results in more panic. Prevent the spread of such infectious feelings by restraining and segregating if necessary.

(3) Involvement in activity helps a service member in three ways; he—

- Forgets himself.
- Has an outlet for his excessive tensions.
- Proves to himself he can do something useful.

c. *Rest.* There are times, particularly in combat, when physical exhaustion is a principal cause for emotional reactions. A unit sleep plan should be established and implemented. When possible, service members should be given a safe and relatively comfortable area in which to sleep. Examples would be an area away from heavy traffic, noise, and congestion or a place that is clean and dry and protected from environmental conditions. The more uninterrupted sleep a service member gets the better he will be able to function in the tactical environment.

d. *Hygiene.* Field hygiene is an important ingredient in a service member's morale. A service member who is dirty and unkempt will not function as well as a service member who has had the opportunity to bathe and put on clean, dry clothing. During combat, unit leaders should stress the importance of personal hygiene. Good personal hygiene not only improves morale, it also is a preventive measure against disease and nonbattle injury (DNBI).

e. *Group Activity.* You have probably already noticed that a person works, faces danger, and handles serious problems better if he is a member of a closely-knit group. Each service member in the team supports the other team members. Esprit de corps is built because the service members have the same interests, goals, and mission, and as a result they are more productive; furthermore, they are less worried because everyone is involved. It is this spirit that takes a strategic hill in battle. It is so powerful that it is one of the most effective tools you have in your *psychological first aid bag*. Getting the service member back into the team or squad activities will reestablish his sense of belonging and security and will go far toward making him a useful member of the unit.

8-12. Reactions and Limitations

Up to this point the discussion has been primarily about the feelings of the emotionally distressed service member. What about your feelings toward him? Whatever the situation, you will have emotional reactions (conscious or unconscious) toward this service member. Your reactions can either help or hinder your ability to help him. When you are tired or worried, you may very easily become impatient with him if he is unusually slow or exaggerates. You may even feel resentful toward him. At times when many physically wounded lie about you, it will be especially natural for you to resent disabilities that you cannot see. Physical wounds can be seen and easily accepted. Emotional reactions are more difficult to accept as injuries. On the other hand, will you tend to be overly sympathetic? Excessive sympathy for an incapacitated person can be as harmful as negative feelings in your relationship with him. He needs strong help, but not your sorrow. To overwhelm him with pity will make him feel even more inadequate. You must expect your buddy to recover, to be able to return to duty, and to become a useful service member again. This expectation should be displayed in your behavior and attitude as well as in what you say. If he can see your calmness, confidence, and competence, he will be reassured and will feel a sense of greater security.

8-13. Stress Reactions

See Tables 8-1, 8-2, and 8-3 for more information.

Table 8-1. Mild Stress Reaction

PHYSICAL SIGNS*	EMOTIONAL SIGNS*
1. TREMBLING, TEARFUL 2. JUMPINESS, NERVOUSNESS 3. COLD SWEAT, DRY MOUTH 4. POUNDING HEART, DIZZINESS 5. INSOMNIA, NIGHTMARES 6. NAUSEA, VOMITING, DIARRHEA 7. FATIGUE 8. THOUSAND-YARD STARE 9. DIFFICULTY THINKING, SPEAKING, AND COMMUNICATING	1. ANXIETY, INDECISIVENESS 2. IRRITABLE, COMPLAINING 3. FORGETFUL, UNABLE TO CONCENTRATE 4. EASILY STARTLED BY NOISE, MOVEMENT 5. GRIEF, TEARFUL 6. ANGER, BEGINNING TO LOSE CONFIDENCE IN SELF AND UNIT

SELF- AND BUDDY AID
1. CONTINUE MISSION PERFORMANCE, FOCUS ON IMMEDIATE MISSION. 2. EXPECT SERVICE MEMBER TO PERFORM ASSIGNED DUTIES. 3. REMAIN CALM AT ALL TIMES; BE DIRECTIVE AND IN CONTROL. 4. LET SERVICE MEMBER KNOW HIS REACTION IS NORMAL, AND THAT THERE IS NOTHING SERIOUSLY WRONG WITH HIM. 5. KEEP SERVICE MEMBER INFORMED OF THE SITUATION, OBJECTIVES, EXPECTATIONS, AND SUPPORT. CONTROL RUMORS. 6. BUILD SERVICE MEMBER'S CONFIDENCE, TALK ABOUT SUCCEEDING. 7. KEEP SERVICE MEMBER PRODUCTIVE (WHEN NOT RESTING) THROUGH RECREATIONAL ACTIVITIES, EQUIPMENT MAINTENANCE.

8. ENSURE SERVICE MEMBER MAINTAINS GOOD PERSONAL HYGIENE.
9. ENSURE SERVICE MEMBER EATS, DRINKS, AND SLEEPS AS SOON AS POSSIBLE.
10. LET SERVICE MEMBER TALK ABOUT HIS FEELINGS. DO NOT "PUT DOWN" HIS FEELINGS OF GRIEF OR WORRY. GIVE PRACTICAL ADVICE AND PUT EMOTIONS INTO PERSPECTIVE.

* MOST OR ALL OF THESE SIGNS ARE PRESENT IN MILD STRESS REACTION. THEY CAN BE PRESENT IN ANY NORMAL SERVICE MEMBER IN COMBAT YET HE CAN STILL DO HIS JOB.

Table 8-2. More Serious Stress Reaction

PHYSICAL SIGNS*	EMOTIONAL SIGNS*
1. CONSTANTLY MOVES AROUND 2. FLINCHING OR DUCKING AT SUDDEN SOUNDS 3. SHAKING, TREMBLING (WHOLE BODY OR ARMS) 4. CANNOT USE PART OF BODY, NO PHYSICAL REASON (HAND, ARM, LEGS) 5. CANNOT SEE, HEAR, OR FEEL (PARTIAL OR COMPLETE LOSS) 6. PHYSICAL EXHAUSTION, CRYING 7. FREEZING UNDER FIRE, OR TOTAL IMMOBILITY 8. VACANT STARES, STAGGERS, SWAYS WHEN STANDS 9. PANIC RUNNING UNDER FIRE	1. RAPID AND/OR INAPPROPRIATE TALKING 2. ARGUMENTATIVE, RECKLESS MOVEMENTS/ACTIONS 3. INATTENTIVE TO PERSONAL HYGIENE 4. INDIFFERENT TO DANGER 5. MEMORY LOSS 6. SEVERE STUTTERING, MUMBLING, OR CANNOT SPEAK AT ALL 7. INSOMNIA, NIGHTMARES 8. SEEING OR HEARING THINGS THAT DO NOT EXIST 9. RAPID EMOTIONAL SHIFTS 10. SOCIAL WITHDRAWAL 11. APATHETIC 12. HYSTERICAL OUTBURSTS 13. FRANTIC OR STRANGE BEHAVIOR

TREATMENT PROCEDURES**

1. IF A SERVICE MEMBER'S BEHAVIOR ENDANGERS THE MISSION, SELF, OR OTHERS, DO WHATEVER IS NECESSARY TO CONTROL HIM.
2. IF THE SERVICE MEMBER IS UPSET, CALMLY TALK HIM INTO COOPERATING.
3. IF CONCERNED ABOUT THE SERVICE MEMBER'S RELIABILITY:
   - UNLOAD HIS WEAPON.
   - TAKE WEAPON IF SERIOUSLY CONCERNED.
   - PHYSICALLY RESTRAIN HIM ONLY WHEN NECESSARY FOR SAFETY OR TRANSPORTATION.
4. REASSURE EVERYONE THAT THE SIGNS ARE PROBABLY JUST STRESS REACTION AND WILL QUICKLY IMPROVE.
5. IF STRESS REACTION SIGNS CONTINUE:
   - GET THE SERVICE MEMBER TO A SAFER PLACE.
   - DO NOT LEAVE THE SERVICE MEMBER ALONE, KEEP SOMEONE HE KNOWS WITH HIM.
   - NOTIFY SENIOR NONCOMMISSIONED OFFICER (NCO) OR OFFICER.
   - HAVE THE SERVICE MEMBER EXAMINED BY MEDICAL PERSONNEL.

Table 8-2. More Serious Stress Reaction (Continued)

TREATMENT PROCEDURES**
6. GIVE THE SERVICE MEMBER EASY TASKS TO DO WHEN NOT SLEEPING, EATING, OR RESTING. 7. ASSURE THE SERVICE MEMBER HE WILL RETURN TO FULL DUTY IN 24 HOURS; AND, RETURN HIM TO NORMAL DUTIES AS SOON AS HE IS READY.
* THESE SIGNS ARE PRESENT IN ADDITION TO THE SIGNS OF MILD STRESS REACTION. ** DO THESE PROCEDURES IN ADDITION TO THE SELF- AND BUDDY AID CARE.

Table 8-3. Preventive Measures to Combat Stress Reaction

1. WELCOME NEW MEMBERS INTO YOUR TEAM, GET TO KNOW THEM QUICKLY. IF YOU ARE NEW, BE ACTIVE IN MAKING FRIENDS.
2. BE PHYSICALLY FIT (STRENGTH, ENDURANCE, AND AGILITY).
3. KNOW AND PRACTICE LIFESAVING SELF- AND BUDDY AID.
4. PRACTICE RAPID RELAXATION TECHNIQUES (FM 22-51).
5. HELP EACH OTHER OUT WHEN THINGS ARE TOUGH AT HOME OR IN THE UNIT.
6. KEEP INFORMED; ASK YOUR LEADER QUESTIONS, IGNORE RUMORS.
7. WORK TOGETHER TO GIVE EVERYONE FOOD, WATER, SHELTER, HYGIENE, AND SANITATION.
8. SLEEP WHEN MISSION AND SAFETY PERMIT; LET EVERYONE GET TIME TO SLEEP.
   - SLEEP ONLY IN SAFE PLACES AND BY STANDING OPERATING PROCEDURE (SOP).
   - IF POSSIBLE, SLEEP 6 TO 9 HOURS PER DAY.
   - TRY TO GET AT LEAST 4 HOURS SLEEP PER DAY.
   - GET GOOD SLEEP BEFORE GOING ON SUSTAINED OPERATIONS.
   - CATNAP WHEN YOU CAN, BUT ALLOW TIME TO WAKE UP FULLY.
   - CATCH UP ON SLEEP AFTER GOING WITHOUT.

APPENDIX A

FIRST AID CASE AND KITS, DRESSINGS, AND BANDAGES

A-1. First Aid Case with Field Dressings and Bandages

Every service member is issued a first aid case (Figure A-1A) with a field first aid dressing encased in a plastic wrapper (Figure A-1B). He carries it at all times for his use. The field first aid dressing is a standard sterile (germ-free) compress or pad with bandages attached (Figure A-1C). This dressing is used to cover the wound, to protect against further contamination, and to stop bleeding (pressure dressing). When a service member administers first aid to another person, he must remember to use the wounded person's dressing; he may need his own later. The service member must check his first aid case regularly and replace any used or missing dressing. The field first aid dressing may normally be obtained from his unit supply.

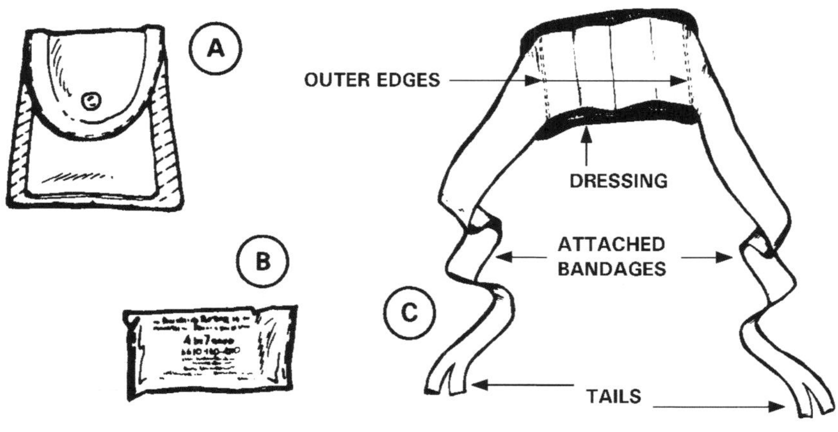

Figure A-1. Field first aid case and dressing (Illustrated A—C).

A-2. General Purpose First Aid Kits

General-purpose first aid kits are listed in the common table of allowances (CTA) 8-100. The operators, crew, and passengers carry these kits on Army vehicles, aircraft, and boats for use. Individuals designated by unit TSOP to be responsible for these kits are required to check them regularly and replace all items used. The general-purpose kit and its contents can be obtained through the unit supply system.

NOTE

Periodically check the dressings (for holes or tears in the packaging) and the medicines (for expiration date) that are in the first aid kits. If necessary, replace defective or outdated items.

A-3. Dressings

Dressings are sterile pads or compresses used to cover wounds. They usually are made of gauze or cotton wrapped in gauze (Figure A-1C). In addition to the standard field first aid dressing, other dressings such as sterile gauze compresses and small sterile compresses on adhesive strips may be available under CTA 8-100.

A-4. Standard Bandages

a. Standard bandages are made of gauze or muslin and are used over a sterile dressing to secure the dressing in place, to close off its edge from dirt and germs, and to create pressure on the wound and control bleeding. A bandage can also support an injured part or secure a splint.

b. Tailed bandages may be attached to the dressing as indicated on the field first aid dressing (Figure A-1C).

A-5. Triangular and Cravat (Swathe) Bandages

a. Triangular and cravat (or swathe) bandages (Figure A-2) are fashioned from a triangular piece of muslin (37 by 37 by 52 inches) provided in the general-purpose first aid kit. If it is folded into a strip, it is called a cravat. Two safety pins are packaged with each bandage. These bandages are valuable in an emergency since they are easily applied.

b. To improvise a triangular bandage, cut a square of available material, slightly larger than 3 feet by 3 feet, and *fold it diagonally*. If two bandages are needed, cut the material along the diagonal fold.

c. A cravat can be improvised from such common items as T-shirts, other shirts, bed linens, trouser legs, scarfs, or any other item made of pliable and durable material that can be folded, torn, or cut to the desired size.

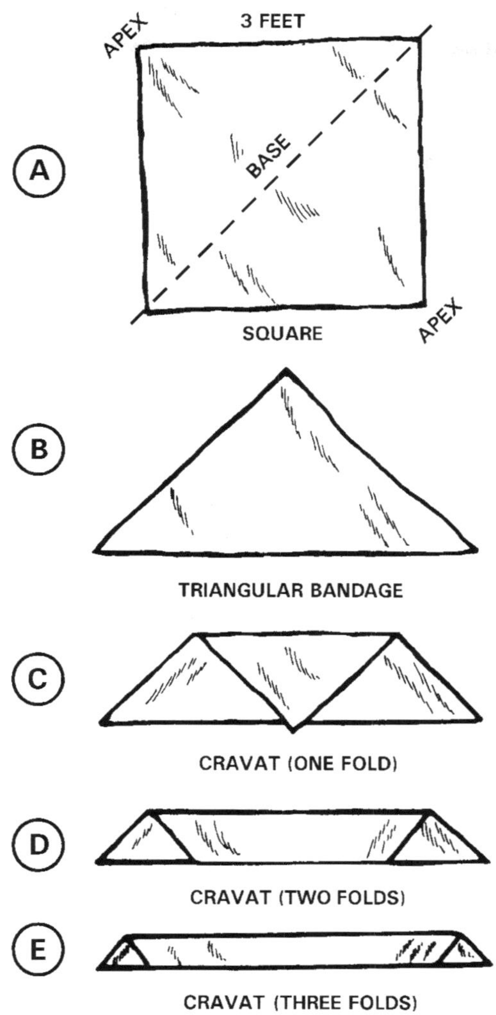

Figure A-2. Triangular and cravat bandages (Illustrated A—E).

APPENDIX B

RESCUE AND TRANSPORTATION PROCEDURES

B-1. General

A basic principle of first aid is to evaluate the casualty's injuries and administer first aid before moving him. However, adverse situations or conditions may jeopardize the lives of both the rescuer and the casualty if this is done. It may be necessary *first to rescue* the casualty before first aid can be effectively or safely given. The life and/or the well-being of the casualty will depend as much upon the manner in which he is *rescued and transported,* as it will upon the first aid and medical treatment he receives. Rescue actions must be done quickly and safely. Careless or rough handling of the casualty during rescue operations can aggravate his injuries.

B-2. Principles of Rescue Operations

a. When faced with the necessity of rescuing a casualty who is threatened by hostile action, fire, water, or any other immediate hazard, DO NOT take action without first determining the extent of the hazard and your ability to handle the situation. DO NOT become a casualty.

b. The rescuer must evaluate the situation and analyze the factors involved. This evaluation involves three major steps:

- Identify the task.
- Evaluate circumstances of the rescue.
- Plan the action.

B-3. Considerations

a. First determine if a rescue attempt is actually needed. It is a waste of time, equipment, and personnel to rescue someone not in need of rescuing. It is also a waste to look for someone who is not lost or needlessly risk the lives of the rescuer(s). In planning a rescue, attempt to obtain the following information:

- Who, what, where, when, why, and how the situation happened?

- How many casualties are involved and the nature of their injuries?

- What is the tactical situation?

- What are the terrain features and the location of the casualties?

- Will there be adequate assistance available to aid in the rescue/evacuation?

- Can first aid and/or medical treatment be provided at the scene; will the casualties require movement to a safer location?

- What specialized equipment will be required for the rescue operation?

- Is the rescue area contaminated? Will decontamination equipment and materiel be required for casualties, rescue personnel, and rescue equipment?

- How much time is available?

b. The time element can play a significant role in how the rescue is attempted. If the casualties are in imminent danger of losing their lives (such as near a burning vehicle or in a burning building) the time available will be relatively short and will sometimes cause a rescuer to compromise planning stages and/or the first aid which can be given. However, if the casualty is in a relatively secure area and his physical condition is strong, more deliberate planning can take place. A realistic estimate of time available must be made as quickly as possible to determine action time remaining. The key elements are the casualty's physical and mental condition, the tactical situation, and the environment.

B-4. Plan of Action

a. The casualty's ability to endure is of primary importance in estimating the time available. Age, physical condition, and extent of wounds and/or injuries will differ from casualty to casualty. Therefore, to determine the time available, you will have to consider—

- Endurance time of the casualty.

- Extent of injuries.

- Type of situation.
- Personnel and/or equipment availability.
- Weather.
- Terrain (natural and man-made).
- Environment (contaminated or uncontaminated).

b. In respect to terrain, you must consider altitude and visibility. In some cases, the casualty may be of assistance because he knows more about the particular terrain or situation than you do. Maximum use of secure/reliable trails or roads is essential.

c. When taking weather into account, ensure that blankets and/or rain gear are available. Even a mild rain can complicate a normally simple rescue. In high altitudes and/or extreme cold and gusting winds, the time available is critically shortened. Be prepared to provide shelter and warmth for the casualty as well as the rescuers.

B-5. Proper Handling of Casualties

a. You may have saved the casualty's life through the application of appropriate first aid measures. However, his life can be lost through rough handling or careless transportation procedures. Before you attempt to move the casualty—

- Evaluate the type and extent of his injuries.
- Ensure that dressings over wounds are adequately reinforced.
- Ensure that fractured bones are properly immobilized and supported to prevent them from cutting through muscle, blood vessels, and skin.

b. Based upon your evaluation of the type and extent of the casualty's injury and your knowledge of the various manual carries, you must select the best possible method of manual transportation. If the casualty is conscious, tell him how he is to be transported. This will help allay his fear of movement and gain his cooperation and confidence.

c. Buddy aid for chemical agent casualties includes those actions required to prevent an incapacitated casualty from receiving additional injury from the effects of chemical hazards. If a casualty is physically unable to decontaminate himself or administer the proper chemical agent antidote, the casualty's buddy assists him and assumes responsibility for his care. Buddy-aid includes—

- Administering the proper chemical agent antidote.
- Decontaminating the incapacitated casualty's exposed skin.
- Ensuring that his protective ensemble remains correctly emplaced.
- Maintaining respiration.
- Controlling bleeding.
- Providing other standard first aid measures
- Transporting the casualty out of the contaminated area.

B-6. Positioning the Casualty

The first step in any manual carry is to position the casualty to be lifted. If he is conscious, he should be told how he is to be positioned and transported. This helps lessen his fear of movement and to gain his cooperation. It may be necessary to roll the casualty onto his abdomen, or his back, depending upon the position in which he is lying and the particular carry to be used.

a. To roll a casualty onto his abdomen, kneel at the casualty's uninjured side.

(1) Place his arms above his head; cross his ankle which is farther from you over the one that is closer to you.

(2) Place your hands on the shoulder which is farther from you; place your other hand in the area of his hip or thigh (Figure B-1).

(3) Roll him gently toward you onto his abdomen (Figure B-2).

b. To roll a casualty onto his back, follow the same procedure described in *a* above, except gently roll the casualty onto his back, rather than onto his abdomen.

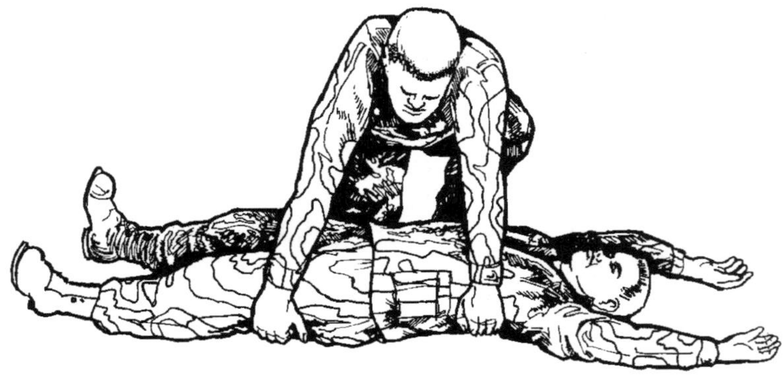

Figure B-1. Positioning the casualty.

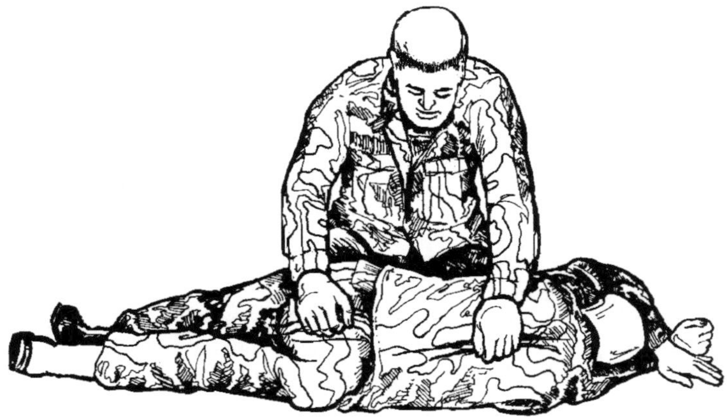

Figure B-2. Rolling casualty onto his abdomen.

B-7. Medical Evacuation and Transportation of Casualties

a. Medical evacuation of the sick and wounded (with en route medical care) is the responsibility of medical personnel who have been provided special training and equipment. Therefore, unless a good reason for you to transport a casualty arises, wait for some means of medical evacuation to be provided. When the situation is urgent and you are unable to obtain medical assistance or know that no medical evacuation assets are available, you will have to transport the casualty. For this reason, you must know how to transport him without increasing the seriousness of his condition.

b. Transporting a casualty by litter (FM 8-10-6) is safer and more comfortable for him than by manual means; it is also easier for you.

Manual transportation, however, may be the only feasible method because of the terrain or the combat situation; or it may be necessary to save a life. In these situations, the casualty should be transferred to a litter as soon as one can be made available or improvised.

B-8. Manual Carries

Casualties carried by manual means must be carefully and correctly handled, otherwise their injuries may become more serious or possibly fatal. Situation permitting, transport of a casualty should be organized and unhurried. Each movement should be performed as deliberately and gently as possible. Casualties should not be moved before the type and extent of injuries are evaluated and the required first aid is administered. The exception to this occurs when the situation dictates immediate movement for safety purposes (for example, it may be necessary to remove a casualty from a burning vehicle); that is, the situation dictates that the urgency of casualty movement outweighs the need to administer first aid. Manual carries are tiring for the bearers and involve the risk of increasing the severity of the casualty's injury. In some instances, however, they are essential to save the casualty's life. Although manual carries are accomplished by one or two bearers, the two-man carries are used whenever possible. They provide more comfort to the casualty, are less likely to aggravate his injuries, and are also less tiring for the bearers. The distance a casualty can be carried depends on many factors, such as—

- Nature of the casualty's injuries.
- Strength and endurance of the bearer(s).
- Weight of the casualty.
- Obstacles encountered during transport (natural or manmade).
- Type of terrain.

a. One-man Carries. These carries should be used when only one bearer is available to transport the casualty.

(1) The *fireman's carry* (Figure B-3) is one of the easiest ways for one individual to carry another. After an unconscious or disabled casualty has been properly positioned, he is raised from the ground, then supported and placed in the carrying position.

(*a*) After rolling the casualty onto his abdomen, straddle him. Extend your hands under his chest and lock them together.

(*b*) Lift the casualty to his knees as you move backward.

(*c*) Continue to move backward, thus straightening the casualty's legs and locking his knees.

(*d*) Walk forward, bringing the casualty to a standing position; tilt him slightly backward to prevent his knees from buckling.

(*e*) As you maintain constant support of the casualty with one arm, free your other arm, quickly grasp his wrist, and raise his arm high. Instantly pass your head under his raised arm, releasing it as you pass under it.

(*f*) Move swiftly to face the casualty and secure your arms around his waist. Immediately place your foot between his feet and spread them apart (approximately 6 to 8 inches).

(*g*) Grasp the casualty's wrist and raise his arm high over your head.

(*h*) Bend down and pull the casualty's arm over and down on your shoulder, bringing his body across your shoulders. At the same time, pass your arm between his legs.

(*i*) Grasp the casualty's wrist with one hand, and place your other hand on your knee for support.

(*j*) Rise with the casualty positioned correctly. Your other hand is free for use.

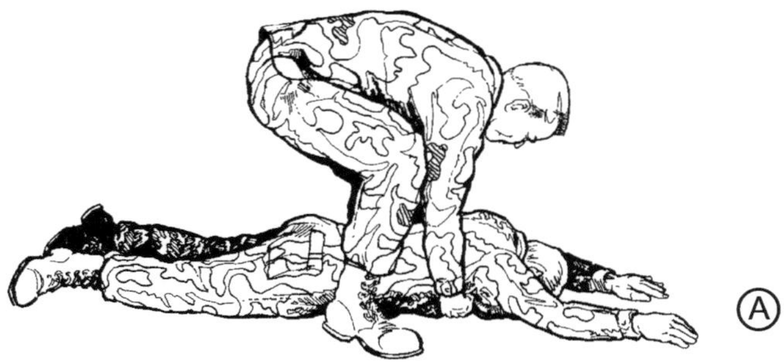

Figure B-3. Fireman's carry (Illustrated A—J).

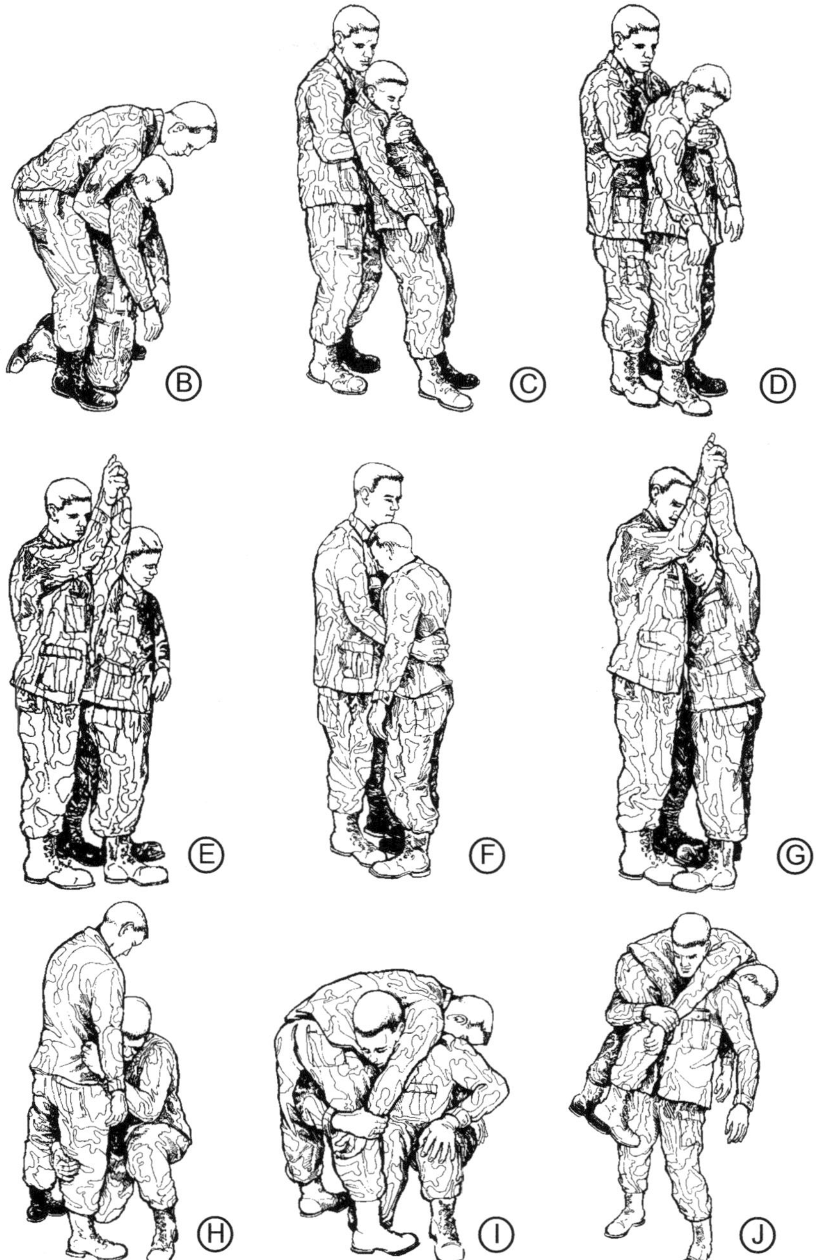

Figure B-3. Fireman's carry (Illustrated A—J) (Continued).

(2) The alternate method of the *fireman's carry* for raising a casualty from the ground is illustrated in Figure B-4; however, it should be used only when the bearer believes it to be safer for the casualty because of the location of his wounds. When the alternate method is used, care must be taken to prevent the casualty's head from snapping back and causing a neck injury. The steps for raising a casualty from the ground for the fireman's carry are also used in other one-man carries.

(*a*) Kneel on one knee at the casualty's head and face his feet. Extend your hands under his armpits, down his sides, and across his back.

(*b*) As you rise, lift the casualty to his knees. Then secure a lower hold and raise him to a standing position with his knees locked.

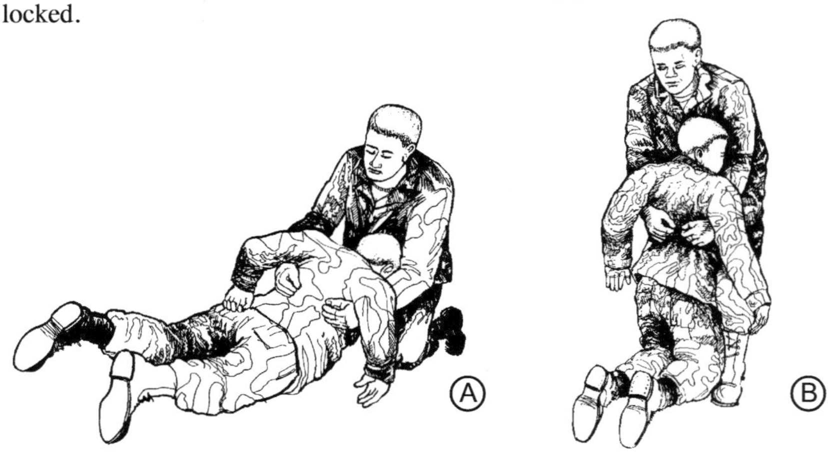

Figure B-4. Fireman's carry (alternate method) for lifting a casualty to a standing position (Illustrated A—B).

(3) In the *supporting carry* (Figure B-5), the casualty must be able to walk or at least hop on one leg, using the bearer as a crutch. This carry can be used to assist him as far as he is able to walk or hop.

(*a*) Raise the casualty from the ground to a standing position by using the fireman's carry.

(*b*) Grasp the casualty's wrist and draw his arm around your neck.

(*c*) Place your arm around his waist. The casualty is now able to walk or hop using you as a support.

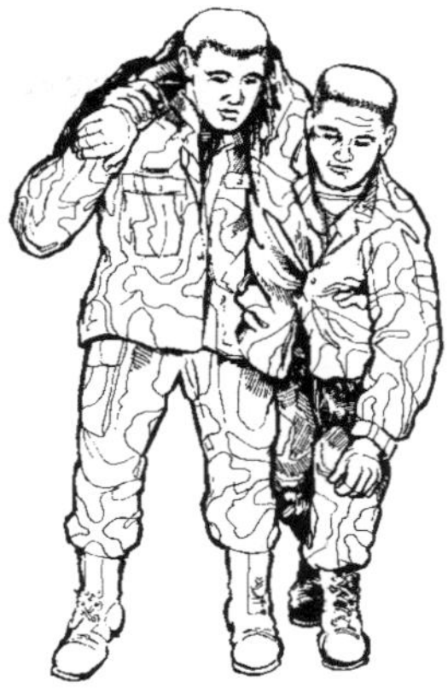

Figure B-5. Supporting carry.

(4) The *arms carry* (Figure B-6) is useful in carrying a casualty for a short distance (up to 50 meters) and for placing him on a litter.

(*a*) Raise or lift the casualty from the ground to a standing position, as in the fireman's carry.

(*b*) Place one arm under the casualty's knees and your other arm around his back.

(*c*) Lift the casualty.

(*d*) Carry the casualty high to lessen fatigue.

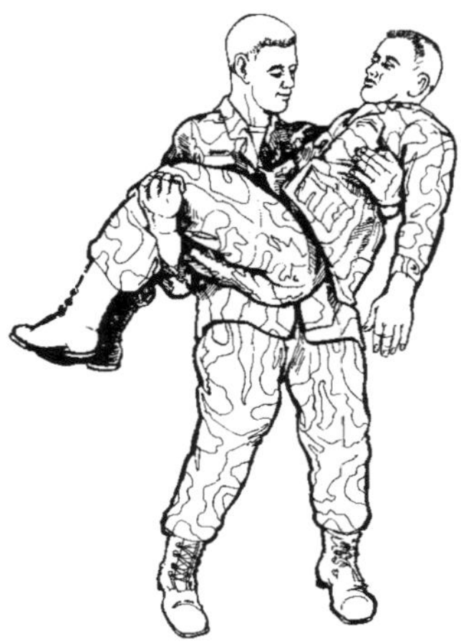

Figure B-6. Arms carry.

(5) Only a conscious casualty can be transported by the *saddleback carry* (Figure B-7), because he must be able to hold onto the bearer's neck. To use this technique—

(*a*) Raise the casualty to an upright position, as in the fireman's carry.

(*b*) Support the casualty by placing an arm around his waist. Move to the casualty's side. Have the casualty put his arm around your neck and move in front of him with your back to support him.

(*c*) Have the casualty encircle his arms around your neck

(*d*) Stoop, raise him on your back and clasp your hands together beneath his thighs, if possible.

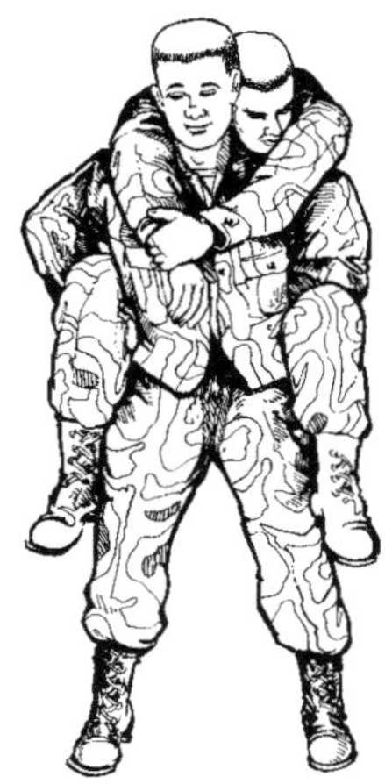

Figure B-7. Saddleback carry.

(6) In the *pack-strap carry* (Figure B-8), the casualty's weight rests high on the your back. This makes it easier for you to carry the casualty a moderate distance (50 to 300 meters). To eliminate the possibility of injury to the casualty's arms, you must hold his arms in a palms-down position.

(*a*) Lift the casualty from the ground to a standing position, as in the fireman's carry.

(*b*) Support the casualty with your arms around him and grasp his wrist closer to you.

(*c*) Place his arm over your head and across your shoulders.

(*d*) Move in front of him while still supporting his weight against your back.

(*e*) Grasp his other wrist and place this arm over your shoulder.

(*f*) Bend forward and raise or hoist the casualty as high on your back as possible so that his weight is resting on your back.

NOTE

Once the casualty is positioned on the bearer's back, the bearer remains as erect as possible to prevent straining or injuring his back.

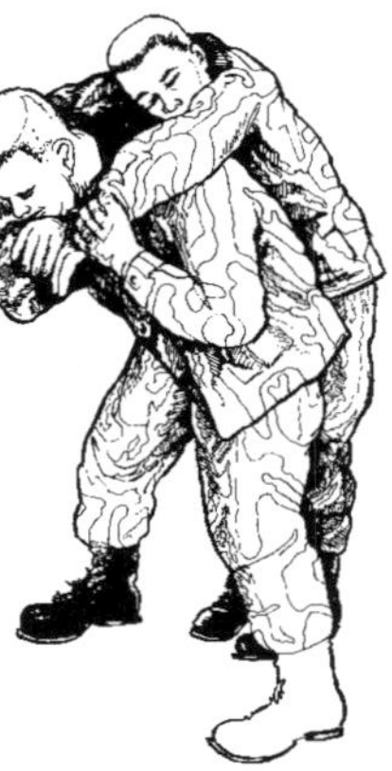

Figure B-8. Pack-strap carry.

(7) The *pistol-belt carry* (Figure B-9) is the best one-man carry for a long distance (over 300 meters). The casualty is securely supported upon your shoulders by a belt. Both your hands and the casualty's (if conscious) are free for carrying a weapon or equipment, or climbing obstacles. With your hands free and the casualty secured in place, you are also able to creep through shrubs and under low-hanging branches.

(*a*) Link two pistol belts (or three, if necessary) together to form a sling. Place the sling under the casualty's thighs and lower back so that a loop extends from each side.

NOTE

If pistol belts are not available for use, other items such as a rifle sling, two cravat bandages, two litter straps, or any other suitable material, which will not cut or bind the casualty may be used.

(*b*) Lie face up between the casualty's outstretched legs. Thrust your arms through the loops and grasp his hands and trouser leg on his injured side.

(*c*) Roll toward the casualty's uninjured side onto your abdomen, bringing him onto your back. Adjust the sling, if necessary.

(*d*) Rise to a kneeling position. The belt will hold the casualty in place.

(*e*) Place one hand on your knee for support and rise to an upright position. (The casualty is supported on your shoulders.)

(*f*) Carry the casualty with your hands free for use in rifle firing, climbing, or surmounting obstacles.

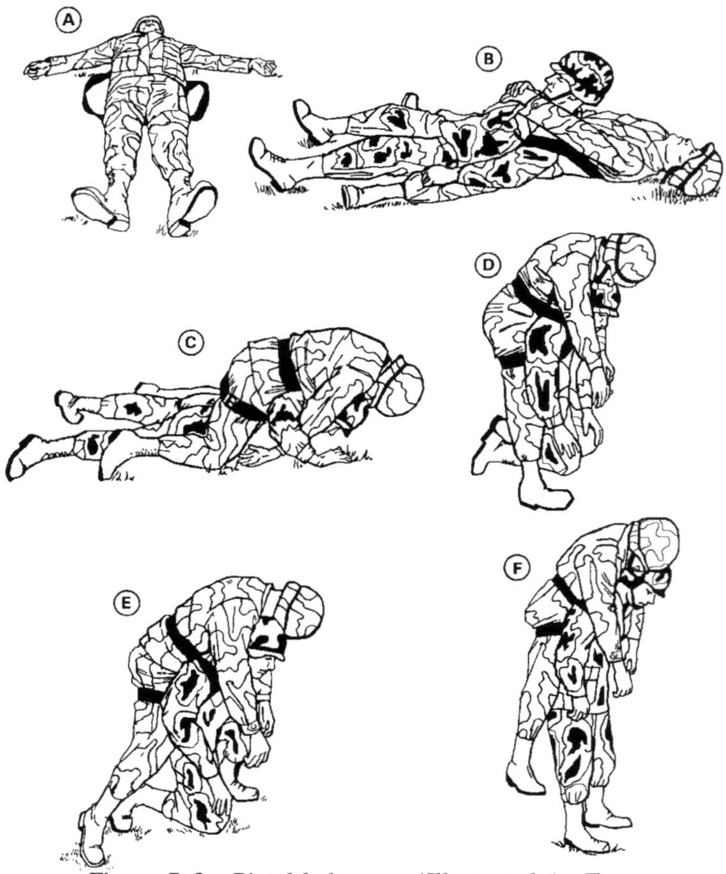

Figure B-9. Pistol-belt carry (Illustrated A—F).

(8) The *pistol-belt drag* (Figure B-10), as well as other drags, is generally used for short distances (up to 50 meters). This drag is useful in combat, since both the bearer and the casualty can remain closer to the ground than in any other drags.

(*a*) Extend two pistol belts or similar objects to their full length and join them together to make a continuous loop.

(*b*) Roll the casualty onto his back, as in the fireman's carry.

(*c*) Pass the loop over the casualty's head, and position it across his chest and under his armpits. Then cross the remaining portion of the loop, thus forming a figure eight. Keep tension on the belts so they do not come unhooked.

(*d*) Lie on your side facing the casualty.

(*e*) Slip the loop over your head and turn onto your abdomen. This enables you to drag the casualty as you crawl.

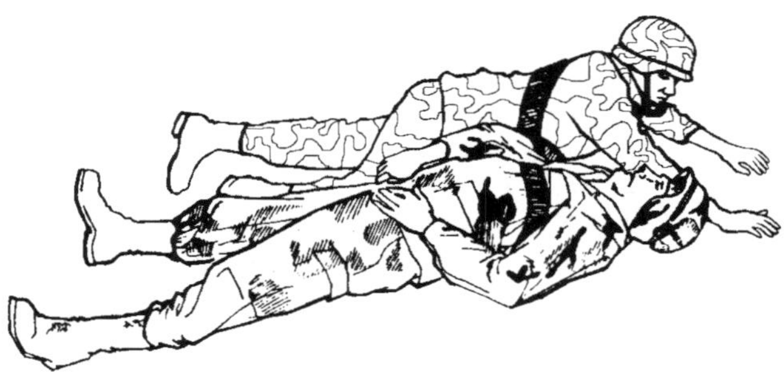

Figure B-10. Pistol-belt drag.

(9) The *neck drag* (Figure B-11) is useful in combat because the bearer can transport the casualty as he creeps behind a low wall or shrubbery, under a vehicle, or through a culvert. If the casualty is unconscious, his head must be protected from the ground. The neck drag cannot be used if the casualty has a broken arm.

NOTE

If the casualty is conscious, he may clasp his hands together around your neck.

(*a*) Tie the casualty's hands together at the wrists.

(*b*) Straddle the casualty in a kneeling face-to-face position.

(*c*) Loop the casualty's tied hands over and around your neck.

(*d*) Crawl forward dragging the casualty with you.

NOTE

If the casualty is unconscious, protect his head from the ground.

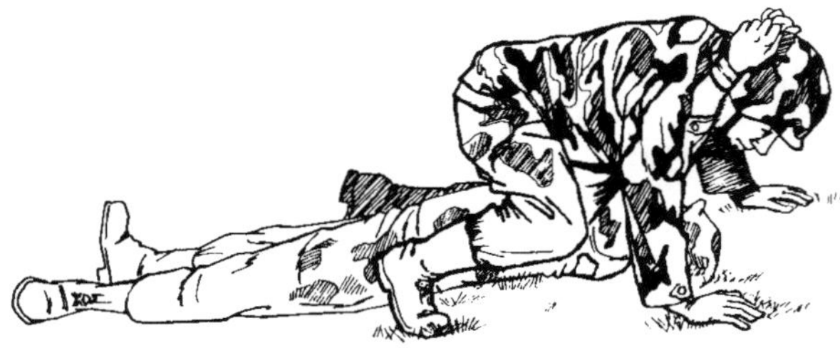

Figure B-11. Neck drag.

(10) The *cradle drop drag* (Figure B-12) is effective in moving a casualty up or down steps.

(*a*) Kneel at the casualty's head (with him lying on his back). Slide your hands, with palms up, under the casualty's shoulders and get a firm hold under his armpits.

(*b*) Rise (partially), supporting the casualty's head on one of your forearms. (You may bring your elbows together and let the casualty's head rest on both of your forearms.)

(*c*) Rise and drag the casualty backward. (The casualty is in a semisitting position.)

(*d*) Back down the steps, supporting the casualty's head and body and letting his hips and legs drop from step to step.

NOTE

If the casualty needs to be moved up the steps, you should back up the steps, using the same procedure.

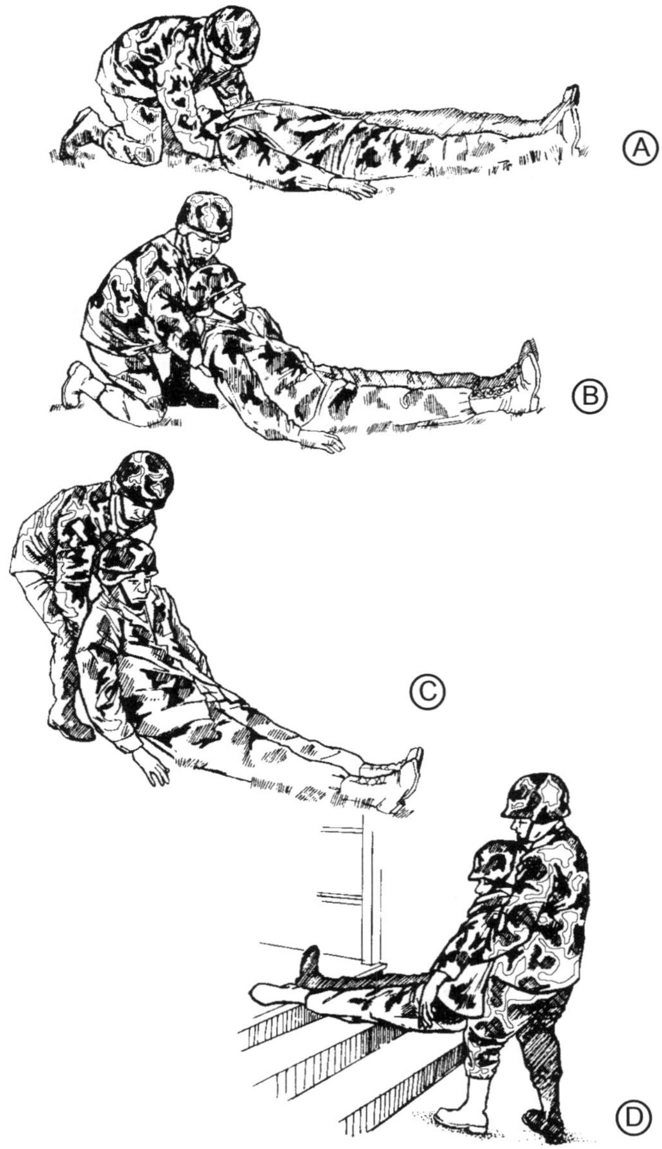

Figure B-12. Cradle-drop drag (Illustrated A—D).

(11) The *LBE carry using the bearer's LBE* can be used with a conscious casualty (Figure B-13).

(*a*) Loosen all suspenders on your LBE.

(*b*) Have the casualty place one leg into the loop formed by your suspenders and pistol belt.

(*c*) Squat in front of the standing casualty. Have him place his other leg into the loop, also.

(*d*) Have the casualty place his arms over your shoulders, lean forward onto your back, and lock his hands together.

(*e*) Stand up and lean forward into a comfortable position.

(*f*) Continue the mission.

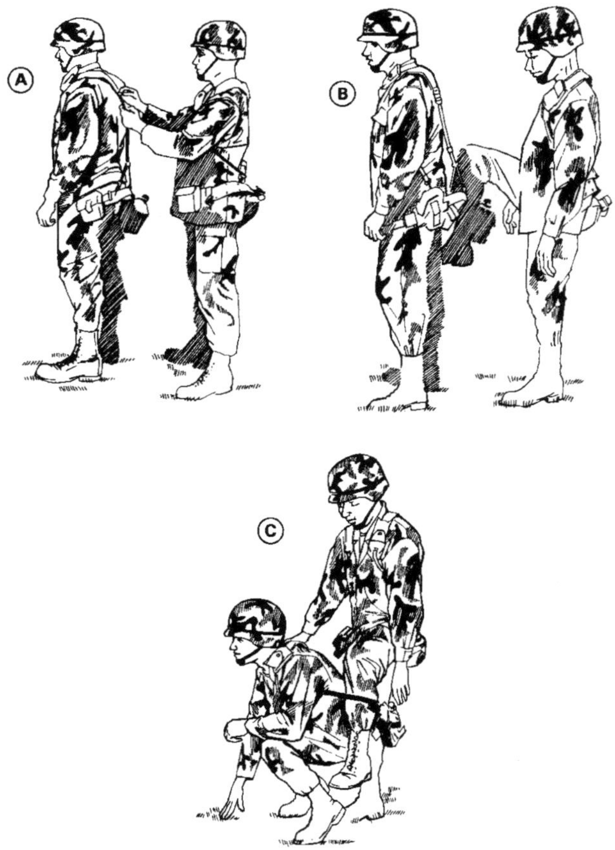

Figure B-13. Load bearing equipment carry using bearer's LBE (conscious casualty) (Illustrated A—F).

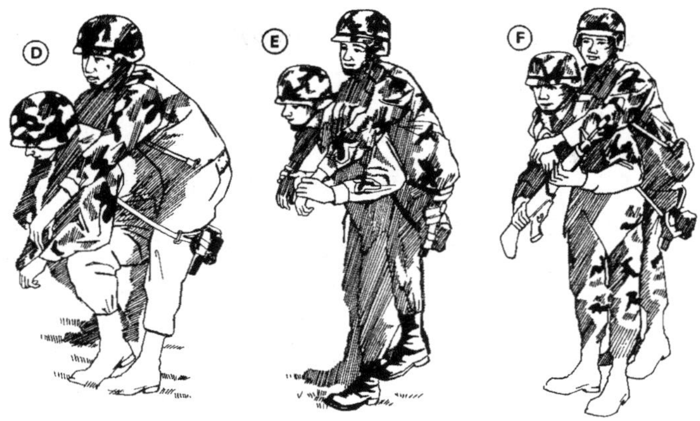

Figure B-13. Load bearing equipment carry using bearer's LBE (conscious casualty) (Illustrated A—F) (Continued).

(12) The *LBE carry using the bearer's LBE* can be used with an unconscious casualty or one who cannot stand (Figure B-14).

(*a*) Position the casualty on the flat of his back.

(*b*) Remove your LBE and loosen all suspender straps.

(*c*) Lift the casualty's leg and place it through the loop formed by your suspenders and pistol belt. Then place the other leg through the same loop. The LBE is moved up until the pistol belt is behind the casualty's thighs.

(*d*) Lay between the casualty's legs; work your arms through the LBE suspenders.

(*e*) Grasp the casualty's hand (on the injured side), and roll the casualty (on his uninjured side) onto your back.

(*f*) Rise to one knee and then push into a standing position.

(*g*) Bring the casualty's arms over your shoulders. Grasp his hands and secure them if the casualty is unconscious. If the casualty is conscious, have him lock his hands in front if he is able to do so.

(*h*) Lean forward into a comfortable position and continue the mission.

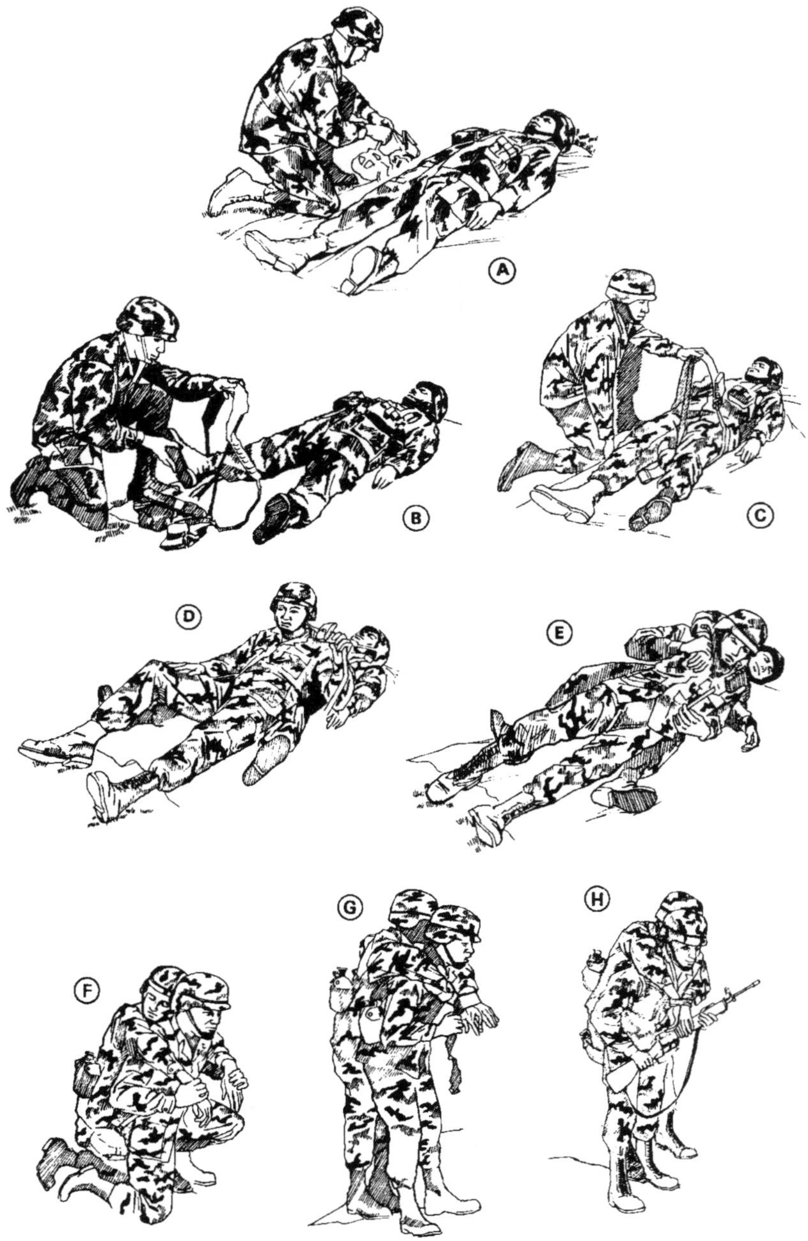

Figure B-14. Load bearing equipment carry using bearer's LBE (unconscious casualty or one that cannot stand) (Illustrated A—H).

(13) The *LBE carry using the casualty's LBE* (Figure B-15) can be used with a conscious or unconscious casualty.

(*a*) Position the casualty on his back with his LBE on.

(*b*) Loosen the casualty's two front suspenders.

(*c*) Position yourself between the casualty's legs, and slip your arms into the casualty's two front suspenders (up to your shoulders).

(*d*) Work his arms out of his LBE suspenders.

(*e*) Grasp the casualty's hand (on the injured side), and roll him (on his uninjured side) onto your back.

(*f*) Rise to one knee, then into a standing position.

(*g*) Grasp the casualty's hands and secure them, if the casualty is unconscious. Have the casualty lock his hands in front of you, if he is conscious.

(*h*) Lean forward into a comfortable position and continue the mission.

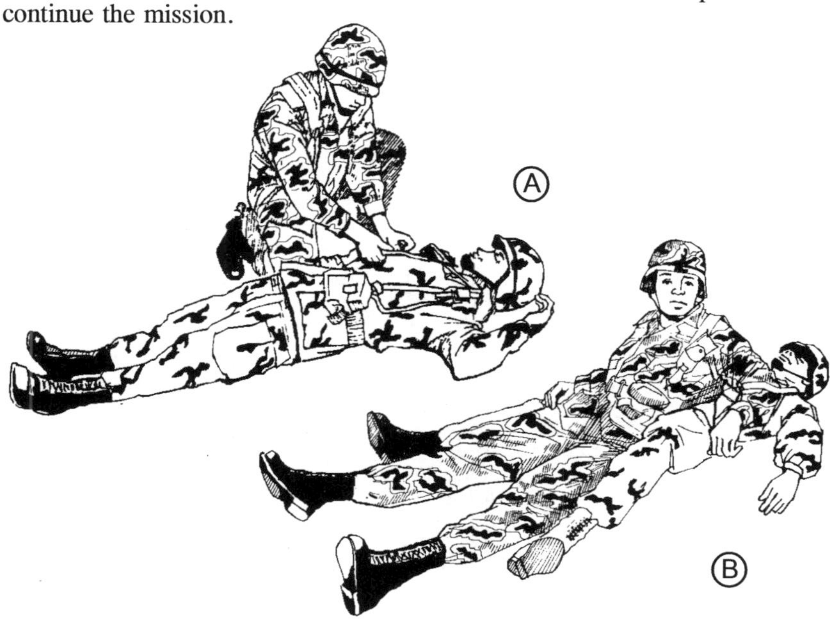

Figure B-15. Load bearing equipment carry using casualty's LBE (Illustrated A—G).

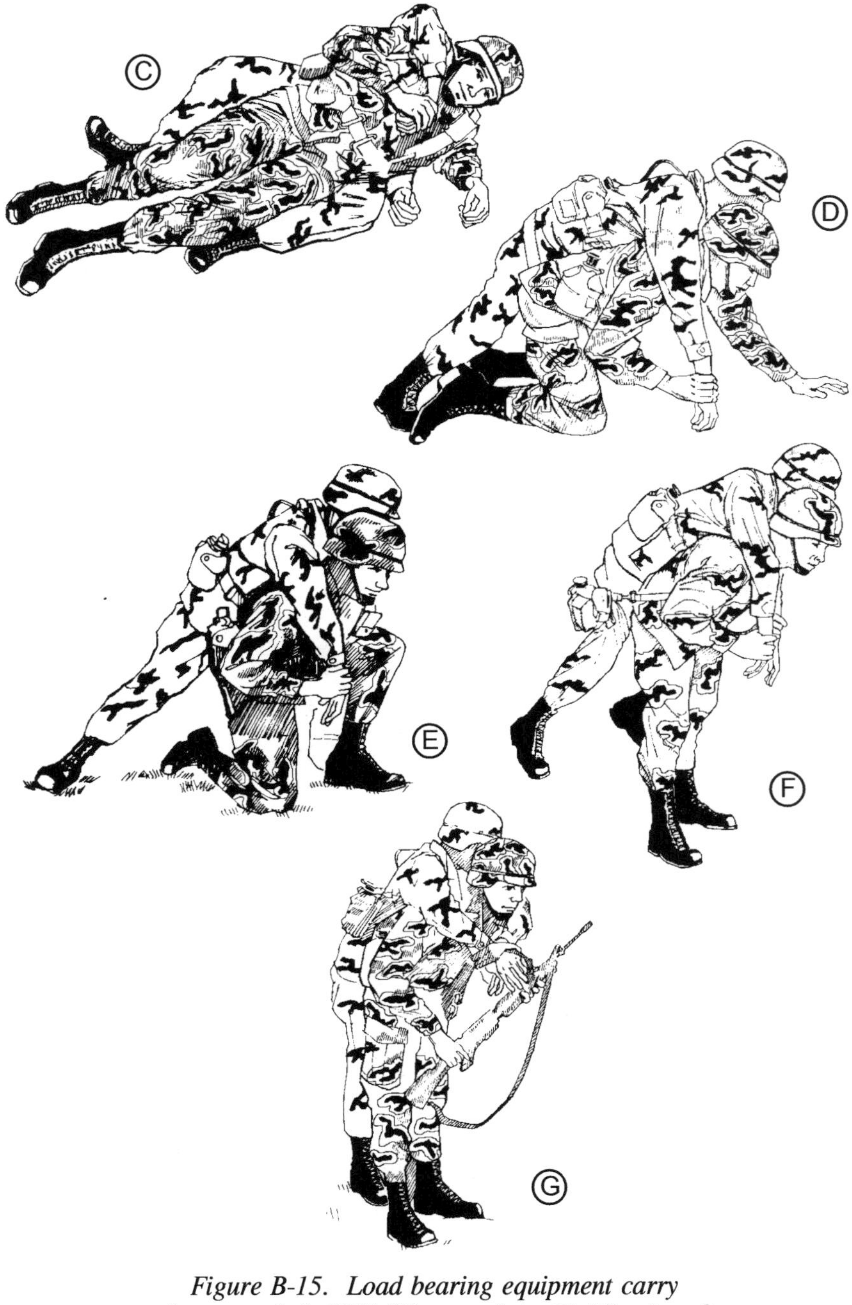

Figure B-15. Load bearing equipment carry using casualty's LBE (Illustrated A—G) (Continued).

b. *Two-man Carries.* These carries should be used whenever possible. They provide more casualty comfort, are less likely to aggravate injuries, and are less tiring for the bearers. Five different two-man carries can be used.

(1) The *two-man support carry* (Figure B-16) can be used in transporting either conscious or unconscious casualties. If the casualty is taller than the bearers, it may be necessary for the bearers to lift the casualty's legs and let them rest on their forearms. The bearers—

(*a*) Help the casualty to his feet and support him with their arms around his waist.

(*b*) Grasp the casualty's wrists and draw his arms around their necks.

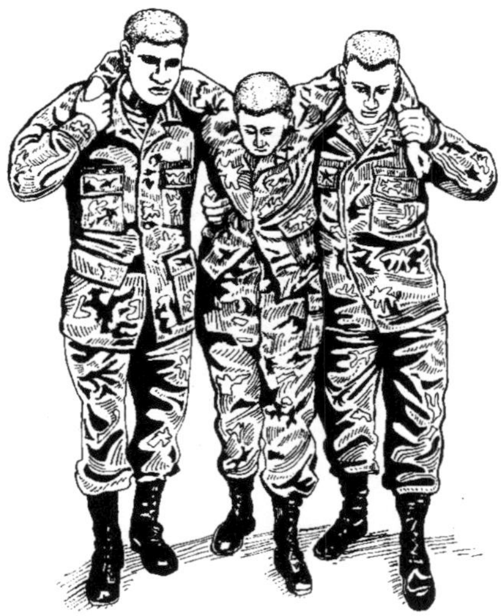

Figure B-16. Two-man supporting carry.

(2) The *two-man arms carry* (Figure B-17) is useful in carrying a casualty for a moderate distance (50 to 300 meters) and placing him on a litter. To lessen fatigue, the bearers should carry the casualty high and as close to their chests as possible. In extreme emergencies when there is no time to obtain a spine board, this carry is the safest one for transporting a casualty with a back injury. If possible, two additional bearers should be used to keep the casualty's head and legs in alignment with his body. The bearers—

(*a*) Kneel at one side of the casualty; then they place their arms beneath the casualty's back, waist, hips, and knees.

(*b*) Lift the casualty while rising to their knees.

(*c*) Turn the casualty toward their chests, while rising to a standing position. Carry the casualty high to lessen fatigue.

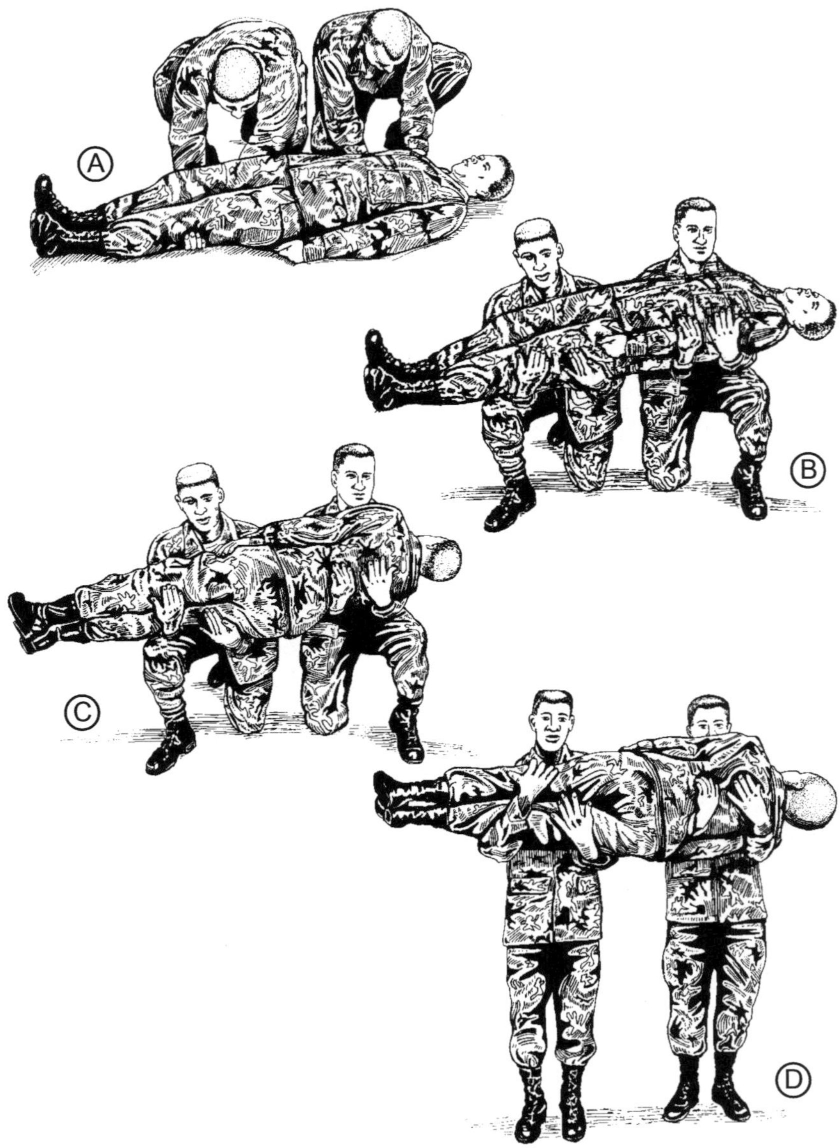

Figure B-17. Two-man arms carry (Illustrated A—D).

(3) The *two-man fore-and aft-carry* (Figure B-18) is a useful *two-man carry* for transporting a casualty for a long distance (over 300 meters). The taller of the two bearers should position himself at the casualty's head. By altering this carry so that both bearers face the casualty, it is useful for placing a casualty on a litter.

(*a*) The shorter bearer spreads the casualty's legs and kneels between them with his back to the casualty. He positions his hands behind the casualty's knees. The other bearer kneels at the casualty's head, slides his hands under the arms, across the chest, and locks his hands together.

(*b*) The two bearers rise together, lifting the casualty.

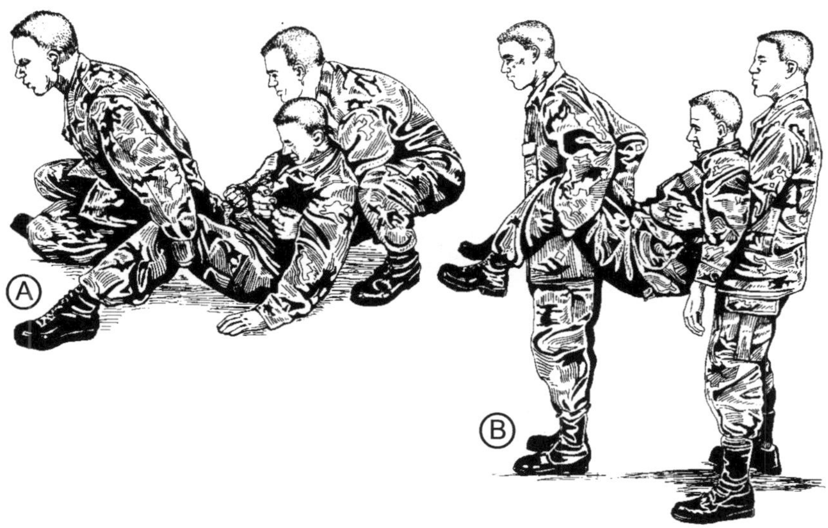

Figure B-18. Two-man fore-and-aft carry (Illustrated A—B).

(4) Only a conscious casualty can be transported with the *four-hand seat carry* (Figure B-19) because he must help support himself by placing his arms around the bearers' shoulders. This carry is especially useful in transporting a casualty with a head or foot injury for a moderate distance (50 to 300 meters). It is also useful for placing a casualty on a litter.

(*a*) Each bearer grasps one of his wrists and one of the other bearer's wrists, thus forming a packsaddle.

(*b*) The two bearers lower themselves sufficiently for the casualty to sit on the packsaddle; then, they have the casualty place his arms around their shoulders for support. The bearers then rise to an upright position.

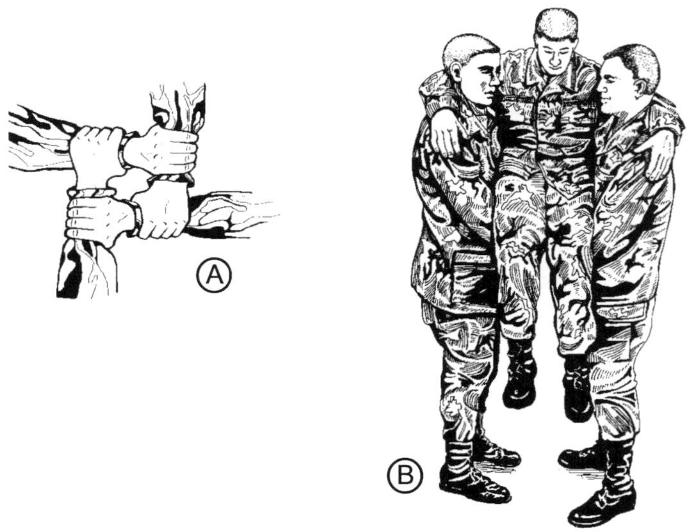

Figure B-19. Four-hand seat carry (Illustrated A—B).

(5) The *two-hand seat carry* (Figure B-20) is used when carrying a casualty for a short distance or for placing him on a litter. With the casualty lying on his back, a bearer kneels on each side of the casualty at his hips. Each bearer passes his arms under the casualty's thighs and back, and grasps the other bearer's wrists. The bearers rise lifting the casualty.

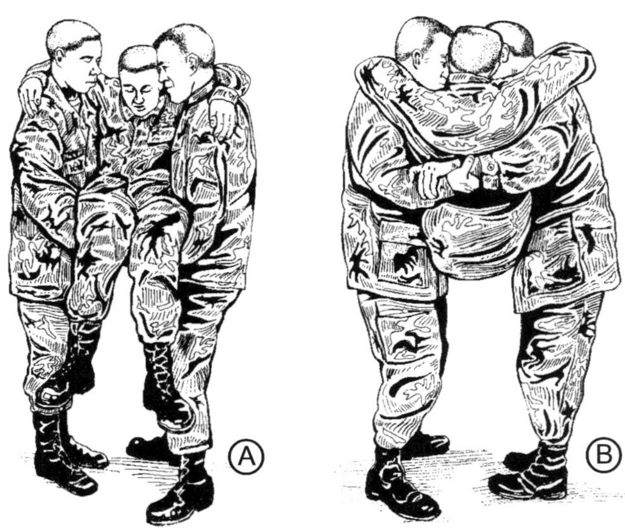

Figure B-20. Two-hand seat carry (Illustrated A—B).

B-9. Improvised Litters

Two men can support or carry a casualty without equipment for only short distances. By using available materials to improvise equipment, the casualty can be transported greater distances by two or more rescuers.

a. There are times when a casualty may have to be moved and a standard litter is not available. The distance may be too great for manual carries or the casualty may have an injury (such as a fractured neck, back, hip, or thigh) that would be aggravated by manual transportation. In these situations, litters can be improvised from materials at hand. Improvised litters must be as well constructed as possible to avoid risk of dropping or further injuring the casualty. Improvised litters are emergency measures and must be replaced by standard litters at the first opportunity.

b. Many different types of litters can be improvised, depending upon the materials available. A satisfactory litter can be made by securing poles inside such items as a blanket, poncho, shelter half, tarpaulin, mattress cover, jacket, shirt, or bed ticks, bags, and sacks (Figure B-18). Poles can be improvised from strong branches, tent supports, skis, lengths of pipe or other objects. If objects for improvising poles are not available, a blanket, poncho, or similar item can be rolled from both sides toward the center so the rolls can be gripped for carrying a patient. Most flat-surface objects of suitable size can be used as litters. Such objects include doors, boards, window shutters, benches, ladders, cots, and chairs. If possible, these objects should be padded for the casualty's comfort.

(1) To improvise a litter using a blanket and poles (Figure B-21), the following steps should be used.

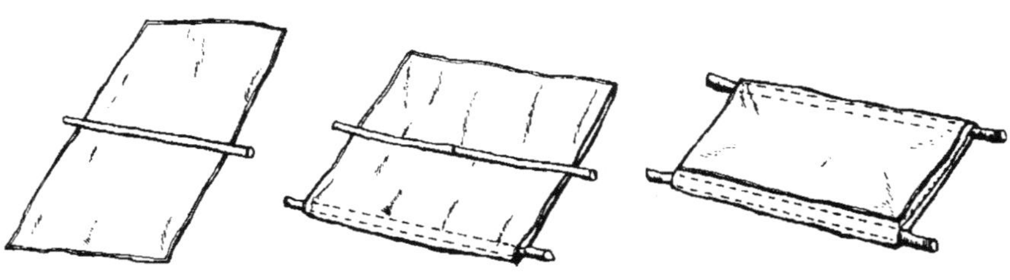

Figure B-21. Litter made with blanket and poles.

(*a*) Open the blanket and lay one pole lengthwise across the center; then fold the blanket over the pole.

(*b*) Place the second pole across the center of the folded blanket.

(*c*) Fold the free edges of the blanket over the second pole and across the first pole.

(2) To improvise a litter using shirts or jackets (Figure B-22), button the shirt or jacket and turn it inside out, leaving the sleeves inside, (more than one shirt or jacket may be required), then pass the pole through the sleeves.

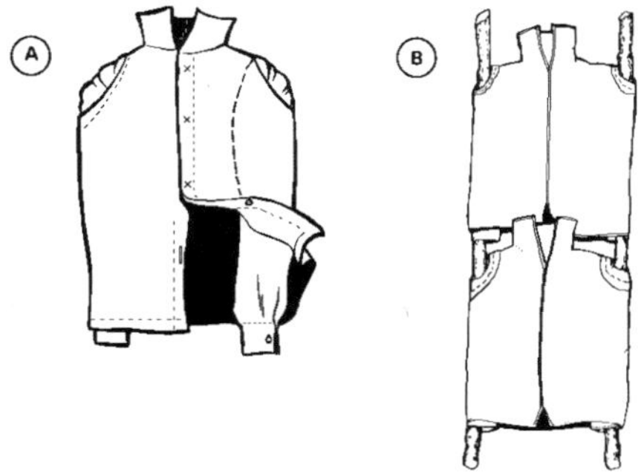

Figure B-22. Litter improvised from jackets and poles (Illustrated A—B).

(3) To improvise a litter from bed sacks and poles (Figure B-23), rip open the corners of bed ticks, bags, or sacks; then pass the poles through them.

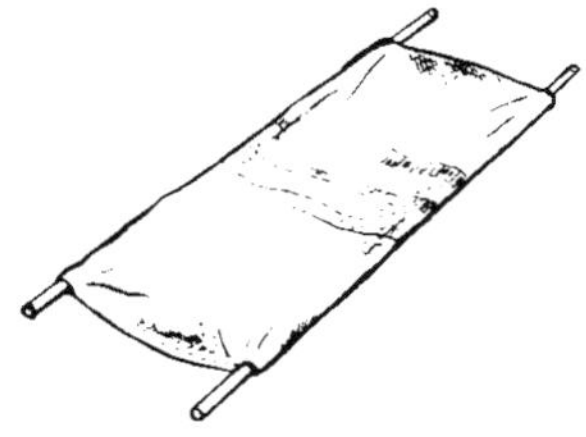

Figure B-23. Litter improvised from bed sacks and poles.

(4) If no poles are available, roll a blanket, shelter half, tarpaulin, or similar item from both sides toward the center (Figure B-24). Grip the rolls to carry the casualty.

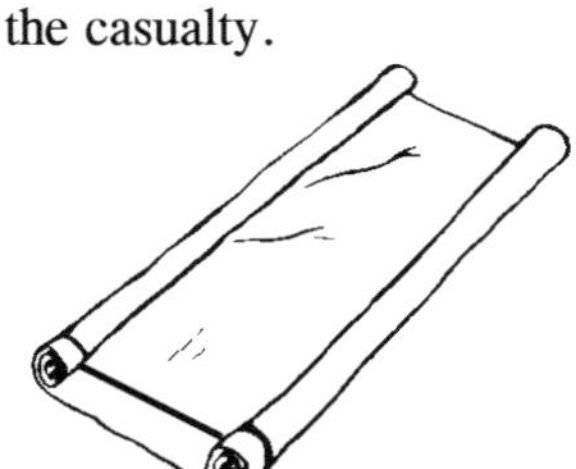

Figure B-24. Rolled blanket used as a litter.

c. Any of the appropriate carries may be used to place a casualty on a litter. These carries are:

- The one-man arms carry (Figure B-6).
- The two-man arms carry (Figure B-17).
- The two-man fore-and-aft carry (Figure B-18).
- The two-hand seat carry (Figure B-20).
- The four-hand seat carry (Figure B-19).

WARNING

Unless there is an immediate life-threatening situation (such as fire, explosion), DO NOT move a casualty with a suspected back or neck injury. Seek medical personnel for guidance on how to transport.

d. Either two or four service members (head/foot) may be used to lift a litter. To lift the litter, follow the procedure below.

(1) Raise the litter at the same time as the other carriers/ bearers.

(2) Keep the casualty as level as possible.

NOTE

Use caution when transporting on a sloping incline/hill.

GLOSSARY

ACRONYMS, ABBREVIATIONS, AND DEFINITIONS

AC hydrogen cyanide
AFMAN Air Force Manual
AOC area of concentration
AR Army regulation
ATM advanced trauma management
ATNAA Antidote Treatment, Nerve Agent, Autoinjector
attn attention

BDO battle dress overgarment
BDU battle dress uniform
BZ anticholinergic drugs

C Celsius
CANA Convulsant Antidote for Nerve Agent
CASEVAC casualty evacuation
cc cubic centimeter
CG phosgene
CHS combat health support
CK cyanogen chloride
Cl chlorine
CLS Combat Lifesaver
CNS central nervous system
CO_2 carbon dioxide
COSR combat and operational stress reactions
CSR combat stress reaction
CTA common table of allowance
CX phosgene oxime

DA Department of the Army
DD Department of Defense
DM diphenylaminochloroarsine (adamsite)
DNBI disease and nonbattle injury
DOD Department of Defense
DP diphosgene
DS direct support

EMT emergency medical treatment

F Fahrenheit
FM field manual

H mustard

HD mustard
HM Hospital Corpsman
HN nitrogen mustard
HSS health service support

IPE individual protective equipment
IV intravenous

JSLIST Joint Services Light Weight Integrated Suit Technology

L lewisite
lasers laser means Light Amplification by Stimulated Emission of Radiation and sources include range finders, weapons/guidance, communication systems, and weapons simulations such as MILES [Multiple Integrated Laser Engagement System].
LBE load bearing equipment
LX lewisite and mustard

MCRP Marine Corps Reference Publication
MILES Multiple Integrated Laser Engagement System
ml milliliter
MOPP mission-oriented protective posture
MOS military occupational specialty
MTF medical treatment facility

NAPP Nerve Agent Pyridostigmine Pretreatment
NATO North Atlantic Treaty Organization
NBC nuclear, biological, and chemical
NCO noncommissioned officer
NTRP Navy Tactical Reference Publication

occlusive dressing air tight transparent dressing used to seal and cover wounds
oz ounce

PAM pamphlet
PS chloropicrin
PTSD post-traumatic stress disorder

QSTAG Quadripartite Standardization Agreement

SOP standing operating procedure
STANAG standardization agreement
STP soldier training publication

2 PAM Cl pralidoxime chloride
TB MED technical bulletin medical
TM technical manual
TSOP tactical standing operating procedure

US United States

WP white phosphorus

REFERENCES

DOCUMENTS NEEDED

These documents must be available to the intended users of this publication.

NATO STANAGs

These agreements are available on request using DD Form 1425 from Standardization Document Order Desk, 700 Robin Avenue, Building 4, Section D, Philadelphia, Pennsylvania 19111-5094.

2122. *Medical Training in First Aid, Basic Hygiene and Emergency Care*. 10 December 1975.
2126. *First Aid Kits and Emergency Medical Care Kits*. 27 September 1983.
2358. *First Aid and Hygiene Training in NBC Operations*. 3 March 1989.
2871. *First Aid Material for Chemical Injuries*. 10 March 1986.

ABCA QSTAGs

These agreements are available on request using DD Form 1425 from Standardization Document Order Desk, 700 Robin Avenue, Building 4, Section D, Philadelphia, Pennsylvania 19111-5094.

535. *Medical Training in First Aid, Basic Hygiene and Emergency Care*. 12 November 1979.

Joint and Multiservice Publications

FM 21-10. *Field Hygiene and Sanitation*. MCRP 4-11.1D. 21 June 2000.

Army Publications

AR 350-41. *Training In Units*. 19 March 1993.
DA PAM 350-59. *Army Correspondence Course Program Catalog*. 26 October 2001.
FM 3-4. *NBC Protection*. FMFM 11-9. 29 May 1992 (Reprinted with basic including Change 1, 28 October 1992; Change 2, 26 February 1996.)
FM 3-5. *NBC Decontamination*. MCWP 3-37.3. 28 July 2000. (Change 1, 31 January 2002.)

FM 3-100. *Chemical Operations Principles and Fundamentals.* MCWP 3-3.7.1. 8 May 1996.

FM 4-02.33 (8-33). *Control of Communicable Diseases Manual* (17th Edition). 3 January 2000.

FM 8-10-6 (4-02.2). *Medical Evacuation in a Theater of Operations—Tactics, Techniques, and Procedures.* 14 April 2000.

FM 4-02.7 (8-10-7). *Health Service Support in a Nuclear, Biological, and Chemical Environment.* 1 October 2002.

FM 8-284 (4-02.284). *Treatment of Biological Warfare Agent Casualties.* NAVMED P-5042; AFMAN (I) 44-156; MCRP 4-11.1C. 17 July 2000. (Change 1, 8 July 2002.)

FM 8-285 (4-02.285). *Treatment of Chemical Agent Casualties and Conventional Military Chemical Injuries.* NAVMED P-5041; AFJMAN 44-149; FMFM 11-11. 22 December 1995.

FM 22-51 (4-02.22). *Leaders' Manual for Combat Stress Control.* 29 September 1994.

CTA 8-100. *Army Medical Department Expendable/Durable Items.* 31 August 1994.

CTA 50-900. *Clothing and Individual Equipment.* 1 September 1994.

STP 21-1-SMCT. *Soldier's Manual of Common Tasks Skill Level I.* 1 October 2001.

Department of Defense Forms

DD Form 1425. *Specifications and Standards Requisition.* March 1986.

READINGS RECOMMENDED

These readings contain relevant supplemental information.

Joint and Multiservice Publications

FM 8-9 (4-02.11). *NATO Handbook on the Medical Aspects of NBC Defensive Operations AMEDP-6 (B), Part I—Nuclear, Part II—Biological, Part III—Chemical.* NAVMED P-5059; AFJMAN 44-151V1V2V3. 1 February 1996.

TB MED 81. *Cold Injury.* NAVMED P-5052-29; AFP 161-11. 30 September 1976.

TB MED 507. *Occupational and Environmental Health Prevention, Treatment and Control of Heat Injury.* NAVMED P-5052-5; AFP 160-1. 25 July 1980.

Army Publications

AR 310-25. *Dictionary of United States Army Terms (Short Title: AD)*. 15 October 1983. (Reprinted with basic including Change 1, 21 May 1986.)

AR 310-50. *Authorized Abbreviations and Brevity Codes*. 15 November 1985.

TM 3-4230-216-10. *Operator's Manual for Decontaminating Kit, Skin: M258A1 (NSN 4230-01-101-3984) and Training Aid, Skin Decontaminating: M58A1 (6910-01-101-1768)*. 17 May 1985. (Change 1, 22 January 1997.)

INDEX

References are to paragraph numbers except where specified otherwise.

FM 4-25.11 (FM 21-11)
23 DECEMBER 2002

By Order of the Secretary of the Army

ERIC K. SHINSEKI
General, United States Army
Chief of Staff

Official:

Joel B. Hudson

JOEL B. HUDSON
Administrative Assistant to the
Secretary of the Army
0233107

By Direction of the Chief of Naval Operations:

Official:

R.G. SPRIGG
Rear Admiral, USN
Navy Warfare Development Command

By Order of the Secretary of the Air Force:

Official:

GEORGE PEACH TAYLOR, JR.
Lieutenant General, USAF, MC, CFS
Surgeon General

DISTRIBUTION:

US Army:Active Army, USAR, and ARNG: To be distributed in accordance with the initial distribution number 110161, requirements for FM 4-25.11.

US Navy: All Ships and Stations having Medical Department Personal.

US Air Force: F

ARMY PIN: 080516-000

MARINE CORPS PCN: 144 000037 00

This page intentionally left blank.

Health Service Support Operations

MCWP 4-11.1

This page intentionally left blank.

MCWP 4-11.1

Health Service Support Operations

U.S. Marine Corps

PCN 143 000040 00

DEPARTMENT OF THE NAVY
Headquarters United States Marine Corps
Washington, D.C. 20380-1775

10 March 1998

FOREWORD

"*Corpsman Up*!" has echoed across numerous battlefields in America's history. To answer this cry, medical personnel assigned to Marine Corps forces (MARFOR) must be knowledgeable, prepared, and able to provide responsive health service support (HSS) so Marines can do what they do best: win battles. Commanders must be aware of HSS requirements and their contributions to mission accomplishment.

Marine Corps Warfighting Publication (MCWP) 4-11.1, *Health Service Support Operations*, disseminates information on the mission, functions, structure, and concept of employment of HSS units. This publication provides overarching doctrine and establishes a practical approach to HSS from the perspective of the commander or staff officer who can apply it without any significant medical background.

This publication establishes general guidance that requires judgment in application. Lower-level tactics, techniques, and procedures for specific application will be published in MCRP 4-22B, *HSS Field Reference Guide*. This MCWP pertains equally to small-unit leaders and senior commanders.

MCWP 4-11.1 supersedes Fleet Marine Force Manual (FMFM) 4-50, *Health Service Support*, dated 19 September 1990.

Reviewed and approved this date.

BY DIRECTION OF THE COMMANDANT OF THE MARINE CORPS

J. E. Rhodes

J. E. RHODES
Lieutenant General, U.S. Marine Corps
Commanding General
Marine Corps Combat Development Command

DISTRIBUTION: 143 000040 00

To Our Readers

Changes: Readers of this publication are encouraged to submit suggestions and changes that will improve it. Recommendations may be sent directly to Commanding General, Doctrine Division (C 42), Marine Corps Combat Development Command, 3300 Russell Road, Suite 318A, Quantico, VA 22134-5021 or by fax to 703-784-2917 (DSN 278-2917) or by E-mail to **smb@doctrine div@mccdc**. Recommendations should include the following information:

- Location of change
  - Publication number and title
  - Current page number
  - Paragraph number (if applicable)
  - Line number
  - Figure or table number (if applicable)
- Nature of change
  - Add, delete
  - Proposed new text, preferably double-spaced and typewritten
- Justification and/or source of change

Additional copies: A printed copy of this publication may be obtained from Marine Corps Logistics Base, Albany, GA 31704-5001, by following the instructions in MCBul 5600, *Marine Corps Doctrinal Publications Status.* An electronic copy may be obtained from the Doctrine Division, MCCDC, world wide web home page which is found at the following universal reference locator: **http://www.doctrine.quantico.usmc.mil**.

Unless otherwise stated, whenever the masculine or feminine gender is used, both men and women are included.

Health Service Support Operations

Table of Contents

Chapter 4 Logistics

Chapter 5 Planning

Chapter 6 Command and Control

Chapter 7 Preventive Medicine

Chapter 10 Combat Casualty Reporting

Chapter 11 Training

Appendices

Chapter 1

Fundamentals

Focus of health service support (HSS) in the past has been on establishing a large and complex system to maximize returns to duty. Our current focus emphasizes the provision of far-forward, mobile, medical and surgical support and stabilization and rapid evacuation of casualties who are unable to quickly return to duty.

HSS is a process that delivers on demand to the warfighter a healthy, fit, and medically ready force; counters the health threat to the deployed force; and provides critical care and management for combat casualties. Aided by technological innovation and logistics, HSS is the employment of medical forces in support of the warfighter.

HSS supports the National Military Strategy of forward presence and power projection. HSS strengthens the warfighting commander by providing essential care in the theater and rapid aeromedical evacuation (AE) of casualties to enhanced medical treatment facilities in the continental United States (CONUS) for definitive care without sacrificing quality of care.

1001. Mission

The HSS mission is to minimize the effects that wounds, injuries, and disease have on units' effectiveness, readiness, and morale. The mission is accomplished by a preventive medicine program that safeguards personnel against potential health risks and by establishing an HSS system. The system provides support from the point of wounding, injury, or illness and evacuation to a medical treatment facility that can provide the level of care required by the patient.

1002. Principles

HSS principles are guides for planning, organizing, managing, and executing Service support. Seldom will all principles exert equal influence; usually, one or two will dominate a given situation. Identifying which ones have priority is essential to establishing effective HSS. Joint Pub 4-02, *Doctrine for Health Service Support in Joint Operations*, states that each Service component has an HSS system that encompasses—

- Conformity—the medical plan must integrate and comply with the commander's plan.
- Proximity—the medical plan must provide HSS as close to combat operations as the tactical situation permits.
- Flexibility—the medical plan must shift HSS resources to meet changing requirements.
- Mobility—the medical plan must anticipate requirements for rapid movement of HSS units to support combat forces during operations.
- Continuity—the medical plan must provide optimum, uninterrupted care and treatment to the wounded, injured, and sick.
- Coordination—the medical plan must ensure that HSS resources in short supply are efficiently employed and used effectively to support the planned operations.

1003. A Healthy and Fit Force

HSS promotes wellness and ensures quality of life to strengthen the human component of military forces against disease and injury. A healthy force ready to deploy anywhere in the world and ready to withstand hardship and deprivation assures warfighting commanders of physical and mental readiness. Wellness requires continuous attention before, during, and after deployment to sustain maximum readiness and warfighting capability.

1004. Casualty Prevention

HSS focuses on both forms of threat: enemy and health. The enemy threat produces combat casualties, whereas the ever-present threat to health produces disease and nonbattle casualties and is a major source of morbidity throughout military history. The enemy threat depends largely on the enemy's intent to use force and to inflict casualties. The health threat depends on a complex set of environmental and operational factors that combine to produce disease and nonbattle injuries. Failure to counter either threat jeopardizes mission accomplishment and ultimately achievement of the operational objective.

1005. Casualty Care and Management

HSS deploys smaller, mobile, and capable elements to provide essential care in the theater. HSS resources are flexible and adaptable and can be tailored to missions ranging from major theater wars to military operations other than war. The major components of casualty care and management are first response, prehospitalization treatment, forward resuscitative surgery, tailorable hospital care, and enroute care.

1006. Functions

Medical plans must include the following functions into the HSS concept of operations:

- Health maintenance—routine sick call, physical examination, preventive medicine, dental maintenance, record maintenance, and reports submission.
- Casualty collection—selection of and manning of locations where casualties are assembled, triaged, treated, protected from further injury, and evacuated.
- Casualty treatment—triage and treatment (self-aid, buddy aid, and initial resuscitative care).
- Temporary casualty holding—facilities and services to hold sick, wounded, and injured personnel for a limited time, usually not to exceed 72 hours. The medical battalion, force service support group, is the only HSS unit staffed and equipped to provide temporary casualty holding.
- Casualty evacuation—movement and ongoing treatment of the sick, wounded, or injured while in transit to medical treatment facilities. All Marine units have an evacuation capability by ground, air, or sea.

1007. The Hague and Geneva Conventions

The conduct of armed hostilities on land is regulated by the law of land warfare, which is both written and unwritten. The law of land warfare is derived from two principal sources: custom treaties and lawmaking treaties such as the Hague and Geneva Conventions. The rights and duties set forth in these conventions are part of the supreme law of the land. Violation of any convention is a serious offense. Under the Conventions, the signatories established the principle of disinterested aid to all victims of war including those who, through wounds, capture, or shipwreck, are no longer enemies but are merely suffering and defenseless human beings. Additional protocols to the Geneva Conventions, accepted and signed in 1977, established the manner in which the victims of war are to be treated. The Conventions established standards of conduct for medical and religious personnel assigned to aid victims. The United States is a signatory to the Geneva Conventions of 1949 and has directed its military forces to abide by its articles. However, future asymmetrical theaters, especially nonstate actions, may not abide—in fact, probably will *not* abide—by the convention accepted by nation states.

Refer to the following sources for principles of international and domestic law and the status and protection of medical personnel under both Conventions.

- NWP 1-14M/MCWP 5-2.1/COMDTPUB P5800.7, *The Commander's Handbook on the Law of Naval Operations.*
- FM 27-10/FMFM 0-25, *The Law of Land Warfare.*
- DA PAM 27-1, *Treaties Governing Land Warfare.*

(reverse blank)

Chapter 2

Intelligence

Accurate and timely intelligence—knowledge of the enemy and the surrounding environment that is needed to support decision-making—is a prerequisite for military success. Intelligence is a fundamental component of command and control that aids the commander in applying combat power at the decisive time and place. Intelligence activity is mission-focused. In MAGTF intelligence operations, intelligence operations are determined by the commander's intelligence requirements. The resulting intelligence effort provides critical knowledge and understanding about the enemy and the environment to help the commander plan and make decisions.

Medical intelligence includes more than just information on disease or other environmental hazards. Raw data must be analyzed and properly acted on to prevent an adverse operational impact. Medical intelligence from all sources—internal and external to the MAGTF—must be assimilated for the commander to have a complete picture of the medical threat.

2001. Internal Medical Intelligence Sources

Preventive Medicine Section

Most preventive medicine assets organic to the Marine expeditionary force (MEF) are found in the preventive medicine section, headquarters and service (H&S) company, medical battalion, force service support group (FSSG). This section provides general support to all MEF major subordinate commands. General support includes identifying information on environmental health, demographics, living conditions, water supply, waste disposal, insects, diseases, and vector issues of military importance, as well as evaluating local food sanitation and sight and hearing conservation programs.

Local Command G-2 Sections

Additional medical intelligence may be requested through G-2 sections of the command element, ground combat element (GCE), aviation combat element (ACE), and combat service support element (CSSE).

Additional information on intelligence support to medical operations can be found in the intelligence series of the Marine Corps warfighting publications (particularly MCWP 2-12, *MAGTF Intelligence Production and Analysis)*.

Health Service Support Element

The health service support element (HSSE) is often the first to receive medical intelligence from on-site care providers due to multiple communications and information links available to sections within the FSSG combat service support operations center (CSSOC).

2002. The Armed Forces Medical Intelligence Center

The Armed Forces Medical Intelligence Center (AFMIC) is a field production activity of the Defense Intelligence Agency. It is the sole producer of medical intelligence in the Department of Defense (DOD). AFMIC provides all-source intelligence on—

- Worldwide infectious disease and environmental health risks.
- Foreign military and civilian health care systems and infrastructure.
- Foreign biomedical developments and life science technologies of military medical significance.

AFMIC maintains extensive data bases; monitors foreign research, development, production, and transitional flow of medical materiel for military interest; and provides intelligence liaison services to key customers. It also conducts in-house and mobile training, including a medical intelligence fellowship program; serves on numerous intelligence committees and working groups; and trains military reservists for mobilization assignments. AFMIC's intelligence products provide direct support to U.S. military customers for operational planning; development of policy, doctrine, and training priorities; and medical research and development.

Queries for medical intelligence support are addressed via the HSS chain or direct from deploying units to—

Defense Intelligence Agency
Armed Forces Medical Intelligence Center
Fort Detrick
Frederick, MD 21701-5004

or via message to—

DIRAFMIC FTDETRICKMD.

Chapter 3

Operations

The Marine Corps organization for combat is based on its unique assigned force structure. HSS is a mission area common to every MAGTF, regardless of the mission. Definitive operational planning for HSS is always an integral part of all MAGTF operations. The inherent flexibility in the MAGTF and the broad spectrum of potential MAGTF missions call for equal flexibility in HSS execution. The size, type, and configuration of HSS capabilities needed to effectively support a MAGTF will be determined by mission, enemy, terrain and weather, troops and support available-time available (METT-T). The following paragraphs provide an organizational framework for command and staff cognizance within which all HSS operations are executed.

3001. Marine Corps Forces

Marine Corps forces (MARFOR) commanders are responsible for coordinating and integrating HSS within their area of operations. The MARFOR surgeon, dental officer, medical planner, and medical administrative officer advise the MARFOR commander on matters relating to the health of the command, medical logistics, patient movement, sanitation, disease surveillance, medical intelligence, and medical personnel issues, as well as current and future HSS planning at the MARFOR level. Additional duties include serving as the liaison for the commander in chief (CINC) and other component surgeons and monitoring HSS aspects of the time-phased force and deployment data flow.

3002. Marine Expeditionary Forces

MEF commanders are responsible for coordinating and integrating HSS within their area of operations. The MEF surgeon, medical planner, medical administrative officer, preventive medicine officer, hospital corpsmen, and dental technicians are responsible for establishing HSS requirements and ensuring the HSS systems established by MEF major subordinate commands form an integrated and responsive network of support.

The surgeon and the staff also advise the MEF commander on matters relating to the health of the command, medical logistics, patient movement, sanitation, disease surveillance, medical intelligence, medical personnel issues, as well as current and future HSS planning at the MEF level. The MARFOR deals with matters more on the operational level of war, but the MEF is more focused toward the tactical level.

HSS beyond the organic capabilities of the GCE and ACE are normally provided by task-organized units of the medical and dental battalions of the FSSG. Additional support may be needed from designated casualty receiving and treatment ships (CRTSs), fleet hospitals, hospital ships, or medical treatment facilities (MTFs) of other Services.

Marine Division

The medical staff of the division headquarters has a division surgeon, medical planner/administrator, a psychiatrist, and hospital corpsmen. Medical staff responsibilities are similar to the MEF's but are more specifically related to the activities of the GCE. When units smaller than divisions deploy as the GCE, the regiment or battalion surgeons assume much of the planning responsibility associated with health services in addition to their clinical responsibilities. Planning occurs on a company or platoon level, with the hospital corpsmen assisting in the planning.

Marine Aircraft Wing

The medical staff of the Marine aircraft wing (MAW) headquarters has a wing surgeon, medical planner/administrative officer, an environmental health officer, industrial hygienist, optometrist, and hospital corpsmen. Medical staff responsibilities are similar to the MEF's but are more specifically related to the activities of the ACE.

A MAW has four Marine aircraft groups (MAGs). Each MAG has a flight surgeon and several hospital corpsmen. Each MAG is supported by a Marine wing support squadron (MWSS) of the Marine wing support group (MWSG). The MWSS medical staff has a flight surgeon and hospital corpsmen. The flight surgeon is the squadron commander's special staff officer responsible for the aeromedical safety and HSS for the squadron.

Force Service Support Group

The group surgeon advises the commander on the health of the command and the adequacy of internal FSSG HSS. The surgeon also has cognizance over the operation of the group aid station. There is also a health service support officer (HSSO) who coordinates FSSG HSS support for GCE and ACE units requiring medical care that exceeds their organic capabilities. The HSSO serves as the officer in charge of the medical section of the CSSOC during exercises or operations. The FSSG has the majority of the MEF's medical capability. It has a medical battalion with three surgical companies (Surg Co) and eight shock trauma platoons (STPs) to provide initial resuscitative care for casualties.

There is a dental battalion to provide field dentistry when deployed and to advise on dental issues. Medical supplies and equipment for the MEF are managed through the medical logistics company (Med Log Co), supply battalion, which issues the authorized medical allowance list (AMAL) and authorized dental allowance list (ADAL) and handles resupply issues. When the Med Log Co or detachment does not deploy with the CSSE, the CSSE supply detachment and/or inter-Service support agreement provides resupply support.

Medical Battalion

The medical battalion, FSSG is organized to execute HSS functions in support of the MAGTF's mission. The medical battalion provides initial resuscitative HSS support to the MEF and is the only source of organic Marine Corps medical support above the aid station level. Its primary mission is to perform those emergency medical and surgical procedures that, if not performed, could lead to death or loss of limb or body function. The battalion's surgical companies provide initial resuscitative surgical intervention, temporary casualty holding, ground evacuation support to forward medical elements, and preventive medicine support.

The battalion structure has 260 holding beds and 9 operating rooms. The medical battalion is made up of an H&S company and three Surg Co. The H&S company contains 8 STPs that have 10 patient holding beds each. Each Surg Co contains 60 beds and 3 operating rooms.

Surgical Company, Medical Battalion, FSSG. The Surg Co (with support from CSS detachments [CSSDs] to provide power, messing, and transportation) supports regimental-size operations and receives casualties from units or individuals providing first response medical treatment. The Surg Co provides MTFs for resuscitative surgery, medical treatment, and temporary holding of casualties from supported forces. They also prepare and evacuate casualties whose medical requirements exceed the established theater evacuation policy.

The Surg Co is composed of a—

- Headquarters platoon.
- Triage/evacuation platoon.
- Surgical platoon—contains three surgical sections, each supporting an operating room, each operating room capable of staffing two 12-hour shifts.
- Holding platoon—contains 3 ward sections, each containing 20 medical/surgical beds.
- Combat stress platoon.
- Services platoon (ancillary)—services two laboratory sections, two pharmacy sections, and two x-ray sections.

Since the Surg Co is a major link in the chain of evacuation, it should be located, whenever possible, in close proximity to an airfield capable of casualty evacuation by fixed-wing aircraft. Components of the Surg Co may be used to reinforce an STP (i.e., surgical section) to provide a far forward resuscitative surgery capability.

Shock Trauma Platoon, H&S Company, Medical Battalion, FSSG. The STP is the smallest, most mobile medical support platoon of the medical battalion. It can serve as a beach evacuation station, reinforce a battalion aid station (BAS), operate as an intermediate casualty collecting and clearing point between forward medical elements and the Surg Co, or serve as the forward element of a surgical company (i.e., triage/evacuation platoon) preparing to relocate. An STP reinforced with preventive medicine, group aid station, and dental personnel may also provide HSS to a CSSD or MEU service support group (MSSG).

Dental Battalion

The dental battalion, FSSG provides dental services to the MEF. By attaching task-organized dental sections and detachments to HSSEs of the MAGTF, battalion personnel maintain dental readiness during exercises, deployments, operations other than war, and combat operations.

In an operational environment, the dental battalion's primary mission is to provide dental health maintenance with a focus on emergency care. Personnel from these detachments may also provide postoperative, ward, central sterilization and supply room support, and other medical support as determined to be appropriate by the medical battalion and Surg Co commanders.

The dental battalion commander has additional special staff officer duties as the MEF and FSSG dental officer. As a special staff officer, the dental officer advises the commanders on all professional, administrative, and operational matters in order to optimize use of dental assets.

Medical Logistics Company

The Med Log Co, Supply Battalion, FSSG is a supply operation directly responsible to the FSSG supply battalion commanding officer. The Med Log Co—

- Maintains medical equipment.
- Maintains centralized acquisition, storing, and stock rotation.
- Constructs medical supply sets (AMAL/ADAL).
- Resupplies AMAL/ADAL and line-items in support of HSS units based on specific mission needs.

3003. Marine Expeditionary Unit

Each MEU element deploys with its own organic HSS capability. HSS above this organic level is provided by an HSS detachment (HSSD) task-organized from the medical and dental battalions, FSSG, as part of the MSSG. HSSD structure may include—

- Shock/trauma platoons.
- H&S company, medical battalion elements.
- Med Log Co detachments.
- Dental detachments.
- Surg Co (e.g., triage/evacuation platoons).

The tactical situation ashore will dictate the size of the HSSE capability ashore. This capability may range from a beach or helicopter evacuation station staffed by a triage/evacuation platoon to an STP reinforced with sections of a Surg Co.

3004. Phasing Support Ashore

During the movement phase of amphibious operations, the commander, amphibious task force (CATF) has overall responsibility for HSS services to embarked personnel.

Landing force (LF) HSS personnel aboard ATF ships augment ATF medical and dental departments by providing care to embarked LF personnel using ship's company medical facilities and supplies. LF Class VIIIA equipment and supplies will not be used aboard ship unless authorized by the MAGTF commander in support of an overwhelming emergency.

The senior medical officer of each ATF ship is responsible to the ship's commanding officer for HSS to *all* personnel. If a ship does not have a medical officer, the embarked LF medical officer will have to provide HSS while embarked.

The stages described in the following paragraphs and shown in figure 3-1 represent only notional phasing. Other variations and combinations resulting from such factors as threat level, mission, terrain, geography, weather, force at risk, opposing forces, etc., are possible.

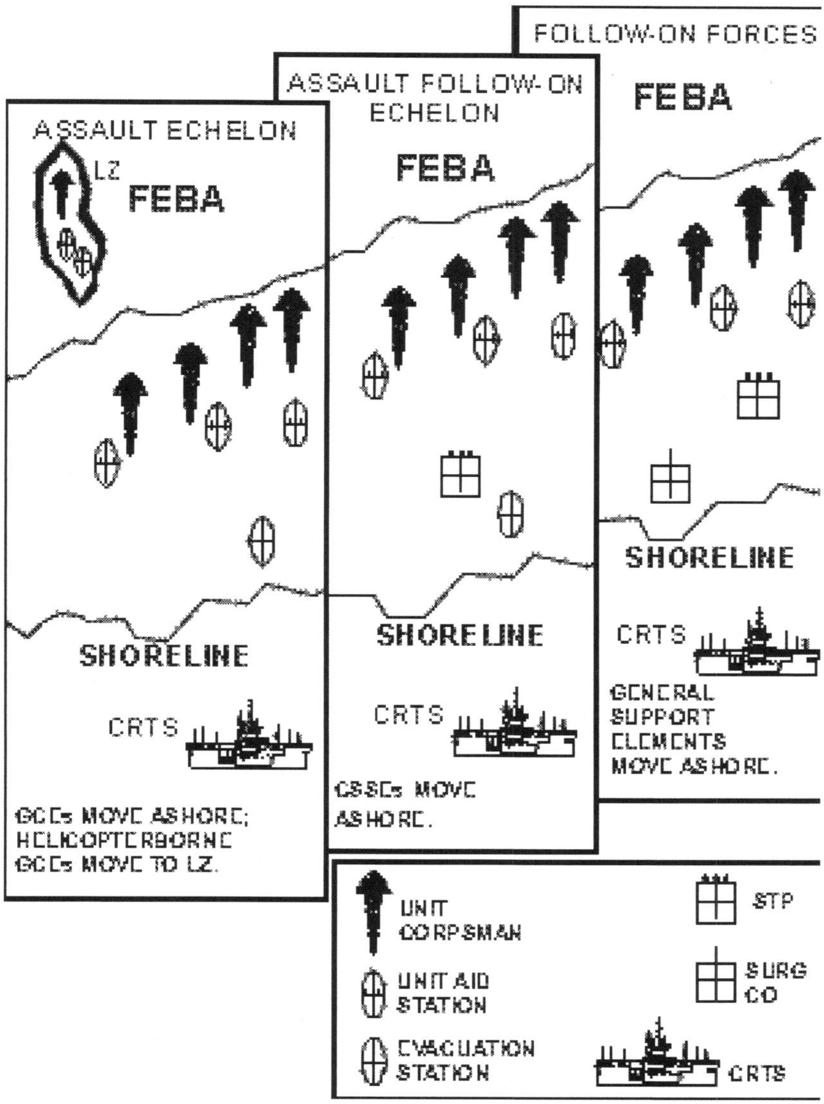

Figure 3-1. Stages of Medical Support in an Amphibious Operation.

Assault Echelon

During the assault phase, HSS ashore is limited to the capabilities of medical sections organic to combat units. First response medical care for assault forces is provided by self-aid, buddy aid, and corpsmen of landed rifle platoons.

When the tactical situation permits, BASs are established and care from a physician is provided. BASs are normally divided into two sections with assigned battalion nonmedical litter bearers divided between the two sections. One section lands with the battalion combat train and provides in-close support to the assault force. The second section lands with the field train and establishes interim evacuation stations until relieved by follow-on HSSEs.

Evacuation stations are then expanded and staffed by the supporting medical battalion, drawing assets from collection and evacuation sections of STPs or triage/evacuation platoons of surgical companies. When established with the landing force support party (LFSP), the supporting medical battalion constitutes the beach evacuation section(s) of the LFSP. The primary role of a beach evacuation station is to evacuate assault force casualties to designated CRTSs.

When evacuation stations attached to the LFSP become operational ashore, established BASs are relieved to conduct their missions in primary support of parent battalions. Following the landing of supporting evacuation stations, expansion of HSS facilities ashore begins.

Assault Follow-on Echelon

While the majority of CSS capabilities during the AFOE continue to be sea-based, projected HSS capabilities ashore will expand along with the FSSG's. Capabilities could be additional STPs with mobile CSSDs.

When progress of assault units is such that the beachhead is relatively secure, HSS is enhanced from follow-on forces.

Follow-on Forces

HSS shifts its posture to achieve shore-based health care consistent with the expected combat intensity and duration of sustained operations ashore, independent of sea-based facilities. This phasing is achieved by upgrading capabilities ashore by consolidating HSS capabilities ashore with those not yet landed.

If a sustained land campaign is envisioned, additional HSS will normally be provided by fleet hospitals (or other Service equivalent facilities) or hospital ships.

3005. Capabilities External to the MAGTF

Casualty Receiving and Treatment Ships

CRTSs have the largest medical capability of any amphibious ship in the ATF. A CRTS's medical spaces include operating rooms, an intensive care unit, a quiet room, ward beds, and overflow beds. Dental spaces include general dental operating rooms, a maxillofacial surgery operating room, and a prosthetics lab. CRTSs require augmentation by Navy medical department personnel to achieve full casualty treatment capability. Casualties are delivered via helicopter and surface craft. ATF ships suitable for use as CRTSs are the LHD, LHA, and LPH. The CATF's Annex Q, *Planning Guidance, Medical Services*, will designate platforms to serve as CRTSs. For medical support capabilities of these vessels and their potential roles as CRTSs, see Fleet Marine Force Reference Publication 1-18, *Amphibious Ships and Landing Craft Data Book.*

Fleet Hospitals

Fleet hospitals are transportable, medically and surgically intensive, and deployable in a variety of operational scenarios. These HSS assets can be used by theater CINCs, Navy component commanders, and joint task force commanders. Although external support requirements exist, fleet hospitals are substantially self-supporting and relocatable. However, relocatability varies with hospital size. An expedient move would require external transportation equipment. See NWP 4-02.4, *Part A, Deployable Health Service Support Platforms—Fleet Hospitals*, for more information.

Hospital Ships (T-AH)

The T-AH is a floating surgical hospital. Its mission is to provide acute medical care in support of combat operations at sea and ashore. Support may be provided to ATFs, joint task forces, and combined forces. The T-AH is designed to receive patients primarily by helicopter. It has limited capacity for receiving patients by surface craft.

Augmentation

Fleet Surgical Teams. Fleet surgical teams (FSTs) are HSS augmentation teams assigned to the fleet CINCs. Combined, the Pacific and Atlantic fleets have nine teams that are considered the fleet CINC's assets in both peacetime and wartime. FSTs provide medical support to the CINC's routine deployment medical requirements. Medical support for other peacetime contingencies that cannot be covered by the FSTs will be provided by mobile medical augmentation readiness teams (MMARTs).

Mobile Medical Augmentation Readiness Teams. MMARTs provide rapid peacetime response teams of pre-identified medical department personnel trained to augment elements of the operating forces. The Commander Naval Medical Command Instruction 6440.2 series contains a detailed discussion of the MMART.

Medical Augmentation Program. The medical augmentation program (MAP) is the means by which operating forces are brought to wartime manning levels by personnel augmentation from CONUS-based activities. MAP is managed by the U.S. Navy Bureau of Medicine and Surgery (BUMED). In special cases, staffing may be above authorized staffing or in addition to authorized billets when directed by the Chief of Naval Operations. Units participating in MAP include CRTSs, MARFOR HSS units, fleet hospitals, and hospital ships.

(reverse blank)

Chapter 4

Logistics

HSS logistics encompasses the procurement, initial issue, management, resupply, and disposition of material required to support medical and dental elements organic to the MARFOR. Requisitions for Class VIIIA (consumable and equipment) material follow the same channels as other classes of supply. Guidance for planning and procuring Class VIIIB (blood products) is found in DOD Instruction 6480.4, *Armed Services Blood Program Operational Procedures*.

As with all classes of supply, careful consideration should be given to stockage levels of Class VIIIA material. Commanders should not be burdened with moving and maintaining excess material, nor should the need for support ever be delayed because of inadequate access or lack of responsiveness. When the medical planner is developing and planning for appropriate levels of Class VIIIA support, the following information is crucial to ensuring that the entire HSS system is responsive to the commander:

- Concept of operation/scheme of maneuver.
- Combat intensity.
- Duration of the operation.
- Casualty estimates.

4001. Allowance and Source of Logistics

The MAGTF surgeon advises the MAGTF commander regarding medical and dental material support. Allocation of material is documented in the table of equipment (T/E); the AMALs/ ADALs; and the normal replenishment supply support. The total T/E and AMALs/ADALs are designed to support a MEF in an estimated worst case scenario for a 60-day period of combat. The quantity of AMALs/ADALs required to support a MEF is determined by the mission requirements of that force. The AMALs/ ADALs are to be allocated to support specific requirements. The authorizing commander is responsible for funding AMALs/ ADALs above the level prescribed by the Marine Corps order 4400 series.

Table of Equipment

A unit's T/E includes items necessary for basic support of the organization. Examples of this type of equipment include—

- Tentage.
- Vehicles.
- Tools.
- Communications equipment.
- Nuclear, biological, and chemical (NBC) gear.
- Specialized clothing.
- Office equipment.
- Other equipment and supplies, as required.

AMALs and ADALs

AMALs and ADALs are specialized equipment and supply assemblages for medical and dental elements to provide combat HSS. The medical and dental elements have the capability to provide the following services:

- Trauma management.
- Resuscitative surgery.
- Expeditionary laboratory.
- Pharmacy.
- X-ray.
- Dental.
- Preventive medicine.
- NBC treatment.
- Patient holding.
- Sick call.
- Environmental supplements.
- HSS test and repair systems.

See appendix B for a detailed description of AMALs and ADALs.

Normal Replenishment Supply Support

HSSEs deploy with their initial issue and the days of supply prescribed by the MAGTF commander. For the first 60 days of operations, Class VIIIA material beyond this level for the MEF is maintained by the CSSE and provided to supported units as required. For operations more than 60 days, medical resupply is generally provided to the using HSS unit by the CINC's designated single integrated medical logistics manager (SIMLM) via the CSSE.

Single Integrated Medical Logistics Manager

HSS logistics is normally a Service responsibility. However, in joint operations, a SIMLM system may be designated to provide central logistical support to all participating Services in the combatant CINC's area of responsibility. As the dominant user, the U.S. Army has been formally tasked by the DOD to perform the peacetime SIMLM mission in the European and Korean theaters. Under wartime or crisis conditions, the U.S. Army will usually be the dominant Class VIII user and must plan for the SIMLM mission.

The SIMLM system encompasses the provision of medical supplies, medical equipment maintenance and repair, blood management, and optical fabrication to all joint forces within the theater of operations, except Navy combatant ships.

HSS logistics can be provided to Navy hospital ships for common, demand-supported medical supplies in the later stages of theater development. Activation of the SIMLM mission depends on the time-phased force and deployment list supporting the contingency. Air delivery of emergency medical supplies can be used where and when tactically supportable. The CSSE supply detachment, which may include portions of Med Log Co, provides Class VIIIA single-item resupply and, eventually, limited medical repair capabilities to all HSS units of the MAGTF. Supporting combat service support detachments provide medical resupply to medical units of other MAGTF elements.

4002. Individual HSS Equipment

Hospital corpsmen assigned to combat support units of the MAGTF are assigned a complete first aid kit as part of their field gear. These kits may be held by the unit organic supply section and issued on an as needed basis. The corpsmen's parent unit supply section is responsible for ensuring that contents of the first aid kit are maintained in good condition, and that medications have not exceeded their shelf life. Dental officers will be issued a dental instrument and supply set (unit-2).

4003. Routine Resupply

HSS personnel needing resupply will forward requisitions to their unit's supply section. The supply section will, in turn, pass the requisition to the supported activities supply system management unit, or if deployed, the supply section of the CSSE. The CSSE orders, receives, and distributes the required material. While HSS personnel may be of help in identifying alternate doses or approved substitutes, care is required in using alternate sources of supply, other than those already approved by the Defense Medical Standardization Board or Navy Medical Logistics Command. HSS personnel may also assist in identifying the location of other U.S. medical facilities where required items may be obtained.

4004. Combat Resupply

During embarkation planning, HSS planners determine the number and type of AMALs/ADALs required to support the assault phase of the operation. Additional Class VIIIA consumable material will be positioned for deployment with the supply section of the CSSE. After the consumable AMALs/ADALs modules are issued and expended, or when directed, resupply will be accomplished by normal line item requisition from the supporting CSSE. When stockpiles of MAGTF Class VIIIA are expended, Class VIIIA will be obtained through the designated SIMLM provider.

4005. Patient Movement Items

Patient movement items (PMI) are the medical equipment and supplies required to support the patient during evacuation, e.g., ventilators, vital sign monitors, and blankets. Handling and return of equipment to the aeromedical evacuation (AE) system requires a reliable supporting logistics infrastructure to ensure that PMI are available and serviceable. The plan for a PMI exchange system and the return of AE equipment and PMI to the originating MTF should be addressed in the respective operation plan (OPLAN).

When a patient requires evacuation, the originating MTF has responsibility to provide the PMI. These items accompany a patient throughout the chain of evacuation from originating MTF to destination MTF, whether it is an intra- or intertheater transfer.

The Services will include and maintain initial quantities of PMI in the appropriate medical assemblages.

4006. Disposal of Materials

Disposal of soiled, contaminated, or other unserviceable Class VIIIA items must be accomplished with due consideration for the safety of U.S. forces and local civilian populations.

Disposal must also be in compliance with local and international laws, ordinances, or customs governing such disposal whenever operations allow. When disposal takes place in the U.S. or its territories, Class VIIIA disposal is coordinated with the local office of the Defense Reutilization Marketing Office. Peacetime disposal overseas is coordinated under the guidance of the Defense Reutilization Marketing Office or supporting CSSE.

When the tactical situation permits during combat operations, the safest method of field disposal is burning, followed by deep burial (over 6 feet). The burial site must be located at a safe distance from watersheds and populated areas. Responsibility for neutralization and disposal of clothing, equipment, and dressings removed during NBC decontamination processes resides with the command's NBC officer.

Disposal of body parts, tissues, and Class VIIIB blood and blood products obtained during operative or diagnostic procedures is, preferably, accomplished in the same manner as used by local medical facilities. Alternative disposal by burning or deep burial requires prior authorization and specific guidance of higher authority. Prior coordination with local health authorities and religious leaders should be accomplished whenever possible.

4007. Protection of Medical Supplies

Medical material and supplies are protected under the law of land warfare and the Geneva Conventions. However, when medical material and supplies are mixed with combat supplies, they lose the protection afforded by these covenants. Marking of medical material and supply storage areas with the red cross of the Geneva Conventions is a tactical decision to be made by the area commander. The Geneva Conventions and the law of land warfare prohibit the destruction of medical material and supplies that must be abandoned in a retrograde movement occasioned by enemy action or other tactical considerations.

Chapter 5

Planning

HSS planning occurs at all levels of command and organizations across the range of military operations. All commanders are responsible for the health and welfare of their troops. All commanders have HSS staffs that plan from the strategic level of war through the tactical level of war.

5001. Joint Guidance

Chairman of the Joint Chiefs of Staff Manual (CJCSM) 3122.03, *Joint Operation Planning and Execution System, Volume II, Planning Formats and Guidance,* sets forth administrative instructions and formats to develop OPLANs of combatant commands, subunified commands, joint task forces, and their subordinate component commands. It may also be applied when significant forces of one Service are attached to forces of another Service.

OPLANs, concept plans (CONPLANs), functional plans, and operation orders (OPORDs) prepared by commanders to fulfill tasks assigned in the joint strategic capabilities plan (or otherwise directed by the Chairman of the Joint Chiefs of Staff) will conform to the guidance contained in CJCSM 3122.03. To facilitate communications on operation planning among military headquarters, commanders will standardize the format and content of other appropriate plans according to CJCSM 3122.03.

5002. Annex Q, Planning Guidance, Medical Services

Guidance for medical services is located in Annex Q, *Planning Guidance, Medical Services*, of OPLANs, CONPLANs, functional plans, and OPORDs. Annex Q identifies requirements and provides guidance to subordinate commanders and their HSS planners. The following are sample HSS appendices to Annex Q:

- Appendix 2, Joint Blood Program.
- Appendix 3, Hospitalization.
- Appendix 4, Patient Movement.
- Appendix 6, Medical Logistics (Class 8A) System.
- Appendix 7, Preventive Medicine.
- Appendix 8, Medical Command, Control, and Communications.

Chapter 6

Command and Control

Command and control (C^2) for HSS is the combination of HSS organizations, people, communications systems, architecture, and medical information which provides the commander timely information to make decisions. C^2 for HSS entails all functions necessary for medical units to rapidly execute HSS functions in response to the needs of the supported unit.

There are four major C^2 areas:

- C^2 organization.
- Communications and information systems.
- Information management.
- MAGTF C^2 centers, agencies, and facilities.

In combination these areas develop, process, and disseminate orders and information to subordinate units and provide the means to receive and implement orders from a higher authority. All of these areas interact to produce effective and harmonious actions.

6001. C^2 Organization

HSS is a part of every level of the MAGTF. Communications assets available vary. HSS shares these assets with other war-fighting functions. In the Marine Corps, the same radios that carry fire support or command information will also carry medical information. The same telephones and switches that commanders use are also used by HSS personnel. There is no "separate" or "dedicated" medical network in the tactical Marine Corps communications architecture. Rather, the architecture supports "common users" who share its resources.

Units responsible for providing detachments which support C^2 for HSS operate under the staff cognizance of the G-6/S-6 (communications and information systems officer) of the supported unit. Marines assigned to these units, in concert with the personnel assigned to the G-6/S-6 sections and HSS organizations, ensure that an effective communications and information systems (CIS) network is planned, installed, operated, and maintained.

6002. Communications and Information Systems

CIS provide management and decision support tools for the HSS commander and staff to collect, transport, process, disseminate, and protect voice, data, and information.

CIS include tactical single channel VHF, SHF, HF, and UHF radios; tactical and commercial telephones; multichannel digital systems; satellite communications; cryptographic equipment; and data systems for classified and unclassified local area network/wide area network (LAN/WAN) connectivity. All of these systems are used by common units and are allocated in accordance with the commander's priorities.

To improve interoperability, increase efficiency, and reduce costs, DOD has mandated that the Services move to a common set of information systems and services. This implementation is occurring with the fielding of the Global Command and Control System (GCCS) and the implementation of the defense information infrastructure (DII) common operating environment (COE).

HSS uses the Joint Operation Planning and Execution System (JOPES) for planning and execution under GCCS. JOPES combines joint policies, procedures, personnel, training, and a reporting structure supported by automated data processing on GCCS. The medical analysis tool (MAT) is the HSS requirements generator and analysis tool supported by GCCS at the Marine Corps component level for planning and execution of HSS.

MEF

CIS support for HSS organizations will be provided by communications battalion. The G-6/S-6 must plan for connectivity among the division, wing, and FSSG as well as external communications with organizations in the joint arena.

Division

CIS support for HSS personnel will be provided by communications company, H&S battalion.

Wing

CIS support for HSS personnel will be provided by the Marine Wing Communications Squadron (MWCS) and Marine Wing Support Group (MWSG).

FSSG

CIS support for HSS personnel will be provided by communications company, H&S battalion and communications platoon, medical battalion.

Deployed MEF

CIS support for HSS personnel will come from both the Navy CIS system and communications battalion.

6003. Information Management

HSS has traditionally been supported by a variety of information systems and procedures that aided the user in the collection, analysis, presentation, and storage of information. Systems used unique hardware and software configurations that performed specialized functions. These systems typically were unable to access or share data and information with other systems. New designs have been developed that consolidate as well as improve accessing and sharing information. This migration has continued under the auspices of the Theater Medical Information Program (TMIP).

TMIP's mission is to provide integrated automation of the theater medical environment. TMIP provides a global capability linking HSS information data bases and integration centers that are accessible to the warfighter while engaged in any mission. The link is essential to aid theater commanders to make time-sensitive decisions critical to the success of their operations. The link is accomplished by integrating the GCCS with the Global Combat Support System. TMIP integrates HSS capabilities under a joint concept of operations to assist the HSS commander/theater surgeon and to support the delivery of responsive combat medical care. TMIP establishes the means to combine existing, developing, and future medical information.

TMIP's C^2 capabilities collect medical information about personnel, medical units, facilities, equipment, supplies, and training during alert/mobilization, deployment/sustainment, and reconstitution/redeployment. Information is received, processed, displayed, and analyzed to generate and publish plans and orders. TMIP enables the assessment of personnel medical status and the readiness and capabilities of the HSS units. The program provides the required information links to HSS organizations and enables rapid decisionmaking on—

- Medical capabilities assessment and sustainability analysis.
- Medical threat/intelligence.
- Combat casualty care.
- Medical logistics.
- Blood management.
- Patient movement.
- Manpower/training.

6004. MAGTF C^2 Centers, Agencies, and Facilities

The main MAGTF C^2 center, agency, or facility for HSS will be found in the combat service support operations center (CSSOC) of the FSSG. The CSSOC is the agency within the CSSE and subordinate CSS units that controls and coordinates the day-to-day operations of the CSS organization. At the FSSG, the CSSOC is operated by the G-3/S-3. Within the ACE, these duties are performed by the G-4/S-4 at the MWSG/MALS/MWSS levels.

The CSSOC's are centrally organized around the functional areas of supply, health services, maintenance, engineer, transportation, and services. The CSSOC controls the CSS radio nets and has direct telephone lines to subordinate units, supported units, and higher headquarters.

Chapter 7

Preventive Medicine

Disease and nonbattle injuries can have a rapid and widespread impact on the effectiveness of our military organizations. The devastation of disease and environmental hazards on personnel is not isolated to the people of a Third World developing nation. Throughout history, military forces have lost more personnel to disease and nonbattle injuries than to wounds sustained in combat. During the Civil War, more Federal soldiers died from disease than wounds. Approximately 44,238 were killed in battle; 49,205 died of wounds; and 186,216 died of disease.

Preventive medicine efforts can dramatically reduce the incidence of disease during military operations. Proactive preventive medicine measures should be incorporated into all levels of care. Real-time disease surveillance data should be used to brief commanders on potential medical and environmental threats and on the effectiveness of preventive medicine measures.

Prevention of disease and nonbattle injuries is a critical function of the HSSE. Naval Medical (NAVMED) P-5010, *BUMED Manual of Naval Preventive Medicine*, prescribes specific preventive medicine measures.

7001. Pre-Deployment

Specific preventive medicine taskings and efforts to be conducted before deployment include—

- Collecting and disseminating environmental and epidemiological information on the theater of operations to the supported commander, HSS units, and MAGTF elements that might be affected, for use in planning and action as changes occur.
- Recommending personnel augmentation requirements to support the OPLAN.
- Recommending immunizations and other preventive measures to counter medical threats within the theater of operations and in-transit staging points.
- Training individuals (through unit training) in personal hygiene, personal protective measures, protection equipment, and field sanitation practices.
- Assisting medical units in completing pre-deployment requirements (immunization, preventive medicine threat briefings, and permethrin treatment of clothing) and in preparing for embarkation of preventive medicine equipment.

7002. Deployment

Specific preventive medicine taskings and efforts to be conducted while deployed include—

- Disseminating militarily significant preventive medicine information to commanders and HSS units in the theater of operation.

- Providing technical oversight on food service operations and procurement.
- Providing oversight and testing at water points and bulk water storage areas.
- Conducting disease vector and pest surveillance and control when feasible.
- Maintaining environmental health and pest control equipment.
- Conducting weekly disease and injury surveillance at all battalions and squadrons.

7003. Marine Expeditionary Force Preventive Medicine Sources

The MEF surgeon's staff includes a physician (the preventive medicine officer) with special expertise in preventive medicine and public health. This physician is responsible to the MEF commander and MEF surgeon for coordinating preventive medicine efforts among the division, the wing, and the FSSG.

Most preventive medicine assets organic to the MEF are found in the FSSG's preventive medicine section of the medical battalions' H&S company. The section is responsible for providing general support to all MEF commands. Support includes identifying information regarding environmental health factors; demographics; living conditions; water supply; waste disposal; insects; diseases and vector issues of military importance, and evaluating local food sanitation, sight, and hearing conservation programs.

7004. Mobile Medical Augmentation Readiness Team

During peacetime, any operational commander may request preventive medicine MMART assistance from the Chief of Naval Operations (N931) via the operational chain of command.

7005. Navy Environmental Health Center

The Navy Environmental Health Center, located in Norfolk, VA, supports operational units. It conducts—

- Risk screening.
- Data evaluation.
- Exposure assessments.
- Toxicity assessments.
- Health risk evaluations.
- Health and safety planning.
- Environmental risk communication workshops and seminars.

The Navy Environmental Health Center and its supporting activities establish and disseminate preventive medicine and environmental protection policy recommendations for BUMED. Field activities in direct support of the Center follow:

- Navy Environmental Preventive Medicine Units—provide updated disease information on areas of the world or specific countries, public health and preventive medicine issues, and occupational health and safety support to military forces.

- Navy Disease Vector Ecology and Control Centers—provide technical and specialized services in the field of disease vector surveillance and control, as well as providing vector control training to various agencies of the federal government. These centers test and evaluate vector control equipment and techniques, collect, summarize, and disseminate disease vector and health threat information. This diverse mission includes a special emphasis on contingency response in the event of armed conflicts, military operations other than war, and operational support of both fleet and shore activities.
- Forward Deployed Laboratory—can quickly identify infectious and biologic threats to the deployed force. During contingency operations, the task force commander may request the support of this deployable, advanced public health laboratory (NWP 4-02, *Operational Health Service Support*).

7006. Additional Resources

The Naval Medical Research and Development Command conducts basic clinical and applied field research directly related to military requirements and operational needs. It is located in Bethesda, MD.

The Naval Medical Research Institute provides research related to immediate operational problems, which include heat stress research that leads to exposure limits for hot-humid shipboard environments; safety equipment, including protective clothing, flight goggles, safety belts, and repellents for insect vectors of disease and sharks. It is also located in Bethesda, MD.

(reverse blank)

Chapter 8

Patient Movement

Patient movement is a casualty management system. It is designed to coordinate the movement of casualties from site of injury or onset of disease through successive levels of care to a facility that can provide the appropriate level of treatment. Prompt movement of casualties through the evacuation system to treatment facilities is essential to decrease morbidity and mortality of battlefield casualties. If casualties occurred at regular intervals, in constant numbers, at predetermined locations, and with predictable injuries, their movement would require little or no coordination. Patient movement is a vital support factor that must be planned. Personnel must be trained on equipment and procedures in advance of operations in the field.

8001. Phases

Coordination of casualty movement is especially critical during operations when casualties must be moved from shore to task force ships. When properly followed, the medical regulating process ensures that patients move only as far rearward in the continuum of care as their health needs dictate which, in turn, assures the efficient and effective use of the limited HSS assets available to the MAGTF. Patient movement may occur in two phases:

- Evacuation—the movement of patients between point of injury or onset of disease to a facility that can provide the necessary treatment capability.

- Medical regulating—the process of selecting destination MTFs with the necessary HSS capabilities for patients being medically evacuated in, between, into, and out of different theaters of geographic combatant commands and CONUS.

8002. Decisionmaking

Degree of care for the sick and wounded in any area of combat is greatly influenced by prevailing tactical situations. Conditions are seldom static, and success in combat must remain the primary goal of combat, combat support, and combat service support units. This environment requires a dynamic casualty management decisionmaking process which must be applied at all HSS units and in the patient movement system.

Casualty Sorting (Triage)

An effective process of casualty sorting, also referred to as triage, is basic to the successful operation of a patient movement system. Rapid evaluations must be made to identify which patients need immediate resuscitation and which patients can tolerate delay in treatment. Deciding which patients should be moved after initial treatment to other medical facilities is of equal importance.

Medical Management

Under combat conditions, the flow of sick and wounded puts variable pressure on capabilities of medical facilities. Incoming casualties necessitate the movement of stable casualties who can be evacuated. Close coordination between clinical and administrative services must be maintained to achieve effective management of individual casualties. Medical officers who are responsible for decisions on movement of individual casualties must work closely with administrative officers charged with implementing patient movement for evacuation. Underlying all considerations is the basic objective of preserving life and limb.

8003. Medical Evacuation Assets

The assigned mission dictates the number and types of aircraft assigned to accomplish all assault support tasks. This mission, along with the limited number of aircraft in the Marine Corps inventory, precludes the assignment of dedicated aeromedical evacuation (AE) aircraft in most cases. All Marine Corps rotary wing transport and utility aircraft have the capability to perform an AE mission. Allocation of aircraft to perform the AE mission would be at the discretion of the MAGTF commander. Assets are designated to perform AE through implied mission tasking or by assuming a standby posture.

Prior planning is essential to ensure proper allocation of aircraft to support AE missions. Within the MEF, the FSSG HSSE, in conjunction with the FSSG logistics movement coordination center (LMCC), plans for medical evacuation aircraft. The LMCC air liaison officer is the direct link to the MAW for identification of medical evacuation missions in the air tasking order. In the absence of an AE capability, casualty evacuation is accomplished using any surface (water or ground) transportation available (ground ambulance, five-ton truck, small boat, landing craft air cushion).

Evacuation concepts used by the Marine Corps are defined as the following:

Dedicated medical evacuation assets are patient movement assets configured for medical evacuation, externally marked with a red cross, and specifically reserved to support the medical evacuation mission. Dedicated medical evacuation assets are authorized protection under the Geneva Conventions.

Designated medical evacuation assets are nonmedical patient movement assets, not externally marked with a red cross, but configured and allocated for patient movement. Designated medical evacuation assets are not afforded protection under the Geneva Conventions.

8004. Aeromedical Evacuation Request Procedures

Normally, when control is seabased, units request AE by radio to the helicopter direction center using the helicopter direction net. When command and/or net control has been passed ashore, units request AE from the direct air support center using the tactical air request/helicopter request net. The air officer will then consult with either the ATF medical regulating control officer when seabased or the LF patient evacuation officer when ashore for a recommendation of the best medical facility to care for the patient.

In operations where dedicated AE assets are assigned, the direct air support center will make liaison with the units responsible to provide AE.

AE missions are classified as preplanned or immediate. Both types of support are delivered in response to specific requests via the assault support request.

AE missions from Marine Corps MTFs to theater hospitals will be coordinated by the patient evacuation/patient movement section, FSSG, in coordination with the HSSE, the CSSOC, LMCC, and the theater patient movement requirements center.

8005. Further Guidance

NWP 4-02.2 Vol. 1, *Patient Movement*, provides a general summary of the HSS system and the specific tactic, techniques, and procedures (TTP) for naval expeditionary force medical regulating. For joint operations, refer to Joint Pub 4-02.2, *Joint Tactics, Techniques, and Procedures for Patient Movement in Joint Operations*.

Chapter 9

Nuclear, Biological, and Chemical Defense

All military personnel must be prepared to operate in a contaminated environment. HSS personnel must also be prepared to provide patient care in an NBC environment. Decontamination of patients and transportation assets causes evacuation delays, making first aid and patient care even more critical. Since the staffing of HSS units is based on conventional warfare requirements, these units will be taxed in their ability to provide effective HSS.

NBC actions cause high casualty rates, materiel losses, obstacles to maneuver, and contamination. Mission-oriented protective posture (MOPP) levels 3 and 4 result in body heat buildup, reduced mobility, and degraded visual, touch, and hearing senses, ultimately reducing unit effectiveness.

Contamination is a major problem in providing HSS in an NBC environment. To maximize the unit's survival and effectiveness, commanders must take action to avoid NBC contamination by making maximum use of alarm and detection equipment and unit dispersion; overhead shelters, shielding materials, and protective covers; collective protection shelters; and chemical agent resistant coatings.

On a contaminated battlefield, the focus is on keeping the Marine in the battle. Effective and efficient triage, emergency treatment, decontamination, and contamination control in the operational area save lives, assure prompt evacuation, and maximize the return-to-duty rate.

9001. Before a Nuclear, Biological, or Chemical Attack

Before an NBC attack, HSS personnel must train to survive the attack, to operate the MTF in the environment, and to effectively care for NBC casualties. HSS personnel must keep their immunizations current, use available preventive treatment against suspected agents, pretreat for suspected agents, and have antidotes and essential Class VIIIA supplies readily available for known or suspected chemical or biological agents.

The best defense for HSS personnel is to protect themselves, their patients, Class VIIIA supplies, and equipment by following contamination avoidance procedures. HSS personnel must ensure that stored Class VIIIA supplies and equipment are in protected areas or in their storage containers with covers in place.

One method of protecting supplies and equipment is to keep them in their shipping containers until needed. When time permits after receiving warnings that an NBC attack is imminent or that a downwind hazard exists, HSS personnel should seek protected areas such as basements, culverts, and ravines for themselves and their patients.

9002. During a Nuclear, Biological, or Chemical Attack

HSS personnel and their patients should remain in the best available protected areas and take up positions within the shelter that are away from windows and other openings. They move out of these positions only when notified that it is safe to do so. In the absence of higher authority, HSS personnel use caution in their movements.

9003. After a Nuclear, Biological, or Chemical Attack

HSS personnel must survey their equipment to determine the extent of damage and their capabilities to continue the mission. Initially, patients from nuclear detonations will be suffering thermal burns or blast injuries. Also, HSS personnel may expect disorientation in patients and other HSS personnel.

Normally, radiation-induced injuries are observed within a few hours or days of the attack. Chemical agent patients manifest their injuries immediately upon exposure to the agent. However, blister agent patients can show signs of exposure immediately or up to 14 days later. Biological agent patients may not show any signs of illness for hours to days after exposure.

All patients receiving treatment must be checked for NBC contamination. Patients are decontaminated before treatment to reduce the hazard to HSS personnel, unless life- or limb-threatening conditions exist. Patients requiring treatment before decontamination are treated in the HSS area of the decontamination station. Cardiac arrest, massive hemorrhage, and respiratory distress are conditions that may require treatment in the decontamination area.

9004. Nuclear Environment

The HSS unit must continue its support mission in a nuclear environment by preparing protective shelters. Well-constructed foxholes with overhead cover and expedient shelters (reinforced concrete structures, basements, railroad tunnels, or trenches) provide good protection from nuclear attacks. Armored vehicles also provide protection against both the blast and radiation effects of nuclear weapons. Casualties generated in a nuclear attack will likely suffer multiple injuries (combinations of blast, thermal, and radiation injuries) which complicate HSS. Nuclear radiation casualties fall into three categories.

The irradiated casualty has been exposed to ionizing radiation but is not contaminated. These casualties are not radioactive and pose no radiation threat to medical care providers. Casualties who have suffered exposure to initial nuclear radiation fit into this category.

The externally contaminated casualty has radioactive dust and debris on clothing, skin, or hair. This presents a "housekeeping" problem to the MTF similar to the lice-infested patient arriving at a peacetime MTF. However, this contamination may present a threat to HSS personnel. The externally contaminated casualty is decontaminated at the earliest time consistent with required medical care. Lifesaving care is always rendered before decontamination.

The internally contaminated casualty has ingested or inhaled radioactive materials, or radioactive material has entered the body through an open wound. The radioactive material continues to irradiate the casualty internally until radioactive decay and biological elimination removes the radioactive isotope. Attending HSS personnel are shielded, to some degree, by the patient's body. Inhalation, ingestion, or injection of quantities of radioactive material sufficient to present a threat to medical care providers is highly unlikely.

9005. Biological Environment

A biological attack may be difficult to recognize because frequently it does not have an immediate affect on exposed personnel. HSS personnel must monitor for biological warfare indicators such as—

- An increase in disease incidences or fatality rates.
- A sudden presentation of an exotic disease.
- Other sequential epidemiological events, especially when presented in lines of communications.

Passive defensive measures (such as immunizations, good personal hygiene, physical conditioning, use of arthropod repellents, use of protective mask, and practice of good sanitation) lessen the effects of most biological intrusions.

Commanders of MTFs must enforce contamination control to prevent injury to HSS personnel and to preserve the MTF's integrity. Incoming patients and equipment must be surveyed for contamination. Ventilation systems in medical treatment facilities without collective protection shelters must be turned off if biological or chemical exposure is imminent.

Decontamination of most biologically contaminated patients and equipment can be accomplished with soap and water.

Patients exposed to a biological agent may require observation and evaluation to determine necessary medications, isolation, or treatment.

9006. Chemical Environment

Handling chemically contaminated patients presents a great challenge to HSS units. The vapor hazard associated with contaminated patients may require HSS personnel to remain at MOPP level 4 for long periods; therefore, HSS personnel must locate clean areas to set up their MTF. The MTF should operate in a contaminated environment only until HSS personnel have the time and means to move to a clean area.

9007. Medical Evacuation

An NBC environment forces the unit commander to consider what evacuation assets will be committed to the contaminated area. If operating forces are in a contaminated area, most or all of the medical evacuation assets will operate there. However, efforts should be made to keep some ambulances free of contamination.

There are three basic modes of evacuating casualties: personnel, ground vehicles, and aircraft. Commanders must recognize the constraints NBC warfare places on casualty evacuation during operations and then plan and train to overcome these deficiencies.

9008. Personnel Considerations

Medical treatment requirements increase when operating in an NBC contaminated environment. As a result, HSS personnel reinforcement and replacement may be necessary. Plans for HSS following an NBC attack must include efforts to conserve available HSS personnel and ensure their best use. HSS personnel provide emergency medical treatment or advanced trauma management and more definitive treatment as time and resources permit. However, to provide definitive care, they must be able to work in a shirt-sleeved environment, not in MOPP levels 3 or 4. Non-HSS personnel conduct search and rescue operations for the injured or wounded; they also provide immediate first aid and decontamination.

(reverse blank)

Chapter 10

Combat Casualty Reporting

Commanders must be thoroughly familiar with combat casualty reporting procedures. The G-1/S-1 section of a command is responsible for submitting prompt, accurate, and complete casualty reports to higher headquarters. In combat operations, unit corpsmen and MTFs are primary sources of individual casualty data. Casualty reporting in the MARFOR is addressed in MCO P3040.42, *Marine Corps Casualty Procedures Manual*, and other local guidance in the 3040 series. The system described in these directives is essentially one in which personnel losses, regardless of cause, are reported through the chain of command to a central location. Figure 10-1 illustrates the flow of casualty information from medical personnel and MTFs upward through the chain of command.

10001. Field Medical Card

Hospital corpsmen at the unit level usually provide the first written information on a casualty through the use of a U.S. Field Medical Card (DD Form 1380). The field medical card (FMC) is a casualty tag printed in a set which provides a tough original copy for attaching to the casualty (whether wounded or deceased). A carbon copy is retained by the hospital corpsman rendering initial treatment.

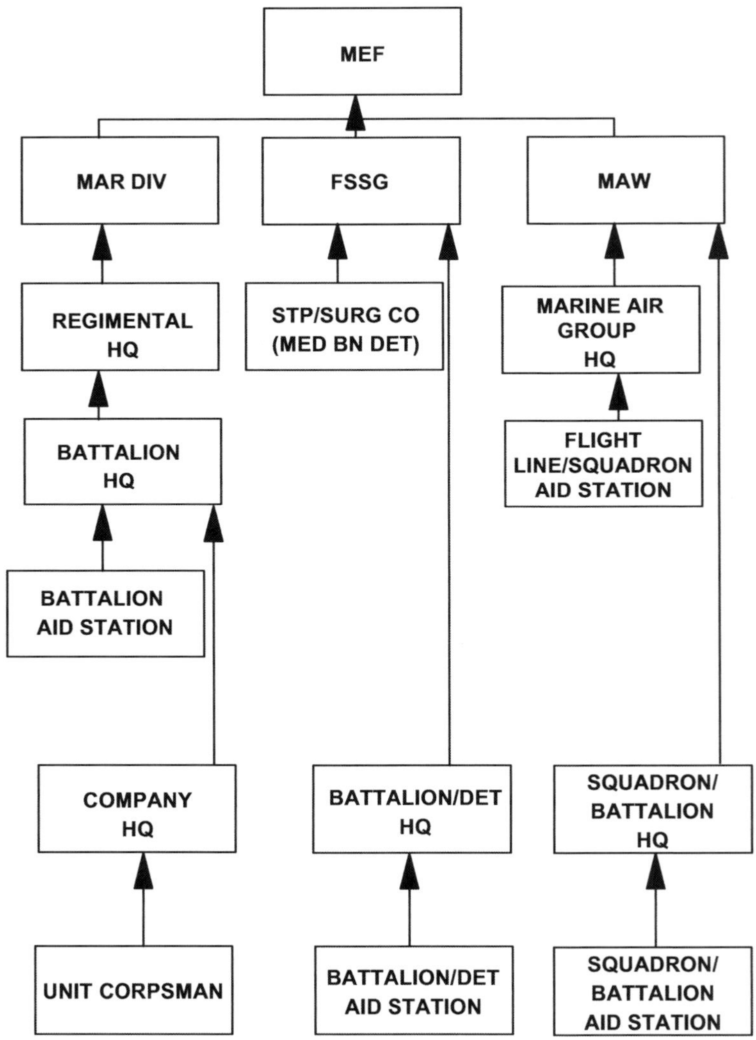

Figure 10-1. Combat Casualty Reporting in the Marine

Expeditionary Force.

The purpose of the FMC is to establish patient accountability and to provide a means to document assessment of condition and treatment rendered by HSS personnel. The FMC is used as an emergency medical tag for all casualties at the time they are initially treated in the field or field medical facility. The completed FMC is an important medical record that will accompany the casualty through the continuum of care. It is also an administrative document that may contain the most dependable information a commanding officer may have regarding a casualty in his unit. Our North Atlantic Treaty Organization allies, by formal agreement, use FMCs containing the same essential information as recorded on the U.S. card.

10002. Identification Tags

Identification tags (dog tags) are essential to casualty identification and recording. Each Service member is issued a chain and two tags to be worn at all times. Tags contain the member's name, social security number, blood type, Service component, religious preference, and protective mask size. The member and the unit are both responsible for ensuring that all information is current and accurate. See BUMED Instruction 6150.35, *Medical Warning Tags*, for more information.

Both identification tags remain with a casualty at all times, except when remains are buried in the combat area. One tag is attached to the grave marker, and the other tag stays with the deceased. Joint Pub 4-06, *Joint Tactics, Techniques, and Proce-*

dures for Mortuary Affairs in Joint Operations, provides detailed procedures for handling deceased personnel.

10003. Automated Medical Record Technology

New automated systems will play a significant role across the range of medical operations. One such device is the portable information carrier (PIC) that stores personal information about its owner. The PIC is a hand-carried, abridged electronic medical record which will serve as the primary repository of individual readiness data such as deployability status, casualty prevention training, medical history, and demographic information. This technology will give the care provider electronic read/write capability to record care given to the patient. This technology will enhance combat casualty care and patient tracking capability by interfacing with command and control systems being developed to track patients' movement, assess logistics requirements, and manage medical surveillance.

Chapter 11

Training

The primary goal of all military training is to achieve and maintain the highest level of preparation possible, thereby developing confidence among the troops and ensuring a high state of readiness. The importance of training as a means of enhancing combat readiness is equally important to HSS personnel. This is especially true given the greatly reduced peacetime staffing of HSS units and the difficulty of obtaining realistic, hands-on trauma training.

Reaching this essential state of readiness requires the medical department to contend with unique circumstances and conditions, including manning levels and the coordinated availability of training. In peacetime, the majority of operating forces' units are manned at slightly more than two-thirds of their mobilization strength, while HSS units are generally manned only with half of the personnel required to carry out their wartime mission. Authorized manning levels fill only about 10 percent of medical corps and nurse corps billets within medical battalions. The end result is that upon mobilization more than half of the medical personnel assigned to operating forces HSS units will be augmentees with greatly varying degrees of field medical skills and experience.

11001. Health Service Support Goals

These manning and training capability constraints require that training efforts be directed toward developing a nucleus of personnel highly skilled in the techniques of establishing and effectively operating HSS facilities in the field. This nucleus, when mobilized, becomes the core of each field medical unit and faces the formidable task of receiving large numbers of augmentees and shaping them into effective health delivery teams. It is not possible to lay out a training program which would be applicable to all HSSEs due to geographic, climatic, and mission variation. Individual commanders of HSS units and other key medical department personnel must structure training in light of achievable goals and limiting factors.

Increased Individual Readiness

Efforts to increase and maintain readiness should extend beyond currently assigned personnel and incorporate augmentees into all training evolutions to the maximum degree funds and scheduling will permit. Surgeons and other key personnel should encourage commanders to involve identified augmentation personnel in exercises when possible. In addition to enhancing individual training, this practice will aid in fostering a sense of unit identity and cohesiveness.

Standardized Methods and Procedures

This is a necessary goal which is elevated to paramount importance because it must be done before mobilization. Augmentees must be familiar with and able to depend on well-developed standing operating procedures in the form of desktop procedures and procedural manuals. The importance of this goal cannot be overly stressed.

Increased Operational Effectiveness Through Higher Levels of Individual and Collective Experience

HSS is basic to all operations. Medical department personnel must, to the maximum degree possible, be involved in all phases of every exercise. The necessity of this involvement is easily and often overlooked in peacetime due to budgetary and time constraints.

11002. Training Pipeline

The following training courses are essential to the development of effective, efficient, and successful HSS personnel. Course quota management and control are under the cognizance of BUMED.

Field Medical Service School

There are two Field Medical Service Schools (FMSSs), one at Camp Lejeune, North Carolina, and the other at Camp Pendleton, California. The mission of these Marine Corps schools is to prepare Navy medical department personnel for service with the MARFOR. Before reporting to the MARFOR, all medical department personnel (officer and enlisted) not having previous field medical service training shall attend an appropriate course of instruction at one of the schools. Both schools teach—

- The role and requirements of HSS units in the field.
- Military tactical and defensive techniques closely related to field HSS.

- HSS planning and concepts for officers and senior petty officers, including medical estimates, medical staff planning, and logistics support.
- MARFOR and MAGTF organization.
- The use and handling of designated table of organization weapons for medical department personnel.

Combat Casualty Care Course

Before reporting to the MARFOR, all medical department officers who are clinical providers (i.e., medical corps, dental corps, nurse corps) shall attend a course of instruction in advanced combat life support. In combat support operations, nonphysician health care providers may be required to assist medical officers in presurgical preparation and wound management. Training is available through the Defense Medical Readiness Training Institute, Fort Sam Houston, Texas.

11003. Commander's Responsibilities

Commander's are responsible for ensuring that all command personnel receive appropriate training in both military and technical subject areas, including emergency medical training of nonmedical personnel and the continued training of medical department personnel in field medical practices and related military subjects. Commanders develop, conduct, and evaluate individual and collective HSS training based on training standards published by the Marine Corps Combat Development Command (MCCDC). When standards have not been published, unit commanders ensure training is based on this MCWP and other doctrinal, tactical, and technical publications approved for Navy and Marine Corps use.

11004. Medical Department Officers and Senior Enlisted

The division and wing surgeons maintain staff supervision of all medical training programs, including exercise planning and execution, for medical department personnel assigned to their respective subordinate commands. Within the FSSG, the group surgeon and dental officer, in coordination with the G-3, exercises staff cognizance of all general medical training programs. Medical and dental battalion commanders are responsible for all battalion training programs including internal planning and execution. The FSSG HSSO exercises staff cognizance of FSSG planning and exercises. All medical department officers and senior hospital and dental corps conduct and/or supervise the training of hospital corpsmen and dental technicians.

11005. Types of Training

Individual Training

Individual training may be conducted in a formal school or at the member's command. This training prepares an individual to perform specific tasks related to general military duties or assigned specialties. Medical department personnel who regularly perform duties of their occupational specialty develop increased confidence and proficiency. Individual training may include first aid and cardiopulmonary resuscitation (CPR) as well as more formal programs such as the Plans, Operations, and Medical Intelligence Course; the Joint Medical Planners Course; the Landing Force Medical Staff Planning Course; and the Medical Regulating Course.

Unit Training

Unit training prepares an individual to function within a unit and as part of a cohesive element. Such elements may include teams, platoons, sections, companies, or whatever size is feasible. MARFOR unit training is normally conducted afloat or in a field environment and involves the entire organization, including assigned HSSEs. Unit training has proven most effective when conducted in a simulated combat environment. These exercises entail setting up treatment facilities in the field and treatment of simulated casualties. Other field units such as infantry battalions, regiments, and combat support and combat service support organizations conduct field training exercises that involve HSS personnel organic to those units.

Exercises

Training exercises provide a realistic training environment, allowing HSS personnel to apply and refine their field medical skills as well as expand their knowledge and skills in the following areas:

- LF organization and communications.
- HSS functions in the field.
- Deployment procedures, including combat loading of HSS equipment.
- Sanitation standards for shipboard and field troops.

- Ship-to-shore operations.
- Casualty evacuation.
- Mass casualty training.
- HSS supply and resupply.
- Operations in severe environments.
- Special problems in the amphibious objective area.

Nuclear, Biological, and Chemical Training

Readiness training for patient decontamination, patient care, and NBC defense may be conducted at individual or unit level. Training in medical procedures associated with NBC casualties cannot be adequately addressed in on-the-job training but requires the participation of instructors specifically trained in the subject area. (See FMFM 11-11, *Treatment of Chemical Agent Casualties and Conventional Military Chemical Injuries*.)

Preventive Medicine Training

HSS personnel in all MARFOR units must receive instruction in the recognition of diseases and environmental hazards that may occur within a specific area of operations. Emphasis should be placed on personal and unit-wide preventive medicine measures at all levels. Division, group, and wing surgeons should periodically review contingency plans, with emphasis on identifying measures necessary to effectively prevent disease and other health hazards. This information should be incorporated into training programs for medical department personnel.

Logistics and Supply Training

The Marine Corps and Navy supply systems are sufficiently different to invalidate most information in Navy training manuals with regard to its applicability to the Marine Corps system. Unit commanders with a health care mission must ensure Navy personnel are sufficiently trained in basic procedures to operate within the Marine Corps supply system.

11006. Dental Personnel

Enlisted dental personnel assigned to the MARFOR receive the same basic FMSS training as hospital corpsmen, but rate specific training for their individual Navy enlisted classification codes. During casualty overload, dental personnel perform roles in combat casualty care. Training emphasis should be placed on increasing skills in combat casualty care and trauma management, including training in the designated roles of preoperative preparation and wound management for dental officers and ward corpsmen duties and central sterilization duties for dental technicians.

11007. Non-Health Service Support Personnel

HSS personnel are responsible for training non-HSS personnel in subjects such as CPR, first aid, buddy aid, personal hygiene, field sanitation, and preventive medicine.

All non-HSS personnel (including chaplains and religious programs enlisted personnel) should receive extensive training in first aid procedures, self-aid, buddy aid, and personal decontamination. Field Manual (FM) 21-11, *First Aid for Soldiers*, and the Marine Corps Institute's *Marine Battle Skills Training Handbook* series list and explain subjects that must be taught.

Personnel should be indoctrinated in specific personal protection and disease prevention topics as described in FM 21-10, *Field Hygiene and Sanitation*, and NAVMED P-5010.

Marine Corps supply personnel in key positions shall be provided training in procedures that enable them to provide medical supply support when deployed. Training should encompass interfacing with the SIMLM system.

Further information on the availability and applicability of specific individual or unit HSS training can be found by addressing Director, Training and Education Division, MCCDC, or Director, Operational Readiness and Training Division, BUMED.

Appendix A

Blood Support

Formally established as the Military Blood Program in 1952 by Presidential Order as part of the National Blood Program, today's Armed Services Blood Program (ASBP) consists of approximately 116 blood banks and blood donor centers worldwide, including 43 Food and Drug Administration (FDA) licensed blood donor centers. The ASBP mission is to provide quality blood products, blood substitutes, and services for all worldwide customers in peace and war. The ASBP is a joint program operated by the military Services and coordinated by the Armed Services Blood Program Office (ASBPO).

The ASBPO is a joint health agency charted to monitor the implementation of blood program policies established by the Assistant Secretary of Defense (Health Affairs) (ASD[HA]) and to coordinate the blood programs of the military Services (Army, Air Force, and Navy) and the unified commands as directed in DOD Instruction 6480.4, *Armed Services Blood Program Operational Procedures.* The ASBPO provides standardization among the Services and enhances the total blood distribution system in peace and war. The U.S. Army Surgeon General, on behalf of the Secretary of the Army, serves as the executive agent for the ASBPO for administrative support and staff supervision. The Joint Chiefs of Staff, by Memorandum of Understanding, are responsible for the review and provision of guidance in all matters regarding blood support in joint operational planning. The ASD(HA) provides policy guidance to the ASBPO. All of the ASBP elements function together to successfully operate the Military Blood Program.

Blood support for the MARFOR is provided by the Navy's Blood Program (NBP). The NBP ensures operational readiness to both the Navy and MARFOR through a viable blood program which meets and exceeds standards of practice. The NBP oversees 30 Navy blood banks worldwide. Of those 30, 19 are with blood donor centers (BDCs). The NBP operates under the FDA License Number 635. The responsible head is the Surgeon General of the Navy/Chief, Bureau of Medicine and Surgery. The alternate responsible head is the Assistant Chief for Operational Medicine and Fleet Support, Bureau of Medicine and Surgery.

Armed Services Whole Blood Processing Laboratory

An Armed Services Whole Blood Processing Laboratory (ASWBPL) is a USAF-managed, tri-service-staffed, central repository for liquid and frozen blood required in peacetime, contingencies, and war. An ASWBPL releases blood to unified commands upon approval by the ASBPO. Theater MTFs may not go directly to the ASWBPL for blood. ASWBPLs—

- Retype blood for A, B, and O blood types and Rh only.
- Pack, ice, and prepare blood for shipment to the theater.
- Maintain a peacetime inventory of 250 units of liquid blood for use as a rapid response requirement.

Joint Blood Program Office

The Joint Blood Program Office (JBPO) is responsible for the joint blood program management in a theater of operations. The

JBPO functions as part of the unified command surgeon's office but may establish an Area Joint Blood Program Office (AJBPO) for regional blood management. The JBPO—

- Works directly for the unified command surgeon. The JBPO may augment the surgeon's staff of the Commander, Joint Task Force.
- Serves as the central point of contact to ASBPO.
- Coordinates joint blood products requirements and capabilities in the theater of operations. Major assessment areas for a JBPO are manpower, training levels, and supplies.
- Coordinates requirements, distribution, and facilities. The JBPO ensures blood is where it's needed. The JBPO quickly determines how to get blood to forward units and Navy ships as well as MTFs.
- Monitors shortfalls within the unified command, including supplies for collection, deglycerolization, distribution, and transfusion of blood/blood products.
- Ensures readiness by having a distribution system, exercises, and training. Other theater staff members (AJBPO, blood support unit [BSU], and MTF officers) may need further training on coordinating with medical planners or transportation officers to anticipate blood/supply needs, making transportation arrangements, or using liquid/frozen products.
- Ensures compliance with ASBP policies, FDA regulations, American Association of Blood Banks standards in peacetime, contingencies, and war.
- Serves as the unified command subject matter expert on determining blood requirements based on Joint Staff casualty pro-

jections and maintaining blood in medical sustainment analysis.

- Provides the joint blood concept; coordinates with logistics, transportation, and communications personnel on the Joint Staff for the unified command; and prepares appendix 2 to Annex Q, *Planning Guidance, Medical Services*.

Area Joint Blood Program Office

AJBPOs can be established within the theater of operations during war or special operations. An AJBPO coordinates requirements and distribution of blood products to support BSUs and MTFs in a specific area, regardless of the Service component. Not all operations will require establishing an AJBPO. An AJBPO may not be a blood bank specialist but will have most of the same responsibilities as the JBPO and may need training and additional guidance from the JBPO.

Blood Transshipment Centers

A blood transshipment center (BTC) is the central receiving point for blood shipments from the ASWBPL and for issue to the BSUs. A BTC can store and process up to 7,200 units of liquid blood daily. A BTC is usually staffed and operated by USAF personnel at a major airhead. BTC blood products are managed by the JBPO or AJBPO (if established). One or more BTCs may be located in each theater of operation. Not all theaters of operations will require the use of a BTC. BTCs—

- Inspect blood received from the ASWBPL or other blood agencies, blood products depots, or other BTCs.

- Store, ice, and re-ice blood and perform quality control.
- Issue blood to BSUs or other component blood users.
- Prepare daily blood reports for JBPO and blood shipment reports for receiving BSU.

Transportable Blood Transshipment Centers

Transportable Blood Transshipment Centers (TBTCs) are mobile, modular, and can be transported into the theater of operations at a site designated by the theater commander. Although TBTCs have the capacity to store frozen blood products, they can deploy with or without those products. Based on theater commanders decisions, the ASBP will have six TBTCs available as blood program elements and one for training deployable personnel.

Blood Products Depots

Blood products depots (BPDs) are located within the unified command to maintain large quantities of frozen blood products for use during armed conflicts or emergencies requiring medical support. These prepositioned stocks of frozen blood products are intended to fulfill initial wartime blood surge requirements until mobilization of CONUS assets can catch up to demand. Subsequent liquid blood supplies will come from CONUS blood donor centers and will be shipped via the ASWBPL and the BTCs.

BPDs are single Service staffed and operated, but the blood products are for use by all components in potential theaters of conflict. Blood maintained at BPDs is managed by the JBPO via the

AJBPO. Not all unified commands and theaters of operations will require or have a BPD. BPDs—

- Store frozen blood products until required.
- Issue blood as directed by the JBPO via the AJBPO.
- Thaw and deglycerolize frozen red cells and distribute to BSUs.

Blood Supply Units

Blood supply units (BSUs) receive, store, and distribute blood within the theater of operations. BSUs are required to provide a 5-day storage supply of blood products based on MTF proposed requirements and blood reports.

BSUs can provide support in a specific geographical area regardless of Service components and can support up to 12 MTFs designated by the JBPO.

The following units/facilities can serve as a BSU: Army blood platoon, Navy fleet hospital, naval amphibious assault vessels, T-AH hospital ships, MTFs, and BPD, when designated.

BSUs provide storage capabilities that maintain temperature requirements for liquid blood.

BSUs can produce ice for shipping and re-icing of blood in the theater. They can also store frozen blood products, including fresh frozen plasma and frozen red cells. A BSU's ability to obtain and store dry ice provides the means to ship fresh frozen plasma to MTFs.

BSUs can collect blood in emergencies, but this is not encouraged due to the lack of capability to perform testing for infectious diseases. Refer to the emergency donor section for protocol regarding blood drawn in theater.

BSUs can support MTFs as designated/determined by the JBPO.

(reverse blank)

Appendix B

Authorized Medical and Dental Allowance Lists

HSS authorized medical allowance lists (AMALs) and authorized dental allowance lists (ADALs) are configured in assemblages such as equipment and supply. The equipment assemblage contains equipment and reusable materiel required to establish the basic function of the assemblage (e.g., an operating room). The supply assemblage contains consumable material to support the function in treating a designated number of casualties or to perform a specific task. For readiness purposes, an equipment module may be stored in combination with its corresponding supply module. The materiel listed in each AMAL/ADAL is the minimum amount to be maintained.

Marine Corps Order 4400 series contains AMAL and ADAL procurement policies and procedures. Policies and procedures include assembly, maintenance, levels of supply, and distribution of materiel. AMALs and ADALs are maintained and resupplied by the medical logistics company, supply battalion, FSSG.

Numbers and Nomenclatures

AMAL 618—Laboratory Equipment. Equipment and reusable materiel required to establish a laboratory capable of hematology, microbiology, urinalysis, and chemical testing.

AMAL 619—Laboratory Supply. Consumable supplies required to perform hematology, microbiology, urinalysis, and chemical testing for 100 patients.

AMAL 627—X-ray Equipment. Equipment and reusable materiel required to establish one x-ray room and processing facility.

AMAL 649—X-ray Supply. Consumable supplies required to provide x-ray support for 100 patients at 10 films per patient.

AMAL 629—Pharmacy Equipment. Equipment and reusable materiel required to establish a pharmacy.

AMAL 630—Pharmacy Supply. Consumable supplies required to provide pharmacy support for 1,000 patients in six 5-day packages for a total of 30 days.

AMAL 631—Shock Surgical Team/Triage Equipment. Equipment and reusable materiel required to establish a basic shock trauma surgical team or triage to receive, resuscitate, sort, and temporarily hold casualties.

AMAL 632—Shock Surgical Team/Triage Supply. Consumable supplies required to receive, resuscitate, sort, and temporarily hold 50 casualties with major wounds and to provide basic line corpsman resupply.

AMAL 633—Ward Equipment. Equipment and reusable materiel required to establish a 20-bed unit.

AMAL 634—Ward Supply. Consumable supplies required to provide ward support for 100 bed days-to-patient.

AMAL 635—Aid Station Equipment. Equipment and reusable materiel required to support one division, wing, group, engineer, or battalion aid station.

AMAL 636—Aid Station Supply. Consumable supplies required to provide aid station support, initial resuscitation, and stabilization of 50 casualties with major wounds prior to evacuation, and to resupply basic line corpsman.

AMAL 637—Preventive Medicine Equipment. Equipment and reusable materiel required to establish a preventive medicine section. The section provides technical preventive medicine advice; inspects food service operations, waste disposal, water potability and sources, and vector control; coordinates control measures required for communicable diseases; and monitors and assists immunization programs.

AMAL 638—Preventive Medicine Supply. Consumable supplies required to provide support of the preventive medicine effort to the MEF in twelve 5-day packages for a total of 60 days.

AMAL 639—Operating Room Equipment. Equipment and reusable materiel required to support an operating room for performing major surgical procedures, administering general anesthesia, sterilizing materiel, and maintaining sterile material.

AMAL 640—Operating Room Supply. Consumable supplies required to provide operating room support for 25 surgical cases.

ADAL 662—Field Dental Operatory. Equipment and reusable materiel required to establish a dental clinic in the field. Consumable supplies required to provide emergency, diagnostic, and preventive maintenance dental care for 400 patients.

AMAL 684—Geographic Supplement. Consumable supplies and reusable materiel required to accommodate special mission- and geographic-related requirements for a MEF in twelve 5-day packages for a total of 60 days.

AMAL 685—Cold Weather Supplement. Consumable supplies and reusable materiel required to accommodate special mission- and geographic-related requirements in areas where cold-related injuries are likely to occur.

AMAL 686—Hot Weather Supplement. Consumable supplies and reusable materiel required to accommodate special mission- and geographic-related requirements into areas where heat-related injuries are likely to occur.

AMAL 687—NBC Individual. Materials required for the individual to conduct primary decontamination and treatment in an NBC environment.

AMAL 688—NBC Unit. Materials required for the units to conduct primary and secondary decontamination and treatment in an NBC environment.

AMAL 691—Med Log Test/Repair Equipment. Equipment and reusable materiel required to perform testing, calibration, and 3d and 4th echelon maintenance of medical/dental equipment.

AMAL 692—Med Log Test/Repair Supply. Consumable supplies required to accommodate a medical repair section in the testing, calibration, and 3d and 4th echelon maintenance of medical/dental equipment.

Appendix C

Glossary

ACE .... aviation combat element
ADAL .... authorized dental allowance lists
AE .... aeromedical evacuation
AFMIC .... Armed Forces Medical Intelligence Center
AJBPO .... Area Joint Blood Program Office
AMAL .... authorized medical allowance lists
ASBP .... Armed Services Blood Program
ASBPO .... Armed Services Blood Program Office
ASD (HA) .... Assistant Secretary of Defense (Health Affairs)
ASWBPL .... Armed Services Whole Blood Processing Laboratory
ATF .... amphibious task force

BAS .... battalion aid station
BDC .... blood donor centers
BPD .... Blood Products Depots
BSSG .... brigade service support group
BSU .... blood support unit
BTC .... blood transshipment center
BUMED .... U.S. Navy Bureau of Medicine and Surgery

CATF .... commander, amphibious task force
CINC .... commander in chief
CJCSM .... Chairman of the Joint Chiefs of Staff Manual
CLF .... commander, landing force
COMDTPUB .... Commandant Publication (U.S. Coast Guard)
CONPLAN .... concept plan
CONUS .... continental United States

CPR .... cardiopulmonary resuscitation
CRTS .... casualty receiving and treatment ship
CSSE .... combat service support element
CSSOC .... combat service support operations center

DOD .... Department of Defense
FDA
Food and Drug Administration
FLAS .... flight line aid station
FM .... U.S. Army field manual
FMC .... field medical card
FMFM .... Fleet Marine Force manual
FMSS .... Field Medical Service School
FSSG .... force service support group
FST .... fleet surgical team

GCCS .... Global Command and Control System
GCE .... ground combat element
GCSS .... Global Combat Support System

H&S .... headquarters and service
HSS .... health service support
HSSD .... health service support detachment
HSSE .... health service support element
HSSO .... health service support officer

JBPO .... Joint Blood Program Office

LAN .... local area network
LF .... landing force
LFSP .... landing force support party
LHA .... amphibious assault ship (general purpose)

LHD ....amphibious assault ship (multipurpose)
LMCC .... logistics movement coordination center
LPH.....................................amphibious assault ship (helicopter)

MAG .... Marine aircraft group
MAGTF .... Marine air-ground task force
MAP...Medical Augmentation Program
MARFOR...Marine Corps forces
MAW... Marine aircraft wing
MCCDC ....Marine Corps Combat Development Command
MCO ....Marine Corps order
MCPP... Marine Corps planning process
MCWP ....Marine Corps warfighting publication
Med Log Co ....medical logistics company
MEF ....Marine expeditionary force
METT-T...................mission, enemy, terrain and weather, troops and support available-time available
MEU..Marine expeditionary unit
MMART................ mobile medical augmentation readiness team
MOPP...................................mission-oriented protective posture
MSSG...MEU service support group
MTF .... medical treatment facility
MWSS.. Marine wing support squadron

NAVMED .... naval medical
NBC ....nuclear, biological, and chemical
NBP.. Navy Blood Program
NWP..naval warfare publication

OPLAN ....operation plan
OPORD ....operation order

PIC .... portable information carrier
PMI .... primary movement items

SHF .... super high frequency
SIMLM .... single integrated medical logistics manager
STP .... shock trauma platoon
Surg Co .... surgical company

TBTC .... Transportable Blood Transshipment Center
T/E .... table of equipment
TMIP .... theater medical information program
TTP .... tactics, techniques, and procedures

USAF .... United States Air Force
USMC .... United States Marine Corps

VHF .... very high frequency

WAN .... wide area network

Appendix D

References and Related Publications

Chairman of the Joint Chiefs of Staff Manual (CJCSM)

3122.03 Joint Operation Planning and Execution System Volume II, Planning Formats and Guidance

Joint Publications

4-02 Doctrine for Health Service Support in Joint Operations

4-02.2 Joint Tactics, Techniques, and Procedures for Patient Movement in Joint Operations

4-06 Joint Tactics, Techniques, and Procedures for Mortuary Affairs in Joint Operations

Department of Defense (DOD) Instruction

6480.4 Armed Services Blood Program Operational Procedures

Navy Publications

Navy Warfare Publications (NWPs)

1-14M Commander's Handbook of the Law of Naval Operations

4-02 Operational Health Service Support

4-02.2 Patient Movement
4-02.4 Part A Deployable Health Service Support Platforms—Fleet Hospitals

NAVMED

P 5010 BUMED Manual of Naval Preventive Medicine

Bureau of Medicine and Surgery (BUMED) Instruction

6150.35 Medical Warning Tags

COMDTPUB

P5800.7 The Commander's Handbook on the Law of Naval Operations

Marine Corps Publications

Marine Corps Doctrinal Publication (MCDP)

2 Intelligence

Marine Corps Warfighting Publication (MCWP)

2-12 MAGTF Intelligence Production and Analysis

5-12.1 The Commander's Handbook on the Law of Naval Operations

Fleet Marine Force Manuals (FMFMs)

0-25	The Law of Land Warfare
4-50	Health Service Support
5-30	Assault Support
11-11	Treatment of Chemical Agent Casualties and Conventional Military Chemical Injuries

Fleet Marine Force Reference Publication (FMFRP)

1-18	Amphibious Ships and Landing Craft Data Book

Marine Corps Handbooks

Marine Battle Skills Training Handbook

Marine Corps Orders (MCOs)

P3040.42	Marine Corps Casualty Procedures Manual
4400	Series Supply/Materiel

Army Publications

Field Manuals (FMs)

21-10	Field Hygiene and Sanitation
21-11	First Aid for Soldiers
27-10	The Law of Land Warfare

Department of the Army Pamphlet (DA PAM)

27-1	Treaties Governing Land Warfare

(reverse blank)

43062404R00199

Made in the USA
Lexington, KY
24 June 2019